D1299226

THE DIAGNOSIS
AND DETECTION
OF BREAST DISEASE

THE DIAGNOSIS AND DETECTION OF BREAST DISEASE

Deborah E. Powell, M.D.

Professor of Pathology and Laboratory Medicine
University of Kentucky College of Medicine
Chair, Department of Pathology and Laboratory Medicine
University of Kentucky Chandler Medical Center
Lexington, Kentucky

Carol B. Stelling, M.D.

Professor of Diagnostic Radiology
University of Kentucky College of Medicine
Director, Breast Diagnostic Center
University of Kentucky Chandler Medical Center
Lexington, Kentucky

With line drawings by **Richard A. Gersony, M.F.A.**

with 576 illustrations

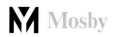 Mosby

St. Louis Baltimore Boston Chicago London Madrid Philadelphia Sydney Toronto

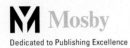
Dedicated to Publishing Excellence

Executive Editor: Susan M. Gay
Developmental Editor: Sandra E. Clark
Project Manager: Linda Clarke
Project Supervisor: Victoria Hoenigke
Illustrations: Richard A. Gersony M.F.A.
Designer: Liz Fett

Copyright © 1994 by Mosby–Year Book, Inc.

All rights reserved. No part of this publication may be reproduced, stored in a retrieval system, or transmitted, in any form or by any means, electronic, mechanical, photocopying, recording, or otherwise, without prior written permission from the publisher.

Permission to photocopy or reproduce solely for internal or personal use is permitted for libraries or other users registered with the Copyright Clearance Center, 27 Congress Street, provided that the base fee of $4.00 per chapter plus $.10 per page is paid directly to the Copyright Clearance Center, 27 Congress Street, Salem, MA 01970. This consent does not extend to other kinds of copying, such as copying for general distribution, for advertising or promotional purposes, for creating collected works, or for resale.

Printed in the United States of America

Mosby–Year Book, Inc.
11830 Westline Industrial Drive
St. Louis, MO 63146

Library of Congress Cataloging-in-Publication Data
The diagnosis and detection of breast disease / Deborah E. Powell,
    Carol B. Stelling.
        p.   cm.
    Includes bibliographical references and index.
    ISBN 0-8016/74875
    1. Breast—Diseases—Diagnosis.   2. Breast—Diseases—Atlases.
I. Powell, Deborah E.   II. Stelling, Carol B.
    [DNLM: 1. Breast Diseases—diagnosis.   2. Breast—pathology—
atlases.   WP 840 D536 1994]
    RG493.D53   1994
    618.1'9075—dc20
    DNLM/DLC
    for Library of Congress   93–49592
                                                                   CIP

94 95 96 97 98 CL/MY 9 8 7 6 5 4 3 2 1

Contributors

Karen S. Baker, M.D.
Assistant Professor of Diagnostic Radiology
Department of Diagnostic Radiology
University of Kentucky College of Medicine
Lexington, Kentucky

Michael L. Cibull, M.D.
Associate Professor of Pathology and Laboratory
  Medicine
Director of Surgical Pathology
Department of Pathology and Laboratory Medicine
University of Kentucky College of Medicine
Lexington, Kentucky

Diane D. Davey, M.D.
Assistant Professor of Pathology and Laboratory
  Medicine
Director of Cytopathology
Department of Pathology and Laboratory Medicine
University of Kentucky College of Medicine
Lexington, Kentucky

C. Darrell Jennings, M.D.
Associate Professor of Pathology and Laboratory
  Medicine
Director of Immunopathology
Department of Pathology and Laboratory Medicine
University of Kentucky College of Medicine
Lexington, Kentucky

Daniel E. Kenady, M.D.
Professor of Surgery
Department of Surgery
University of Kentucky College of Medicine
Lexington, Kentucky

Patrick C. McGrath, M.D., F.A.C.S.
Assistant Professor of Surgery
Department of Surgery
University of Kentucky College of Medicine
Lexington, Kentucky

Deborah E. Powell, M.D.
Professor of Pathology and Laboratory Medicine
University of Kentucky College of Medicine
Chair, Department of Pathology and Laboratory
  Medicine
University of Kentucky Chandler Medical Center
Lexington, Kentucky

Carol B. Stelling, M.D.
Professor of Diagnostic Radiology
University of Kentucky College of Medicine
Director, Breast Diagnostic Center
University of Kentucky Chandler Medical Center
Lexington, Kentucky

To Rosemary, Jean, Nancy, Sandi, Doris,
Abby, Betty, Virginia, Scotty, Ann, Mary,
Rosie, Kelley, Janet and all the women
with breast disease who have taught
us so much, we dedicate this book.

Preface

This book represents for us the culmination of a longstanding collaboration predicated on the belief that patients are best served when physicians work as a team. We have therefore written this book to emphasize the importance of the team approach to the diagnosis of breast diseases. We believe that it is important for the treating physicians from different disciplines to be aware of the diagnostic pitfalls that each face. This is both the purpose in writing this type of book and what we hope is its most important message. The completion of this book is difficult for us. The relocation of one of us (CBS) to a new institution marks the end of a professional collaboration begun in 1980. While our working relationship will of necessity be diminished by this move, our personal respect and friendship will endure.

This book is also the product of the work of a large number of individuals besides ourselves. We are extremely grateful to all of them for their help and their expertise which has enabled us to complete this project. We would like to thank our co-authors for their hard work in producing chapters that make the book truly a team effort. Thanks are extended to Diana Kimball, Debra Martin, and Retha Higgs for capable secretarial help with numerous manuscript revisions. Joy Stoll and Sandi Jaros were generous with their help in finding cases and materials for photographs and in literature searches. We are indebted to Richard Geissler, Gary McClure and William Gill for excellent photographic support. Richard Gersony is responsible for the magnificent illustrations that we feel enhance the book greatly. The staff of the film library in the Department of Diagnostic Radiology helped identify and find cases, and Sylvia Valle, one of our supervisory histotechnologists, willingly prepared high-quality slides from old blocks. A number of colleagues contributed unusual cases that we did not have in our own departments. We are extremely grateful to these individuals, whose names are cited in the book with their cases. We would also like to thank our colleagues at the University of Kentucky Medical Center and particularly the cytotechnologists, histotechnologists, and radiologic technologists who have worked with us over the years in the diagnosis of breast disease for the patients at our medical center. We would also like to thank our editors at Mosby, Susan Gay, Sandra Clark, and Vicki Hoenigke, who worked with us on this project from initial conception to final product with help when needed and nudging when appropriate. Most especially we would like to thank our families, and in particular our husbands, Dr. Michael Stelling and Dr. Ralph Powell. Without their understanding and support this book could not have been written.

Finally, as the dedication states, we would like to thank and pay tribute to our patients with breast disease. They are responsible for teaching us much of what we write here and are indeed the reason for this book.

Deborah E. Powell, M.D.
Carol B. Stelling, M.D.

Contents

PART I

Technical and Clinical Aspects of Breast Diagnosis

The Normal Breast: Structure, Function, and Epidemiology

Deborah E. Powell

The human mammary gland arises in the embryo along two lines, called the milk lines, which extend on the anterior chest from the level of the axillae to the groin. Usually only two glands develop, one on each side of the anterior thorax. However, accessory breast tissue may be found at any point along the milk line, and in rare instances tumors can arise in this accessory tissue or the tissue can respond to hormonal stimulation with hypertrophy and formation of a mass (Fig. 1-1, A and B).

The human breast is a type of apocrine sweat gland, modified for the secretion of milk. It is a hormonally responsive tissue that usually develops identically in both the male and female until puberty. At this time, stimulated by hormones primarily from the pituitary gland and ovary, the female breast develops and the male breast does not undergo similar developmental changes.

STRUCTURE OF THE FEMALE BREAST

The mammary glands are located in the superficial fascia of the anterior chest wall.[3-5] The suspensory ligaments of Cooper anchor the breast to the underlying pectoralis major muscle fascia and to the overlying dermis. A lateral projection of the gland, the axillary tail of Spence, may extend for a variable distance into the axilla (Fig. 1-2, A and B).[1] The blood supply to the breast is primarily from the internal mammary and lateral thoracic arteries. The lymphatic drainage is to pectoral, axillary, and subclavicular lymph nodes predominantly; however, internal mammary lymph nodes may drain medial portions of the breast. Occasion-

ally, lymph nodes are found within the mammary parenchyma, especially laterally (Fig. 1-3).

The female breast, after puberty, is composed of glandular and ductal elements embedded within varying amounts of fibrous and adipose tissue. The glandular elements or lobules consist of small secretory ductules and acini. These are the terminal units of a system of branching ducts that ramify as subdivisions from the large lactiferous ducts.[4] Approximately 20 to 25 major lactiferous ducts empty into the nipple. Before opening into the nipple, each lactiferous duct dilates to form the lactiferous sinus, located approximately 1 cm beneath the nipple. The nipple and areola are covered by pigmented epithelium. These structures are richly supplied by nerves and blood vessels and contain bands of smooth muscle. In the nipple these bands are oriented parallel to the lactiferous ducts and in a circular pattern near the base of the nipple. Contraction of this smooth muscle causes erection of the nipple. On the areola are found small, raised nodules referred to as tubercles of Montgomery. These nodules contain sebaceous glands not associated with hair follicles and glands of Montgomery.[2] The glands of Montgomery function during lactation and represent true secreting structures, similar to the secretory units found in the breast. Their ducts are coiled, however, before they dilate into a lactiferous sinus. These lactiferous ducts, often accompanied by sebaceous glands, form the tubercles of Montgomery on the areolar surface (Fig. 1-4).

At their point of origin at the nipple, the lactiferous ducts are lined by a keratinizing squamous epithelium. Usually the opening of the ducts in the nonpregnant female is blocked by a keratin plug. At or above the level of the lactiferous sinus, the duct lining becomes a cuboidal epithelium with a prominent underlying basement membrane. Between the epithelium and the basement membrane is a discontinuous layer of myoepithelial cells (Fig. 1-5). This lining of cuboidal lumi-

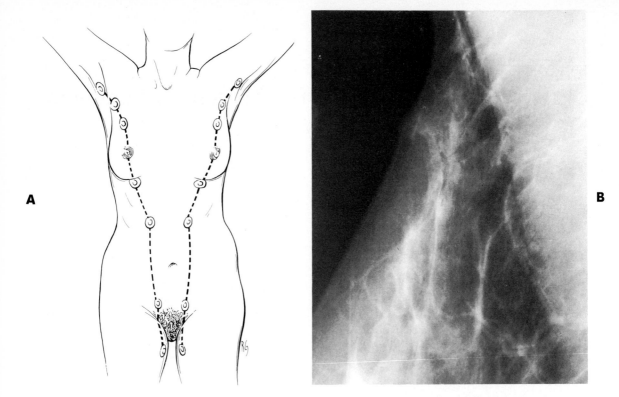

Fig. 1-1 A, Diagrammatic representation of the embryonic milk lines illustrating sites at which accessory breast tissue and supernumerary nipples can arise. **B,** A supernumerary nipple projects from the skin surface in the tail of the breast in this oblique projection. A ductal structure extends from the axillary parenchyma to the nipple.

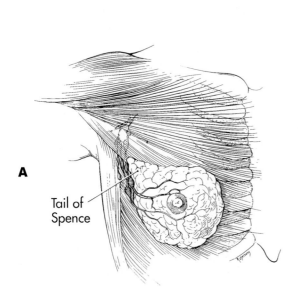

Tail of Spence

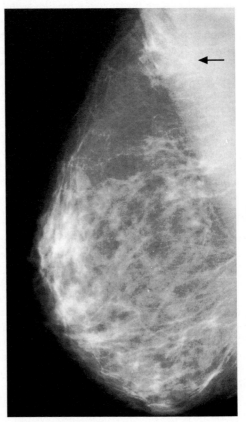

Fig. 1-2 A, Diagrammatic representation of the axillary tail of Spence. Note the location of the lymph nodes which may occasionally be found within the breast parenchyma in this region. **B,** Breast parenchyma in the low axillary area represents normal axillary breast tissue (*arrow*).

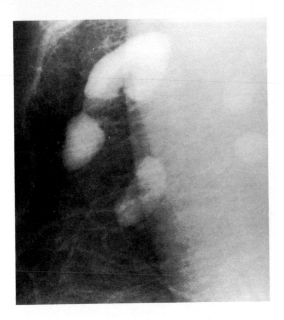

Fig. 1-3 Normal lymph nodes with fatty hilum located in breast tissue and projected over pectoral muscle.

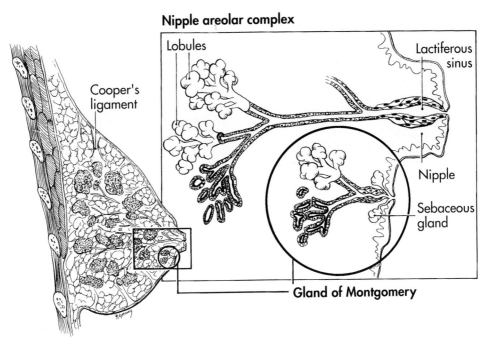

Fig. 1-4 Diagrammatic representation of the breast and the nipple-areolar complex. Both the main duct system extending from the nipple to the lobular units and the glands of Montgomery, which terminate on the areola, are illustrated. The main lactiferous ducts dilate beneath the nipple epithelium to form the lactiferous sinus. To this point, the duct is lined by stratified squamous epithelium. More distal, the ducts are lined by a double layer of epithelial and myoepithelial cells. The ducts of the glands of Montgomery are associated with sebaceous glands as they empty onto the surface of the areola at the tubercle of Montgomery. The most superficial portion of this duct structure is coiled and then dilates slightly before branching. The glands of Montgomery terminate in small secretory structures, similar to the true lobules.

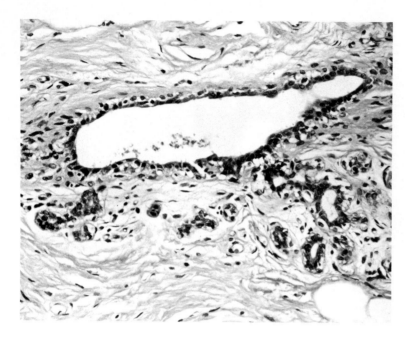

Fig. 1-5 Photomicrograph of small mammary ducts illustrates the two-layered cell lining. The darker stained epithelial cells are located closer to the lumen, whereas the pale staining vacuolated myoepithelial cells are located adjacent to the surrounding stroma.

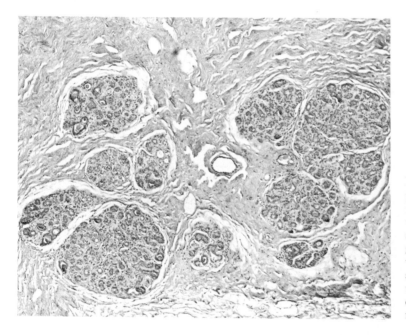

Fig. 1-6 This low-power photomicrograph of a lobule illustrates the centrally located terminal duct and the peripherally arranged clusters of small glandular structures grouped within a loose fibrovascular stroma. The stroma exterior to the lobule and the terminal duct is composed of collagen-rich connective tissue.

nal epithelium, myoepithelium, and basement membrane extends down to the level of the secretory units of the breast.[3] The epithelium may undergo changes under the influence of hormones, particularly estrogen and progesterone, in a cyclic fashion during the female reproductive years, as will be discussed later. The terminal acinar units of the breast are also lined by cuboidal epithelium, underlying myoepithelium, and basement membrane. These small groupings of acinar structures

are referred to as lobules, and an alveolar or terminal duct is usually identified centrally within the lobular unit (Fig. 1-6). The individual terminal units of the lobule are contained within a specialized connective tissue, which is loose and highly cellular, termed the perilobular stroma. This lobular connective tissue has a rich capillary network but contains little to no fat (Fig. 1-7,A–C). Outside the lobule, the parenchyma of the breast consists of a mix of dense fibrous paucicel-

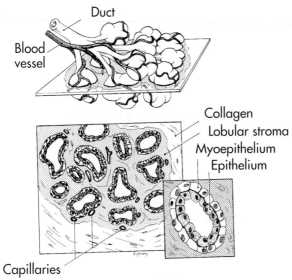

A

Duct

Blood
vessel

Collagen
Lobular stroma
Myoepithelium
Epithelium

Capillaries

Fig. 1-7 A, Diagrammatic three-
dimensional cross-sectional represen-
tations of the lobule, emphasizing
the stromal vascularity and the preservation of the double-layered epithelium into the most distal lobular
units. Low (**B**) and higher power
(**C**) photomicrographs of the lobule
illustrate these features histologically.

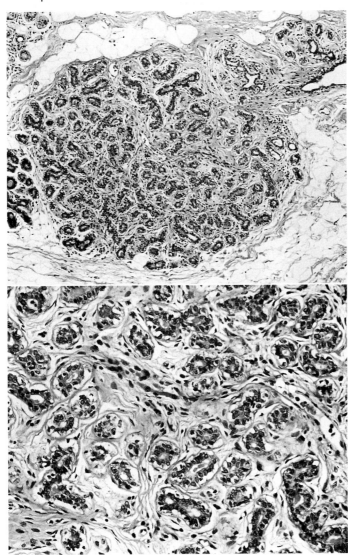

B

C

lular connective tissue and mature adipose tissue in which small blood vessels can be identified.

FUNCTION OF THE FEMALE BREAST

The female breast undergoes striking hormonally mediated changes at menarche or shortly before.[8,13] The production in the ovaries of estrogen followed by progesterone stimulates the growth of the breast parenchyma. Other hormones such as growth hormone, thyroxine, and insulin also play a role in this process. There is elongation and branching of the duct system with the development of terminal buds into rudimentary lobular structures. Fat deposition, vascularization, and change in volume of the connective tissue parenchyma also occur at this time, and these latter changes are important for increase in size and protrusion of the breast disk. Changes in nipple and areola also occur, consisting mainly of increased size and pigmentation. Occasionally there is a marked increase in volume of one or both breasts during puberty, which is referred to as pubertal hyperplasia. This is contrasted with giant fibroadenoma in Chapter 9. The formation of the lobule is accentuated by pregnancy when the lobules become fully differentiated.

Several studies have been published on changes that occur in the epithelial cells and in the perilobular stroma during the menstrual cycle.[6,10,14] In the follicular phase of the cycle the acini are small, with no evidence of active secretion by the radially oriented cells lining the lumina. The lobular stroma is compact, with relatively few lymphocytes and little edema or metachromasia. Epithelial cells are shown to undergo some evidence of cytoplasmic blebbing during the early luteal phases of the menstrual cycle without evidence of active secretion, whereas myoepithelial cells become strikingly vacuolated. True apocrine secretion into a distended lumen is seen in the latter half of the luteal phase. There is an increase in epithelial mitotic figures close to the beginning of menstruation followed by an increase in cell death (apoptosis) at the time of menses, which extends into the early part of the follicular phase. During the luteal phase the perilobular stroma becomes more edematous, and lymphocytic infiltration and metachromasia peak at the time of menses (Fig. 1-8).

The breast becomes fully differentiated during pregnancy and lactation, and the terminal lobular units are most affected during this physiologic state. Several histologic changes occur in the terminal ducts and lobules with enlargement and formation of new lobular units early in pregnancy. By the end of the second trimester of pregnancy, secretory changes are well developed and the cuboidal luminal epithelial cells show evidence of vacuolization. Accumulation of fat droplets occurs within the cytoplasm of the epithelium of the lobules during the third trimester. The lobules undergo striking hyperplasia to occupy most of the breast parenchyma during this time, with a decrease in the interlobular connective tissue. Finally, the expanded lobular units show marked distention of their lumina by colostrum (Fig. 1-9, A–C).

After lactation, the breast undergoes involutional changes, which may take several months. Some of these changes are probably due to a reduction in prolactin levels, but the role of mechanical and vascular stimuli on this involution is not understood well. However, the lobular units become more compact and lose the luminal secretions, and the interlobular stroma once again becomes more prominent.[3] This pattern is referred to as the resting lobule. Some patients who are not pregnant or lactating have been found to have these same secretory changes in breast biopsies, often in a focal distribution.[11,12] These changes, often referred to as focal pregnancy-like changes, may be associated with exogenous hormones such as oral contraceptives as well as other medication.[7]

After menopause, the breast undergoes involution and atrophy, which involves primarily parenchymal elements of the breast, particularly the lobule (Fig. 1-10). Parenchymal cells undergo atrophy and fibrosis, and hyalinization of the stroma of the lobule as well as the lobular elements themselves is seen. Concomitantly, there is an increase in adipose tissue within the breast and a decrease in both fibrous connective tissue and elastic tissue (Fig. 1-11, A and B). Ultimately, much of the breast consists of adipose tissue and some hyalinized fibrous stroma with small ductal elements and occasionally a few lobular units, which may show microcystic change of the terminal ductules. Occasionally, persistence of lobules is seen in breasts of postmenopausal women who are not receiving exogenous hormones.[9] This latter finding is considered by some to represent evidence of endogenous hormone secretion. It is considered to be a risk factor for subsequent development of carcinoma by some authors.[15]

HORMONES AND THE FEMALE BREAST

As mentioned, the mammary gland is a hormonally responsive organ. The female breast is most impressively influenced by estrogen and progesterone, but several other hormones also affect the mammary gland, especially during lactation. Estrogen produced chiefly by the ovary is important for the increased size of the breast during puberty

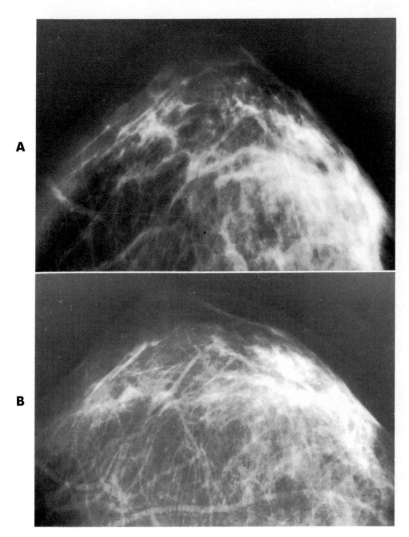

Fig. 1-8 Monthly cyclic changes. Numerous vague densities in the breast become more prominent in the premenstrual phase (A) as compared with midcycle (B). This variability is seldom noted radiographically.

and again in pregnancy, when estrogen is produced by the placenta as well. Estrogen promotes fat deposition and growth of both stroma and the duct system of the breast. Progesterone, also from the ovary, stimulates growth of the lobules and acini. Progesterone also causes an increase in interstitial fluid in the breast, particularly in the perilobular stroma. During pregnancy, progesterone from the placenta stimulates marked increase in lobules, in both size and number, and is responsible for secretory modifications in the cytoplasm of the acinar cells. Other hormones (insulin, growth hormone, glucocorticoids, and prolactin) are important for the growth of the duct system of the breast.

Although the lobule of the breast is prepared for lactation by progesterone, prolactin is necessary for lactation to occur. Lactation in the pregnant female is inhibited by estrogen and proges-terone produced by the placenta, despite the fact that serum prolactin levels rise during pregnancy to 10 times that of the nonpregnant state. However, after delivery, with loss of placental estrogen and progesterone, lactation is stimulated by the high serum prolactin. Growth hormone, glucocorticoids, and parathyroid hormone are required for proper composition of the milk, and oxytocin, which stimulates myoepithelial cell contraction, permits the ejection of milk from the acini.

At the cellular level, estrogen and progesterone function by binding to specific receptor proteins.[20] These, with other steroid hormone receptor proteins, are members of a supergene family—the nuclear hormone receptor family—which in addition to the steroid receptors includes receptors for vitamin D, thyroid hormone, and retinoic acid.[17] The estrogen and progesterone receptors are con-

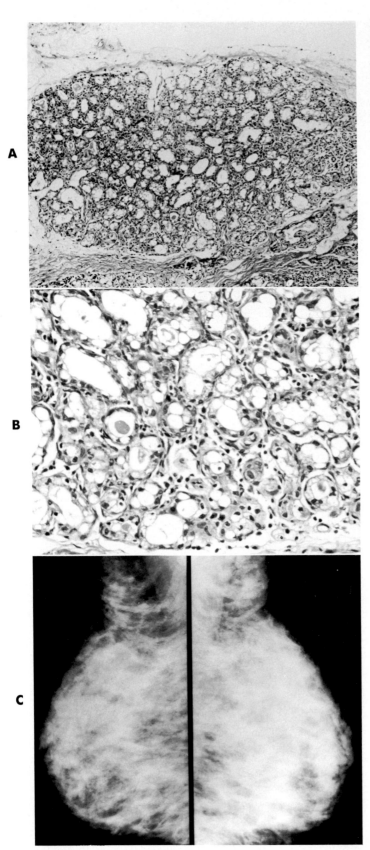

Fig. 1-9 A, During the last trimester of pregnancy there is marked hyperplasia of the lobules, with striking expansion in their size. **B,** The vacuolization of the cytoplasm of the lobular epithelial cells that occurs during the third trimester is illustrated in this photomicrograph, which also illustrates the distention of the gland lumens by secretory material. **C,** During pregnancy the mammary parenchyma is extremely dense, lowering the sensitivity of mammography. Note presence of axillary breast tissue.

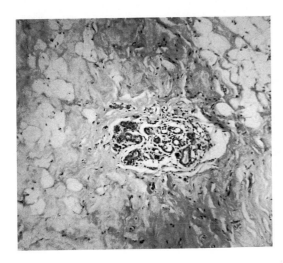

Fig. 1-10 Atrophic lobule. The atrophic breast is composed predominantly of fat and dense fiburous tissue. Lobules are small and contain a few small acinar units as seen in the center of this photomicrograph. Contrast the size of this lobule with the one illustrated in Fig. 1-16 from a premenopausal patient.

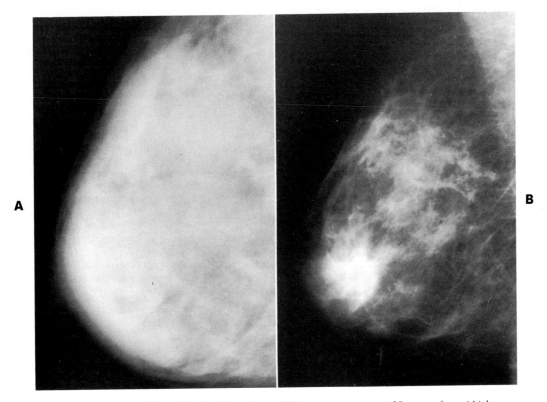

Fig. 1-11 Extremely dense fibroglandular tissue of this young woman at 28 years of age **(A)** became heterogeneously dense as fatty tissue replaced glandular stroma by age 36 years **(B).**

centrated to a large extent within the cell nucleus, where they bind their ligands and function as nuclear transcription factors to enhance the expression of specific genes. Some receptor protein is also present in the cytoplasm.[19] Target tissues such as the breast generally contain elevated levels of these receptors, which are phosphorylated proteins containing sulfhydryl groups required for ligand interactions. All of these receptors contain a ligand-binding region, a DNA domain, and variable regions that contribute in some way to optimal function. In its resting or unactivated state, the estrogen receptor is complexed with a 90 kd heat shock protein (Hsp 90). This complex in some way prevents the binding of the unactivated estrogen receptor to DNA, but the association of the estrogen receptor and Hsp 90 is broken during ligand binding and receptor activation. Binding of receptor to hormone activates the receptor and increases its affinity for DNA, and the receptor-ligand complex becomes tightly associated with the nuclear compartment of the cell. In the case of the estrogen receptor, the activated receptor then binds to DNA estrogen response elements (EREs), which function as enhancers of transcription.[16] EREs, like other hormone response elements (HREs), may be clustered to form highly active hormone response units. This clustering may be particularly marked in the vicinity of some hormonally regulated genes. The mechanisms by which HREs activate gene transcription are incompletely understood at this time, and some inhibitory HREs have also been identified.

Although estrogens are thought to be implicated in the development of many carcinomas of the breast, the exact mechanism is unknown. Estrogenic stimulation at critical stages of mammary development or involution may be an important factor.[18] Even though the exact role of steroid hormones in mammary carcinogenesis is unclear, identification and quantification of levels of estrogen and progesterone receptors in breast tumor tissue are important for the management and development of treatment plans for patients with breast cancer. A variety of methods, both qualitative and quantitative, are available for analysis of estrogen and progesterone receptors. This is discussed further in Chapter 8.

MAMMOGRAPHIC PATTERNS OF THE NORMAL BREAST

The mammographic appearance of the normal adult female breast has been classified into subtypes. The impetus for this classification by John Wolfe[32,33] was initially to determine whether certain mammographic patterns were associated with an increased risk for breast cancer. The four clas-

sic Wolfe categories were titled N1, P1, P2, and DY. Later, a fifth classification, QDY, was suggested, but this classification has not been widely used. Briefly, criteria for these categories are as follows:

N1 or normal — A pattern of islands of radiolucent fat with a delicate trabeculated appearance.

P1 — Prominent duct pattern, again showing a breast predominantly composed of radiolucent fat but with up to one fourth of the volume exhibiting cord-like structures or a beaded appearance of ducts. This prominent duct pattern is most apparent in the subareolar area but may be seen extending to one quadrant.

P2 — In this pattern more than one fourth of the breast volume is involved by prominent ducts where dense linear structures involve, in some instances, all of the parenchyma.

DY — A markedly dense appearance of the breast. The prominent duct pattern is absent and most of the lucent fat is replaced. Many breasts with a DY pattern show a homogeneous radiodense pattern.

QDY — A breast pattern seen in women less than 40 years of age exhibiting a considerable DY pattern but with small islands of radiolucent fat.

These changes are illustrated in Fig. 1-12. Correlations have been made between histopathology and Wolfe's mammographic parenchymal patterns.[22,30] One study[30] used mammograms and breast biopsy specimens from 143 patients to attempt to define histopathologic changes associated with each of the four Wolfe's patterns. On the basis of this study, it was shown that the N1 classification showed normal ducts, lobules, and stroma, and the P1 pattern showed prominent periductal and perilobular fibrosis. Also in this P1 pattern, some focal nodular lesions were identified that were usually classified as low-grade epithelial atypias. The P2 pattern likewise demonstrated histopathologic evidence of periductal and perilobular fibrosis, but this was frequently more marked than in the P1 patterns. In addition, breasts with the P2 pattern showed more nodular and focal lesions of the terminal lobular units with increasing

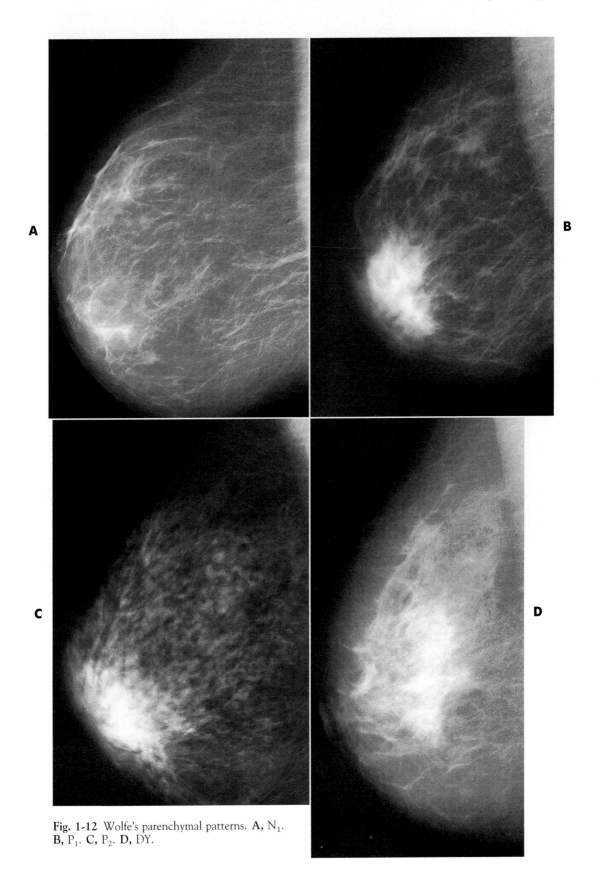

Fig. 1-12 Wolfe's parenchymal patterns. **A,** N_1.
B, P_1. **C,** P_2. **D,** DY.

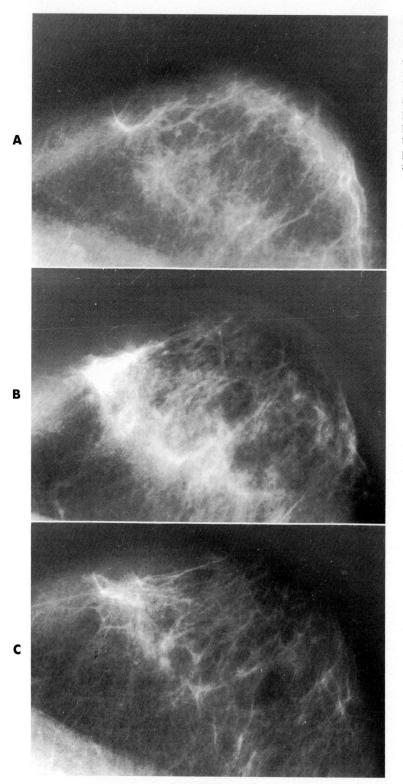

Fig. 1-13 Effect of hormonal replacement therapy. **A,** The breast consists almost entirely of fat tissue. **B,** Twenty-four months later the patient is on hormonal replacement therapy and there are numerous vague parenchymal densities. **C,** The parenchyma has atrophied to fatty tissue 1 year later, after patient stopped hormonal therapy.

grades of atypia. The DY pattern showed marked confluent fibrosis. In addition, it showed within the dense fibrous tissue increased numbers of atypical lobules having high-grade epithelial atypia. Studies by Wolfe suggested that these parenchymal patterns were associated with varying degrees of cancer risk, as discussed further in this chapter.[33] Wolfe[31] also demonstrated that the radiographic parenchymal patterns could change with aging in the breast, and this finding was later confirmed by Flook and others.[23] Most breasts initially classified as having low-risk N1 or P1 patterns did not show evidence of significant change during periods of follow-up, which averaged 7.5 years in Wolfe's study and slightly less than 15 years in Flook's study. However, both studies confirmed that a significant percentage of patients initially showing DY parenchymal patterns changed with aging, usually to a high-risk P2 pattern but at least in some patients to lower risk P1 or N1 patterns.

Mammographic patterns are also known to change with hormonal status of the patient. Recent studies[21,28,29] have all suggested that in a certain percentage of women receiving postmenopausal hormonal replacement either with estrogen alone or more frequently with estrogen and progesterone combinations there is an increase in density and occasionally in cyst formation within breast parenchyma that has been shown to regress when hormone treatment is withdrawn (Fig. 1-13, A–C.) Pathologic studies have shown some evidence of epithelial hyperplasia and of persistence or development of new lobules in women receiving hormonal replacement therapy.[7,25] Whether oral contraceptive use in premenopausal women alters the appearance of the breast mammographically is still somewhat controversial. Studies by Gravelle and others[24] suggested an increased number of low-risk (N1 and P1) patterns and a lower number of high-risk (P2 and DY) patterns in women who used or had previously taken oral contraceptive pills. However, studies by Leinster and Whitehouse,[27] while confirming the finding of a decrease in the proportion of patients with P2 patterns and an increase in the proportion with N1 patterns, also showed a slight increase in the incidence of DY pattern in both premenopausal and postmenopausal patients who had taken oral contraceptive pills.

In addition to parenchymal patterns in the breast, criteria for benign examination include symmetry of the breast tissue (Fig. 1-14). Although in some textbooks, asymmetry of breast tissue has been considered an indication of malignancy, this rationale is not supported in a study by Kopans and others.[26] Their study of 8408 mammograms demonstrated 3% of patients to show some type of asymmetric breast tissue, including asymmetric volume, asymmetry in density, or asymmetry in prominent ducts without evidence of a mass. Twenty of the 221 patients showing asymmetry underwent biopsy, with three having malignant lesions. All three of the lesions were associated with palpable masses, leading the authors to conclude that asymmetry was not in itself a reason for biopsy and represented a normal variation, whereas asymmetry in the presence of a

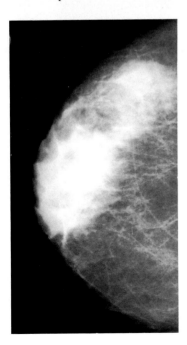 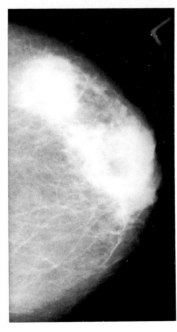

Fig. 1-14 Bilateral symmetry of heterogeneously dense parenchyma on craniocaudad projections.

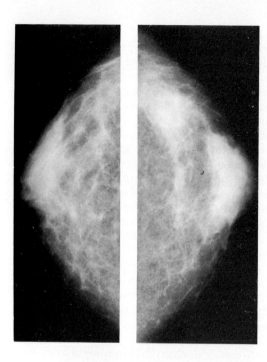

Fig. 1-15 Asymmetric breast tissue in the left axillary tail relative to the right axillary tail. There was no palpable asymmetry and no radiographic change over 3 years.

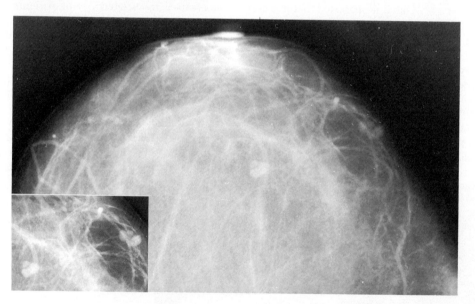

Fig. 1-16 Normal small intramammary lymph nodes showed no change over 3 years.

palpable mass should, of course, lead to a biopsy procedure (Fig. 1-15). Other examples of normal breast patterns on mammography include accessory axillary breast tissue, which may be unilateral or bilateral and which is distinct from the axillary tail of Spence (Fig. 1-2B). It has been suggested that this tissue is best visualized on oblique and exaggerated craniocaudad views.[1] Finally, intramammary lymph nodes represent a normal variant finding (Fig. 1-16).

EPIDEMIOLOGY AND RISK FACTORS FOR BREAST DISEASE

Numerous epidemiologic studies have dealt with potential risk factors for the development of breast cancer (Box 1-1 and Box 1-2). Excellent recent reviews such as those of Kelsey and Gammon[49,50] provide a good summary of present knowledge. Most of the epidemiology data is available for breast cancer; fewer studies have been done for benign breast disease.

BOX 1-1 RISK FACTORS FOR BREAST CANCER[44,49,50]

Female over 40 years of age
Prior history of breast cancer
Early menarche, before age 12 years
Late menopause, after age 50 years
Late first pregnancy (after age 30 years)
Nulliparity
Obesity[46]
High socioeconomic status
Daily alcohol consumption[56]
P_2 or DY Wolfe parenchymal pattern[38]
History of more than one breast operation
Atypical hyperplasia on biopsy
Personal history of other adenocarcinoma
Ionizing radiation exposure[34,40,45,52]
Genetic predisposition[39,44,48,58]

BOX 1-2 FACTORS THAT HAVE NO EFFECT ON BREAST CANCER RISK[48]

Breast feeding
Number of children
Breast size
Caffeine[53]
Cysts and nonhyperplastic breast disease
Thyroid medications[37,57]

Most epidemiologic studies of benign breast disease have considered only biopsy-diagnosed cases. As pointed out by numerous authors, this research by no means represents the entire population of women with benign breast disease.[43] The term *benign breast disease* can encompass the multiple histologic patterns of fibrocystic change as well as other benign lesions (radial scars) and benign tumors such as fibroadenomas and intraductal papillomas. Fibrocystic disease and fibroadenomas represent the most common of these entities but are very different in terms of their age incidences and possibly their epidemiology. Moreover, although the most common patterns of fibrocystic change are not associated with an increased risk of breast cancer, a few low-incidence proliferative subgroups do show an increased cancer risk.[42]

A review by Ernster published in 1981 assessed current epidemiologic studies of fibrocystic disease to that time.[43] Many of the risk factors reported were those shown to be important for breast cancer risk. However, some of the risk factors most strongly associated with breast cancer (e.g., family history) show no significant association with benign breast disease. Likewise, reproductive factors known to be associated with increased breast cancer risk showed inconsistent or weak associations with benign breast disease. These include nulliparity and low parity as well as late menopause. Late age at first childbirth and early menarche showed no association with benign breast disease in this review. A negative association of obesity with benign breast disease has been reported in several studies. This is in direct contrast to the increased association with obesity reported for breast cancer. Several studies summarized reported a protective effect of oral contraceptive pills on benign breast disease.

More recently other reports have examined possible associations of cigarette smoking,[55] alcohol consumption,[54] and estrogen therapy[35,47,59] with benign breast disease. No significant association of either alcohol or cigarette use was found. In contrast, conjugated estrogen replacement therapy was associated with benign breast disease in several studies. However, all the patients in these studies were treated with estrogen alone and not estrogen-progesterone combination therapy.

For breast cancer, the factors associated with most significantly increased risk are age, country of birth, and family history.[49,50] It has long been known that breast cancer incidence increases with age despite the fact that more cases are now being detected in young women. Likewise, the increased incidence of breast cancer in North America and northern Europe and the relatively low incidence in Asia and Africa have been known for some time. Finally, although recent studies on heredity are interesting and have produced some slightly different data, it has long been accepted that there is an increased relative risk of two to three times for women who have an affected first-degree relative with breast cancer.

Numerous breast cancer risk factors are related to either endogenous or exogenous hormonal status. These include the increased relative risk associated with nulliparity and older age at first birth. There is a relative risk of approximately 1.4 for women whose age is greater than 35 years at the time of their first full-term pregnancy. Correspondingly, for women whose breast cancers are diagnosed after 50 years of age, there seems to be a decreased risk with increased number of pregnancies. This, however, does not hold true for women with breast cancer diagnosed before the age of 45 years. Although the older literature suggested a protective effect of lactation and new studies are producing some controversial data, the effect of lactation, if any, is probably not strongly protective. Early age at menarche and late age at menopause also increase a woman's risk for the subsequent development of breast cancer. There has been shown to be a decreased risk in women who undergo bilateral oophorectomy before the age of 40 years. Exogenous hormones in the form of replacement estrogens or oral contraceptive pills continue to be of interest to investigators concerned with their possible role in the development of breast cancer. Despite numerous studies on women who have used oral contraceptive pills, there have been no consistent data showing an increased risk for the subsequent development of breast cancer. One exception may be a subgroup of women who have used contraceptive pills for relatively long periods starting at an early age, specifically before their first full-term pregnancy. This finding, however, needs to be substantiated, and this group of women needs to be studied as they enter the higher risk age groups. Replacement estrogen therapy may be associated with a slightly increased risk of developing breast cancer, specifically in women who have long-term (greater than 20-year) use of exogenous estrogens or who have used relatively high doses. This question needs to be further studied, and particularly women who are receiving both estrogen and progestational agents as replacement therapy need to be assessed for the possible protective role of progestins. Finally, a slightly increased risk of subsequent breast cancer development has been shown in women who received diethylstilbestrol during pregnancy.

Life-style variables have also been of intense interest to epidemiologists studying breast cancer risk. It is well accepted that the risk of breast cancer is greater with increasing weight in postmenopausal patients. Some recent studies have also suggested that increased height may be an independent risk factor, but this information needs to be confirmed in other studies. Although the role of dietary animal fats was for a time thought to be an important risk factor for breast cancer, primarily based on animal data and data from other populations, recent, more sophisticated studies have failed to show convincingly that increased dietary animal fat is significantly related to increased breast cancer risk. Total caloric intake may be more important as a risk factor than dietary fat.[60] Several studies to date have shown some increased risk for subsequent breast cancer development with alcohol consumption, but there are still unanswered questions about whether this is related to moderate or heavy drinking and

whether the type of alcohol ingested is important in the assessment of risk.[56,61] No good associations of cigarette smoking and subsequent breast cancer development have been shown, and likewise other factors that have been investigated, including stress, depression, and hair dyes, have not shown convincing evidence of increased breast cancer risk. Some recent studies suggest the possible relationship of moderate physical activity to modest decreases in breast cancer risk. Recently, there has been a suggestion that exposure to electromagnetic fields may increase risk, but to date relatively few studies have addressed this issue.

Hereditary factors have been shown to be very important, as previously mentioned. Relative risks of breast cancer for women who have one primary first-degree relative with breast cancer are 1.5 to 2,[44] and the risks are markedly increased for women with both a mother and a sister who develop breast cancer. It has been reported that for this latter group the relative risk may approach 5.0 by age 65. Although in the past studies emphasized the importance of a family history of premenopausal bilateral breast cancer, this may not be as important as previously thought. Some recent studies of families with ataxia telangiectasia and other large family cohorts have suggested the possibility of a dominantly inherited susceptibility gene.[39,58] While this finding probably involves relatively few families, it provides added impetus for research that may lead to the discovery of breast cancer susceptibility genes. It has been known for some time that women who have had carcinoma of the ovary or endometrium are at slightly increased risk to develop carcinoma of the breast. Certainly a history of previous breast cancer is significant risk to the subsequent development of a second primary tumor. Women with one breast cancer have a three- to four-fold increased risk of developing a second cancer of the breast, and this is exacerbated in women with a positive family history.

Certain mammographic patterns in the breast have been associated with increased risk for the subsequent development of breast cancer. These were discussed earlier in this chapter. Specifically, patients with P2 and DY patterns have been shown by several studies to have a slight increased risk for breast cancer.[32] Studies of possible relationships between known risk factors for breast cancer and the Wolfe's mammographic patterns[51] showed some differences between premenopausal and postmenopausal patients. However, for both groups a rise in the incidence of the high-risk patterns was noted to be associated with late age at first pregnancy and a history of breast biopsy. Conversely, also for both groups, a decrease in incidence of the high-risk patterns was noted with increasing weight and increasing breast size. Although the role of fibrocystic disease as a breast cancer risk factor has long been considered, recent studies have defined the groups of women with fibrocystic disease who are truly at risk for the subsequent development of breast cancer. Studies by Dupont and Page have shown convincingly that the risk of breast cancer is most significant for the very small group of women who are shown to have proliferative fibrocystic disease with atypia on breast biopsy.[41] This finding is unusual in the entire universe of women who undergo breast biopsy and probably constitutes less than 5% of all biopsies for fibrocystic disease. The much more common proliferative patterns of fibrocystic disease that do not show atypia and constitute approximately 25% of breast biopsies for fibrocystic disease convey a risk of a much lower magnitude. The same authors have also shown that these proliferative changes are more significant in women with a family history of breast cancer. The relative risks of either proliferative fibrocystic disease or proliferative fibrocystic disease with atypia are magnified by the addition of a positive family history.

The role of radiation in the subsequent development of breast cancer is of considerable interest, and numerous studies have been conducted to assess this. It has convincingly been shown that there is an increased risk of subsequent breast cancer if the breast tissue is exposed to radiation before the age of 40.[52] This is true whether the radiation dose is administered as one large dose (for example, in survivors of the atom bomb explosions) or in multiple small doses received over time. It is also known that this increased risk persists for a very long time, certainly greater than 35 years and possibly for the entire life of the patient. Recent studies have also shown that this risk can begin if the breast is exposed to radiation in infancy and appears to be important in all patients exposed to radiation under age 40.[45] In contrast, women who receive radiation to the breast after age 40 have no or at best only minimal increased risk of the subsequent development of breast cancer. Recent studies[36] looking at the possibility that radiation therapy for breast cancer may increase the risk of development of a second primary tumor of the breast have shown that, in general, radiation therapy contributes little to the subsequent development of breast cancer. The only patient group in whom some increased risk attributable to radiation therapy rather than the primary tumor itself could be shown is women who undergo such treatment at a young age, that is, less than 45 years.

REFERENCES

Structure of the female breast

1. Adler DD, Rebner M, Pennes DR: Accessory breast tissue in the axilla: mammographic appearance, *Radiology* 163:709, 1987.
2. Montagna W, Yun JS: The glands of Montgomery, *Br J Dermatol* 86:126, 1972.
3. Page DL, Anderson TJ: *Diagnostic histopathology of the breast*, London, 1987, Churchill Livingstone.
4. Vorherr H: *The breast: morphology, physiology and lactation*, 1974, Academic Press.
5. Wheater PR, Burkitt HG, Daniels VG: *Functional histology*, ed 2, London, 1987, Churchill Livingstone.

Function of the female breast

6. Anderson TJ, Ferguson DJP, Raab GM: Cell turnover in the "resting" human breast: influence of parity, contraceptive pill, age and laterality, *Br J Cancer* 46:376, 1982.
7. Fechner RE: Benign breast disease in women on estrogen therapy: a pathologic study, *Cancer* 29:273, 1972.
8. Guyton AC: *Textbook of medical physiology*, ed 6, Philadelphia, 1981, WB Saunders.
9. Hutson SW, Cowen PN, Bird CC: Morphometric studies of age related changes in normal human breast and their significance for evolution of mammary cancer, *J Clin Pathol* 38:281, 1985.
10. Longacre TA, Bartow SA: A correlative morphologic study of human breast and endometrium in the menstrual cycle, *Am J Surg Pathol* 10:382, 1986.
11. Mills SE, Fechner RE: Focal pregnancy-like change of the breast, *Diagn Gynecol Obstet* 2:67, 1980.
12. Tavassoli FA, Yeh I: Lactational and clear cell changes of the breast in non-lactating, non-pregnant women, *Am J Clin Pathol* 87:23, 1987.
13. Topper YJ, Freeman CS: Multiple hormone interactions in the developmental biology of the mammary gland, *Physiol Rev* 60:1049, 1980.
14. Vogel PM and others: The correlation of histologic changes in the human breast with the menstrual cycle, *Am J Pathol* 104:23, 1981.
15. Wellings SR, Jensen HM, DeVault MR: Persistent and atypical lobules in the human breast may be precancerous, *Experientia* 32:1463, 1976.

Hormones and the female breast

16. Beato M: Gene regulation by steroid hormones, *Cell* 56:335, 1989.
17. Evans RM: The steroid and thyroid hormone receptor superfamily, *Science* 240:889, 1988.
18. Korenman SG: The endocrinology of breast cancer, *Cancer* 46:874, 1980.
19. Nelson J, Clarke R, Murphy RF: The unoccupied estrogen receptor: some comments on localization, *Steroids* 48:121, 1986.
20. Parker MG, editor: *Nuclear hormone receptors*, London, 1991, Academic Press.

Mammographic patterns of the normal breast

21. Berkowitz JE and others: Hormonal replacement therapy: mammographic manifestations, *Radiology* 174:199, 1990.
22. Fisher ER and others: The histopathology of mammographic patterns, *Am J Clin Pathol* 69:421, 1978.
23. Flook D and others: Changes in Wolfe mammographic patterns with aging, *Br J Radiol* 60:455, 1987.
24. Gravelle IH and others: The relation between radiographic features and determinants of risk of breast cancer, *Br J Radiol* 53:107, 1980.
25. Huseby RA, Thomas LD: Histological and histochemical alterations in the normal breast tissues of patients with ad-

vanced breast cancer being treated with estrogenic hormones, *Cancer* 7:54, 1954.

26. Kopans DB and others: Asymmetric breast tissue, *Radiology* 171:639, 1989.

27. Leinster SJ, Whitehouse GH: The mammographic breast pattern and oral contraception, *Br J Radiol* 59:237, 1986.

28. Peck DR, Lowman RM: Estrogen and the postmenopausal breast. Mammographic considerations, *JAMA* 240:1733, 1978.

29. Stomper PC and others: Mammographic changes associated with postmenopausal hormone replacement therapy: a longitudinal study, *Radiology* 174:487, 1990.

30. Wellings SR, Wolfe JN: Correlative studies of the histological and radiographic appearance of the breast parenchyma, *Radiology* 129:299, 1978.

31. Wolfe JN: Breast parenchymal patterns and their changes with age, *Radiology* 121:545, 1976.

32. Wolfe JN: Breast patterns as an index of risk for developing breast cancer, *AJR Am J Roentgenol* 126:1130, 1976.

33. Wolfe JN: Risk for breast cancer development determined by mammographic parenchymal pattern, *Cancer* 37:2486, 1976.

Epidemiology and risk factors for breast disease

34. Anderson N, Lokich J: Bilateral breast cancer after cured Hodgkin's disease, *Cancer* 56: 2092, 1985.

35. Berkowitz GS, Kelsey JL, Holford TR: Estrogen replacement therapy and fibrocystic breast disease in postmenopausal women, *Am J Epidemiol* 121:238, 1985.

36. Boice JD and others: Cancer in the contralateral breast after radiotherapy for breast cancer, *N Engl J Med* 326:781, 1992.

37. Brinton LA, Rogers R, Hoover RN. Breast cancer risk factors among screening program participants, *J Natl Cancer Inst* 62:37, 1979.

38. Carlile T, Thompson DJ, Kopecky KJ, et al: Reproducibility and consistency in classification of breast parenchymal patterns, *AJR Am J Roentgenol* 140:1, 1983.

39. Coles C, Thompson AM, Elder PA, et al: Evidence implicating at least two genes on chromosome 17p in breast carcinogenesis, *Lancet*, 336:761, 1990.

40. Cook KL, Adler DD, Lichter A, et al: Breast carcinoma in young women previously treated for Hodgkin disease, *AJR Am J Roentgenol* 155:39, 1990.

41. Dupont WD, Page DL: Risk factors for breast cancer in women with proliferative breast disease, *N Engl J Med* 312:146, 1985.

42. Dupont WD and others: The epidemiological study of anatomic markers for increased risk of mammary cancer, *Pathol Res Pract* 166:471, 1980.

43. Ernster VL: The epidemiology of benign breast disease, *Epidemiol Rev* 3:184, 1981.

44. Harris JR, Lippman ME, Veronesi U, Willett W: Breast cancer, New Engl J Med, 327:319, 1992.

45. Hildreth NG, Shore RE, Dvorestsky PM: The risk of breast cancer after irradiation of the thymus in infancy, *N Engl J Med* 321:1281, 1989.

46. Ingram D, Nottage E, Siobhan N, et al: Obesity and breast disease: the role of the female sex hormones, *Cancer* 64:1049, 1989.

47. Jick SS, Walker AM, Jick H: Conjugated estrogens and fibrocystic breast disease, *Am J Epidemiol* 124:746, 1986.

48. Kelly PT, Anderson DE: Familial breast cancer: new data show lower risks for some sisters and daughters, *Your Patient & Cancer* May:25, 1981.

49. Kelsey JL, Gammon MD: Epidemiology of breast cancer, *Epidemiol Rev* 12:228, 1990.

50. Kelsey JL, Gammon MD: The epidemiology of breast cancer, *CA* 41:146, 1991.

51. Leinster SJ and others: Factors associated with mammographic parenchymal patterns, *Clin Radiol* 39:252, 1988.

52. Miller AB and others: Mortality from breast cancer after irradiation during fluoroscopic examination in patients being treated for tuberculosis, *N Engl J Med* 321:1285, 1989.

53. Phelps HM, Phelps CE: Caffeine ingestion and breast cancer, *Cancer* 61:1051, 1988.

54. Rohan TE, Cook MG: Alcohol consumption and risk of benign proliferative epithelial disorders of the breast in women, *Int J Cancer* 43:631, 1989.

55. Rohan TE, Cook MG, Baron JA: Cigarette smoking and benign proliferative epithelial disorders of the breast in women: a case-control study, *J Epidemiol Community Health* 43:362, 1989.

56. Schatzkin A and others: Alcohol consumption and breast cancer in the epidemiologic follow-up study of the first national health and nutrition examination survey, *N Engl J Med* 316:1169, 1987.

57. Shapiro S, Slone D, Kaufman DW, et al: Use of thyroid supplements in relation to the risk of breast cancer, *JAMA* 244:1685, 1980.

58. Swift M, Reitnauer PJ, Morrett D, et al: Breast and other cancers in families with ataxia-telangiectasia, *N Engl J Med* 316:1289, 1987.

59. Trapido EJ and others: Estrogen replacement therapy and benign breast disease, *J Natl Cancer Inst* 73:1101, 1984.

60. Willett WC and others: Dietary fat and the risk of breast cancer. *N Engl J Med* 316:22, 1987.

61. Willett WC and others: Moderate alcohol consumption and the risk of breast cancer, *N Engl J Med* 316:1174, 1987.

Mammography for Asymptomatic and Symptomatic Patients

Carol B. Stelling

INTRODUCTION

In the late 1980s the trend to separate screening mammography from problem-solving or diagnostic mammography began to take hold in many centers in North America. This trend is expected to increase, particularly in those regions where a high-volume screening mammography program is economically feasible. The separation of these two types of examinations (screening from problem-solving mammography) is not only a reflection of the fact that screening mammography is now covered by many third-party payers and by Medicare, but also a reflection of the fact that an armamentarium of special mammography views and problem-solving maneuvers has been developed for the diagnostic situation. This chapter provides an overview of both screening mammography and diagnostic mammography with appropriate references.

SCREENING MAMMOGRAPHY
Definition and guidelines

Screening mammography as it is defined in North America is the use of two-view mammography in asymptomatic women 40 years of age and older for the detection of unsuspected breast cancer. Screening mammography is one part of a compre-

hensive breast screening program that also includes monthly breast self-examination by the patient (BSE) and regular physical examination of the breast by a health care professional. The current guidelines recommended by the American Cancer Society for the initiation and interval performance of this three-pronged protocol for breast health are presented in Box 2-1.

The guidelines were modified in 1983 to include mammography every 1 to 2 years for women aged 40 to 50 years.[4] Before this recommendation, women were advised to have a baseline mammogram between the ages of 35 and 40 years and to consult their personal physician for his or her recommendation for the frequency of subsequent mammography to be based on personal risk factors.[3] Because the American Cancer Society/National Cancer Institute Breast Cancer Detection Demonstration Projects found that one third of the breast cancers were detected in women between the ages of 35 and 49 years, that most of these lesions were either in situ or did not involve the lymph nodes, and that most of these were detected by mammography, the guidelines were updated in 1983.[1,6]

In the mid-1980s, however, there remained different opinions on appropriate screening guide-

BOX 2-1 CANCER-RELATED CHECKUP GUIDELINES FOR BREAST CANCER DETECTION RECOMMENDED BY THE AMERICAN CANCER SOCIETY (1993)

For the early detection of cancer in people without symptoms. TALK WITH YOUR DOCTOR. Ask how these guidelines relate to you.

CANCER-RELATED CHECKUP should include the procedures listed below plus health counseling. Some people are at higher risk for certain cancers and may need to have tests more frequently.

Age 18-39: BREAST GUIDELINES
- Examination by a health care professional every 3 years
- Self-examination every month

Age 40 and over: BREAST GUIDELINES
- Examination by a health care professional every year
- Self-examination every month
- Screening mammogram (breast x-ray) at age 40. Every 1-2 years, ages 40-49. Every year age 50 and older.

Remember, these guidelines are not rules and only apply to people without symptoms.

BOX 2-2 CONSENSUS STATEMENT

The undersigned organizations are in agreement concerning the components and frequency of a breast screening program; differences in wording or presentation in previous official statements should not be construed as departing from the following consensus:

Clinical examinations of the breasts and mammography are the basic detection methods. The examinations are complementary, and both are necessary to achieve maximum detection rates.

It is recommended that the screening process begin by age 40 years and consist of annual clinical examination with screening mammography performed at 1- to 2-year intervals.

Beginning at age 50 years, both clinical examination and mammography should be performed on an annual basis.

The recommendations apply to women without signs or symptoms of breast cancer; the frequency and type of examination will vary for the individual with symptoms and should be determined by the responsible physician.

American Academy of Family Physicians
American Association of Women Radiologists
American Cancer Society
American College of Radiology
American Medical Association
American Society of Internal Medicine
American Society for Therapeutic Radiology and Oncology
College of American Pathologists
National Cancer Institute
National Medical Association
American Osteopathic College of Radiology

From Mammography screening urged, *ACR Bulletin* 45:1, 1989.

lines by various health organizations. Discrepancies of detail were confusing to physicians and to the public. On June 27, 1989, 11 of the nation's largest health care and medical research organizations reached a consensus on mammography screening guidelines. Their joint statement is reproduced in Box 2-2.[5] The statement not only covers screening mammography but also addresses mammography for women with symptoms for which the frequency and type of examination will vary and should be determined by the responsible physician. This consensus statement indicates that screening mammography should begin by age 40 years and is consistent with the 1991 recommendation to drop the baseline examination.

There is an increasing trend to recommend annual screening for women 40 to 49 years of age in Europe and in some centers in the United States.[2] The rapid growth rate of some cancers in young women gives a short lead time for detection, resulting in a breakthrough of interval cancers between 2-year screening intervals.[7]

Risk factors

There are instances in which asymptomatic women are considered at special risk for developing breast cancer (Box 2-3). These women are frequently referred for screening mammography beginning at an earlier age or with a particular recommendation for annual examinations. An individual practice must decide whether to give these women who are at special risk diagnostic mammographic examinations or screening mammograms. Women who are particularly anxious or

BOX 2-3 WOMEN AT SPECIAL RISK FOR DEVELOPING BREAST CANCER

Strong family history of breast cancer:
  Mother or sister with breast cancer before menopause[9]
  Mother or sister with bilateral breast cancer[8]

Personal history of breast cancer

Ductal or lobular hyperplasia with atypia diagnosed by breast biopsy[18]

Carcinoma of the breast associated with other tumors in patient or family, including soft-tissue sarcoma, osteosarcoma, glioma, leukemia, and adrenocortical carcinoma[12,14,15]

---

cancerphobic would probably appreciate an early report, such as is often provided in a diagnostic mammography practice. In our practice we schedule women who have had a mastectomy for breast cancer to have a diagnostic mammogram. We then can take special projections at the same time and provide an early report for the woman to carry to her surgeon, who completes the evaluation with a physical examination.

A personal history of breast cancer is a significant risk factor for subsequent development of breast cancer.[13] Up to 16% of women who have had a diagnosis of breast cancer develop a second primary cancer. Half of these asynchronous cancers develop during the first 6 years after the initial biopsy. In large groups, a second primary breast cancer is diagnosed at a rate of approximately 0.5% to 1% per year.[19]

We prefer that young women who are less than 35 years old and whose mother had breast cancer before the menopause be scheduled for a diagnostic mammogram for their first examination. We believe it is worthwhile to spend extra time explaining that the concept of breast cancer screening includes monthly breast self-examination (BSE) and annual physical examination in addition to mammography. We explain that the complementary role of clinical palpation is particularly valuable in women with dense breast parenchyma. We try to give the patient confidence in a long-term program of breast health maintenance with all three modalities (i.e., BSE, physical examination of the breasts by a health care professional, and mammography).

It is recommended that daughters of women who have had breast cancer begin screening mammography 10 years before the age at which the mother was diagnosed.[17] For instance, a daughter would begin mammography screening at age 32 years if her mother was 42 years old when breast cancer was detected. This recommendation is based on the understanding of tumor biology to date. There is a difficulty, however, in that mammography is generally considered to be of minimal value in young women, age 25 years and younger. Not only is the breast parenchyma frequently very dense in these young women, but also the risk from radiation exposure is estimated to be higher for this age group than for women over 35 years of age. Therefore, it is usual to begin mammography screening for women with a very strong family history at age 28 or 30 years, but not before age 25 years.

A definition of a strong family history for breast cancer requires a female blood relative, mother or sister, who had breast cancer before the menopause, or a maternal relative who had bilateral breast cancer. This strong family history should indicate the need for extra vigilance on physical examination and annual mammography. A history of breast cancer on the father's side or in an elderly relative on the mother's side is of moderate risk but is not considered a strong family history. These women with moderate risk should follow the American Cancer Society Guidelines for BSE, physical examination, and mammography for early cancer detection.

Women with a biopsy-proven diagnosis of lobular and/or ductal hyperplasia with atypia are also at special risk (five times that of the general population) for subsequent development of breast cancer.[18] A history of breast cancers in a mother, sister, or daughter increases this risk to eight to ten times that of the general population.[18] In our practice these women usually are observed yearly by mammography and are seen every 6 months for a physical examination of the breasts by their surgeon. We usually perform diagnostic mammography and provide early reports to the woman and her physician. Any questionable mammographic change merits further evaluation by magnification spot films, targeted physical examination, close mammographic follow-up, or biopsy as indicated by the mammographic findings.

Other risk factors for developing breast cancer are discussed in Box 1-1. Most of these are not considered sufficiently strong to begin screening mammography before age 35 years. Factors that have no known effect on breast cancer risk are listed in Box 1-2. The risk of exogenous hormone replacement therapy remains a complex issue.[10,11,16,20]

Screening mammography technique

Screening mammography as practiced in the United States in the 1990s is a quality two-view examination of each breast. There is an increasing trend for women to seek mammography centers that have applied for and received accreditation from the American College of Radiology (ACR). Some of the technical concerns addressed in this section include number of views, film-screen mammography versus xeromammography, dedicated units with optimal compression and grids, processor developing, and quality assurance.

Number of views. Although some centers in Europe have advocated using a single oblique mammographic projection for breast cancer screening,[30] there is considerable evidence that two views of each breast are preferable for breast cancer detection.[22,23,31,32,34] In fact, two views per breast are the only accepted norm in the United States, even for the second screening mammogram.[26] Not only does the combination of the craniocaudal view and the mediolateral oblique projection detect more cancers than a single view, but also the combination results in a lower recall rate for problem-solving views.

In one report, single-view mammography would have required additional views in 26% of cases to further evaluate potential abnormalities as compared to a recommendation for additional views in only 7% of cases when two views of each breast were available for interpretation.[34] The mediolateral oblique view is superior to a true lateral projection to include the maximal amount of breast tissue.[29] A true lateral projection does not replace an oblique view but may be added as a supplementary projection.[21]

Dedicated mammography units and processing. The use of a conventional tungsten tube for mammography is only of historical interest. Throughout the 1980s the few remaining such units were replaced by dedicated mammography units with either a molybdenum target tube and molybdenum filter or a specially designed tungsten target tube with appropriate filtration for mammographic imaging.[25] Additional features on dedicated mammography equipment include excellent breast compression, grid capability, and automatic exposure control. According to a nationwide survey in 1988, film-screen examinations were performed on dedicated mammography equipment in 99% of the facilities.[24]

There has also been an increase in the routine use of grids, with a resultant 30% increase in the average mean glandular dose and an increase in average image quality scores.[24] Stationary grids require more exposure than reciprocating grids.[25]

In addition, the value of excellent compression cannot be overemphasized in the context of technical improvements in film-screen mammography in the last decade (Fig. 2-1).[25] Vigorous compression is necessary and, when explained to the patient, is accepted by 94% of women.[27] Inadvertent cyst rupture may occur but should not dissuade the continued use of firm compression.[33]

Another national trend is the shift from xeromammography toward the use of film-screen mammography. The higher dose, higher cost, and need for more frequent preventive maintenance and repair for xeromammography as contrasted to film-screen mammography are all reasons that more facilities have chosen to use film-screen receptors. In 1985 approximately 38% of facilities used xeromammography. By 1988 this percentage had dropped to 17%.[24] The need to provide low-dose quality screening mammography at an affordable cost for hundreds of thousands of women has accelerated this trend toward film-screen receptors.

Emphasis on proper film processing has been stressed to optimize image quality at an acceptable radiation dose.[25] For some single-emulsion films radiation exposure can be reduced approximately 30% by extended-cycle processing.[35,36] Extended-cycle processing requires optimizing the processor replenishment rate, development time, and temperature for the film-screen combination used so that the processor becomes dedicated to mammography films. New film-screen combinations can produce superior phantom images at a reduced radiation dose.[28] Additional references related to technical issues and radiation dose are provided for the reader at the end of the chapter.

Quality assurance

A wide variability of dose and image quality for mammography has been documented.[40] Because of concern for quality at an acceptable dose, the ACR began the voluntary ACR accreditation program of screening mammography units in October 1986. The number of accredited units has steadily increased (e.g., 647 in early 1989, 2,410 units in January 1991 and 6,237 units in January 1993). This program is expected to be ongoing and to include site visits for verification.

The accreditation process has four components: (1) a survey form, (2) typical mammography images, (3) a phantom test image, and (4) a phantom dose measurement. Testing to include processor performance as a component of the program has begun.[42] Participation rate has proved to be higher in states where participation in American Cancer Society Breast Cancer Awareness Screening Programs or reimbursement requires accreditation as a prerequisite. Some states have passed legislation mandating that reimbursement be tied

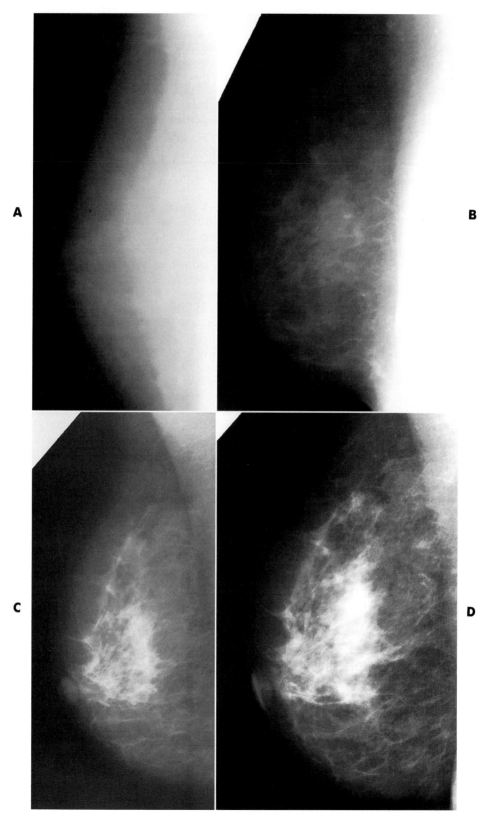

Fig. 2-1 A series of oblique film-screen mammograms of one woman over a period of 16 years illustrates improvement in image quality. **(A)** 1973; **(B)** 1984; **(C)** 1986; **(D)** 1989.

BOX 2-4 REASONS FOR FALSE-NEGATIVE MAMMOGRAMS[43,44]

Lesion not visualized

Dense fibrous and glandular breasts
Subareolar location
Located outside breast
Poor technique

Lesion misinterpreted

Lesion had no malignant criteria
Obvious oversight
Subtle radiographic sign(s) not recognized
Palpating one lesion, imaging another
Nonbelief

to a quality assurance program such as the ACR voluntary program. Sites that fail the accreditation process are encouraged to correct the problem or problems and reapply.

In addition to programs that evaluate image quality and dose, professional quality assurance programs are strongly encouraged.[37,48,50] Establishing the sensitivity and specificity of one's own practice is valuable as evidence of a reasonable approach for any given case.[38,39,49] In such a practice audit, a review of the false-negative mammographic interpretations is recommended to determine if the reason for the "miss" is correctable (Box 2-4). Double reading of screening mammograms is practiced by some centers to increase sensitivity.[38,41] An understanding of how the prevalence of disease in the population affects the positive predictive value of a test is essential in assessing one's statistics for a screening, diagnostic, or mixed population.[45-47]

BSE instruction

Instruction in BSE is recommended by the American Cancer Society as part of a total breast health program. Many mammography centers provide BSE instruction as a routine part of the screening mammogram evaluation. It is usually presented as a public education video, which is provided for patient and/or family review. The video can be efficiently introduced as a continuous tape in the waiting area or played in individual carrels. A supplementary instructional program using trained volunteers may allow the patients to practice on a model of a breast containing lumps and/or to have their personal questions answered. Methods and role of BSE instruction in detection of early breast cancer are discussed in more detail in Chapter 4.

Self-referral screening mammography

Annual physical examination of the breast by a health care professional is recommended by the American Cancer Society beginning at age 40 years as part of the cancer-related checkup guidelines. Traditionally, patients are referred for mammography by their personal physician, who also provides the physical examination of the breast. Women who have discussed the advisability of having a screening mammogram with their physician and who call and schedule their own appointment may be called patient-initiated physician referrals.[55]

Self-referral by patients themselves for screening mammography is gaining some ground in the United States. The issues that such a practice raise are not simple.[52-55] A thorough understanding of the added responsibilities and costs for providing screening mammography to self-referred patients is encouraged before making the difficult decision of how to handle the self-referred patient (Box 2-5). Practice settings that accept self-referred women may attempt to convert as many as possible into patient-initiated physician referrals, thereby reducing the costs of self-referral (Box 2-6). Practices that accept women by referral only may make it easier for a self-referred patient to obtain a physician referral by providing a list of physicians who will accept follow-up responsibility.[55] If southern California is any indication of national trends, acceptance of self-referred patients will increase in the 1990s across North America.[51]

High-volume, low-cost screening mammography*

Efforts to find ways to reduce the costs of screening mammography resulted in the planning and implementation of quality high-volume screening mammography programs.[58,59,61,65-67] These programs recommend ways to streamline the examination of large numbers of normal women to optimize use of resources and pass on cost savings of high volume to the consumer (Table 2-1). Central to the premise of high volume is the concept that the role of screening mammography is to detect a lesion that is then further evaluated by clinical examination, problem-solving mammography, breast ultrasonography, cyst aspiration, fine-needle aspiration biopsy, or biopsy. Patient throughput is maximized by the use of standard views and the plan to recall any findings that need special evaluation. A radiologist is not present in the screening center. The films are read at a viewer later, preferably with the use of a computer to generate "canned" reports. The value of using a com-

---

*NOTE: Additional selected references concerning screening mammography are grouped at the end of this chapter.

BOX 2-5 ADDED RESPONSIBILITIES FOR RADIOLOGISTS WHO ACCEPT SELF-REFERRED PATIENTS

1. Radiologist must obtain adequate history and perform or arrange for a breast physical examination.

2. Radiologist must discuss findings and concerns with patient and be sure she understands.

3. Radiologist must make specific recommendations regarding management and follow-up and arrange referral to a physician who will accept full clinical responsibility for management of patient's breast care.

4. Patient must be informed that mammography is only a part of a total breast health program, which also includes BSE and physical examination.

5. Patient should be encouraged to seek general medical attention elsewhere.

6. Radiologist must provide necessary follow-up to ensure patient is obtaining recommended care (e.g., phone calls or even registered letters).

7. Radiologist may offer supplementary services: ultrasound, cyst aspiration, fine-needle aspiration cytology, if coordinated with her personal physician.

Modified from Eklund GW, Brenner RJ: The self-referred patient: a challenge to breast imaging practices, *Admin Radiol* IX:133, 1990.

BOX 2-6 ADDED COSTS OF ACCEPTING SELF-REFERRED WOMEN

Radiologists' time to properly notify patient and guarantee follow-up care

Potential for increased malpractice premiums

Costs of triage

Modified from Sickles EA: Mammography screening and the self-referred woman. *Radiology* 166:271, 1988.

puter to manage a screening mammography program has been emphasized.[64,68] A desktop microcomputer stores and retrieves records of prior screening mammograms, directs entry of the film interpretation data by the radiologist, prints reports automatically, schedules future examinations up to a year in advance, and tracks follow-up procedures.[61] The computer should be user-friendly with self-help screens and should accommodate multiple users, particularly if the center is growing.[56] Random selection is preferred for data input by the radiologist so that he or she does not have to review every sequential entry. The option of adding free text should also be available to supplement the canned report for abnormal findings.[57] Tracking of biopsy results or repeat mammographic examination is also desirable.[62] A simple report classification system can be developed to make long-term tracking by computer more effective.[63] Standardization of mammographic reporting is facilitated by the development of the American College of Radiology Breast Imaging Database and Reporting System.

Separation of screening mammography from problem-solving mammography is gaining acceptance. In the Los Angeles area, the trend for differentiating screening and problem-solving examinations occurred as a result of an American Cancer Society–sponsored community-wide low-cost mammographic screening project. In January 1986, only 3.5% of facilities separated screening from diagnostic mammography ($45 to $55). This had increased to 29% of the centers by July 1988 ($50 to $118). Screening fees were significantly lower in office-based practices as compared to hospital-based practices.[51] In rural areas, efficient volume may be difficult to achieve, resulting in higher charges for screening mammography.[70]

In centers where only one mammography unit is available, it is still possible to separate screening from problem-solving (diagnostic) mammography by designating different time segments on the schedule.[69] This concept can be expanded by providing diagnostic mammography only during those hours when a radiologist is on duty to monitor the examination and by scheduling screening mammography at all other times, including evenings and weekends.

Initially, as some centers began offering a two-tiered level of mammographic service, the third-party payers did not cover screening mammography. As soon as a CPT-4 code was developed for screening mammography, a mechanism was in place for reimbursement for screening mammography as distinct from diagnostic mammography (January 1990). Legislation in most states encourages the value of screening mammography. Some

Table 2-1 **Methods to reduce screening mammography costs**

Method	Procedure
Accept only referred patients	Require referring physician's to triage and follow-up abnormal reports
Eliminate billing	Require payment in advance
Reduce examination time	Limit to CC and oblique views
Increase throughput	Batch process at end of day, providing technical recall rate is low
Reduce costs of reporting	Generate "canned" normal reports, print mailing envelopes, and verify report by computer
Reduce interpretation fees	Detect lesions, do not characterize them; use automated viewers and review off-site
Reduce salaries	Cross-train personnel, retain personnel, use volunteers
Increase accessibility	Provide convenient parking, evening and weekend hours, mobile vans, marketing
Keep startup costs low	Buy dedicated equipment for screening only (e.g., not magnification)

states even mandate coverage of screening mammography by third-party payers. In January 1991, Medicare began reimbursement for screening mammography every other year for women aged 65 years and older. Thus, the trend to separate screening from diagnostic mammography is also finding support from third-party payers.

Recall and compliance

Patients and physicians will be more accepting of a two-tiered service structure if they are preinformed of the possibility of a callback for further evaluation. The reasons for callback may vary considerably with the age of the population being screened and the experience of the radiologist.[74,92] The rate of recall for problem-solving views will be higher for first-time screenings than for repeat screenings.[75,87] Most reported recall rates for problem solving after first-time screenings are in the range of 5% to 8%.[87,90,91] One of the most common causes of false suspicion on a screening mammogram is a simulated spiculated mass caused by superimposition of normal tissue.[71] An abnormal report should indicate the type of lesion, its location, and a specific recommendation for further evaluation (Table 2-2). In general, these recommendations include additional views, breast ultrasonography, correlative physical examination, follow-up mammogram in 4 to 6 months, or surgical referral. These added "down-

stream" costs may be added to any cost-benefit analysis of screening mammography.[74]

To keep the level of anxiety generated by an abnormal screening report to a minimum, certain steps are recommended. The patient's letter or report should be delayed for 4 or more days so that her physician may first receive notification of an abnormality. If the lesion is suggestive of cancer, it is also advisable to telephone the referring physician personally before the report is mailed. It is valuable to provide a clear indication as to the next course of action in the report to allow an expedient work-up. Most patients would also like to know the reason for recall in words they can understand. The reason can be easily phrased in a letter if sufficient computer support is available. Delays in the recommended follow-up have been reported to include:

1. Failure to receive the report or misplacement of the report by office personnel
2. Report misunderstood
3. Report sent to wrong address
4. Report filed before acted on by clinician
5. Difficulty with patient communication; for example, patient moved, had no phone, did not speak English
6. Patient refused surgical referral

Direct reporting to the patient should help decrease delays in diagnosis.[85] Cost accounting of

Table 2-2 **Recall for problem-solving maneuvers**

Problem	Procedure
Question skin Ca^{++}	Spot localization using grid
Characterize calcifications	Focal coned spot magnification views
Occult circumscribed mass,[82] cyst or solid?	Breast ultrasonography
Mass, uncertain if palpable	Targeted physical examination
Mass, to characterize margin	Focal compression with magnification
Mass, uncertain of location	Targeted physical examination and true lateral views
Asymmetric breast tissue[83,86]	Targeted physical examination Follow-up mammography Fine-needle aspiration or ultrasonography as needed
Lesion seen on one view only[91]	Change beam 5 to 10 degrees and use focal spot compression with magnification to determine if lesion is pseudomass or real lesion

screening programs should include the costs of following up on a recommendation so that patients do not fall through the cracks.[90]

Despite the major technical advances in screening mammography over the past 10 years, this tool is still underused.[76,77,81,84] Strategies to increase use are many.[80,88] Reduction in cost is perhaps the most successful strategy.[93] Education of patients, referring physicians, and medical staff is strongly encouraged.[73] If a woman believes that her physician believes in regular mammography, this has been found to be an important predictor of compliance.[79,89] The radiologic technologist should be encouraged to function as an educator to reduce anxiety, increase understanding of the procedure, and underscore the importance of screening mammography.[78] A warm and empathic technologist can do a great deal toward enhancing subsequent screening compliance.[72]

PROBLEM-SOLVING (DIAGNOSTIC) MAMMOGRAPHY
Definition and indications

Problem-solving or diagnostic mammography is mammography practiced with a radiologist monitoring the examination at the time of service (Box 2-7). It is indicated for women with a new problem, question of a problem, or the need to know her results in the same day, whether because of anxiety, history of breast cancer, biopsy-proven

hyperplasia with atypia, a follow-up appointment in the clinic, and so on. These women do not want to wait the 7 to 10 days it may take to receive the results of a screening mammogram. In our practice we feel free to talk to our patients about the outcome of their mammogram or ultrasonogram in general terms. The referring physician retains the role of directing appropriate surgical referral.

Problem-solving mammography differs from screening mammography in several aspects. The patients are frequently more anxious about their condition, already having had a problem or requiring a new evaluation. The history form is more detailed for a problem-solving mammogram, and the radiologist has the opportunity to supplement the form with direct questioning (Table 2-3). Additional projections are often used to evaluate questionable abnormalities, particularly those detected on a prior screening mammogram. Sufficient time is allocated for the examination (usually 30 minutes) to permit a thorough evaluation, including special views and a correlative physical examination of the breast as needed.

Correlative physical examination

The practice of a correlative physical examination of the breast is particularly advisable in women who have dense glandular tissue and who present with the question of a lump or thickening in ei-

BOX 2-7 DEFINITION OF SCREENING AND DIAGNOSTIC MAMMOGRAPHY[94]

Screening mammography

Screening mammography is a radiological examination utilized to detect unsuspected breast cancer at an early stage in asymptomatic women. The intent of the examination is to separate women into groups of low and high probability of breast cancer. Screening mammography is a radiological examination of the breast ordinarily limited to craniocaudal and mediolateral oblique views. It may be performed in settings where a physician is not in attendance. A definitive diagnosis may not be rendered. Where pathology is suspected, a recommendation for additional imaging studies, diagnostic mammography, or biopsy may be warranted.

Diagnostic mammography

Diagnostic mammography is a comprehensive radiologic examination and consultation. In addition to the standard craniocaudal and mediolateral oblique views, the examination may include multiple specialized views which may be indicated as part of the examination. Correlation with patient history, symptoms, physical findings, or referring physician examination and/or concerns is part of the total examination. It is performed under the direct, on-site supervision of a physician qualified in mammography.

Diagnostic mammograms are performed on patients who have a variety of signs and symptoms, such as breast mass, discharge, pain, dimpling, augmented, reconstructed or otherwise altered breast structure, or have abnormal screening mammography. It may also be performed on women who have a personal or family history of breast cancer or who desire for other reasons to have the more comprehensive examination with physician interaction.

(From Council adopts definition of screening and diagnostic mammography. *ACR Bulletin* 48(10):27, 1992.)

BOX 2-8 MAMMOGRAPHIC ARTIFACTS

Body part related to positioning
Hair
Eyeglasses
Nose[99]
Ear[99]
Hand
Other nipple[98]
Pectoral muscle[96,102]
Rib[100]
Shoulder

Metallic density:
Deodorant
Adhesive tape
Shrapnel
Pacemaker
Ca^{++} catheter[95]
Tattoo[97]

Film handling
White fingerprint (before exposure)
Black fingerprint (after exposure)
Static
Fungus in processor
Roller marks
Dirty screens
Scratches (feeder tray)
Light leak
Film loaded backwards

Soft tissue/water density
Drop of discharge
Skin tag
Mole
Keloid[103]
Skin fold

ther breast. Some artifacts can be more easily explained after the patient is seen (Box 2-8). The physical examination helps assure the radiologist that the area has been included in the routine views or may indicate that additional views are required. For instance, in a dense breast, a "lumpogram" of the mass performed with a focal compression device and an x-ray beam tangential to the skin surface closest to the mass is recommended (Fig. 2-2). Such a view may profile the edge of the palpable lesion against the subcutaneous fat and allow characterization of the border, e.g., circumscribed versus indistinct. Without the physical examination and the tailored lumpogram, the palpable mass in the dense breast would be hidden by the surrounding dense tissue. For this clinical problem, ancillary ultrasonography could also be used to differentiate a cyst from a solid mass, but ultrasound examination may not be necessary for a palpable lesion since direct needle aspiration is just as effective, is cheaper, and may be therapeutic. Practices that add ultrasonography for a palpable mass may wish to include the ultra-

Table 2-3 **Specialized history for diagnostic mammography**

Heading	Examples
Procedure and date	Augmentation mammoplasty Reduction mammoplasty Cyst aspiration Fine-needle aspiration cytology Biopsy Lumpectomy Quadrantectomy Lymph node dissection Modified mastectomy Radical mastectomy Radiation therapy
Medications	Hormone replacement therapy Chemotherapy Drugs associated with gynecomastia Drugs associated with galactorrhea Drugs associated with bleeding disorder
Nonsurgical trauma	Horse bite Insect bite Shoulder restraint injury Direct blow Knife or gunshot wound
Medical condition associated with lymphadenopathy	Infection Sarcoidosis Rheumatoid arthritis Lymphoma or Hodgkin's disease Lymphoproliferative disorder Collagen vascular disease

Medical condition that may be associated with breast masses	Malignancies including
	    Small cell carcinoma
	    Melanoma
	    Renal cell carcinoma
	Wegener's granulomatosis
	Other

sound charge as part of a total diagnostic evaluation.

Another type of patient in whom physical examination is helpful is the woman with a history of lumpy breasts whose mammogram shows only fat. Normal fatty tissue may feel very lumpy. These women with large, tender breasts sometimes have so many lumps as to be told they have fibrocystic disease. A correlative physical examination helps to reassure these women that they have normal fatty tissue on physical examination as well as on mammography.

This last example raises another advantage of diagnostic mammography (e.g., patient counseling). By demonstrating the mammogram directly to the patient, the radiologist can reinforce the value and limitations of mammography. In the presence of a small, nondiscrete palpable finding, the radiologist can advise the patient to continue monthly BSE and report any interval change to

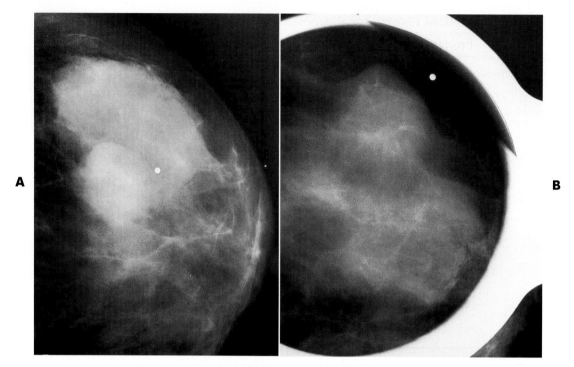

Fig. 2-2 Lumpogram of a palpable mass in a 46-year-old woman. A palpable mass (bb) is obscured by dense tissue on the craniocaudal view (**A**). A tangential view with focal compression (**B**) delineates the smooth margin of the mass against subcutaneous fat. Diagnosis: cyst proven by aspiration.

her referring physician. The correlative physical examination is a great help in a diagnostic setting in keeping the radiologist from overlooking a palpable mass, and thereby it results in a more appropriate and accurate assessment (Table 2-4).

In addition, there are several other clinical settings deserving special discussion. First, it is not uncommon for a woman to seek a breast checkup after a period of marked weight loss or weight gain. The breast texture has changed and she becomes unsure of her normal texture, particularly if she has not been practicing BSE regularly. Close questioning often reveals a stressful situation such as a severe illness, divorce, job loss, or death or illness of a loved one. These women may appear cancerphobic and can greatly benefit by a diagnostic evaluation, including instruction in BSE, with the knowledge that their mammogram is normal.

The physical examination can also help determine whether the lesion that is visualized by mammography is in fact the same lesion that is palpable in the breast. Disconcordance between the palpable finding and the mammographic appearance is not unusual.

For the complaint of nipple discharge, the correlative physical examination of the breast is extremely valuable. It is important to characterize the spontaneity, color, and distribution of the discharge. If spontaneous, the fluid discharges on its own without the requirement of manual expression. The patient may see spontaneous discharge on her clothing. Nonspontaneous discharge is elicited only on physical examination and may be most marked premenstrually. Spontaneous nipple discharge that is caused by an intraductal growth comes from a single duct opening. Hormonally related discharge can usually be elicited from more than one ductal system in the breast and is frequently bilateral. Therefore, careful physical examination for nipple discharge includes a *bilateral* examination. If the discharge is from a single duct and is spontaneous, a surgical consultation is recommended to excise the suspected intraductal growth. A duct injection study (galactogram) may be helpful to demonstrate the location and depth of the process relative to the nipple if the physical examination fails to localize the source to a particular breast segment. The reader is referred to Chapter 3 for a discussion of galactography.

Correlative breast physical examination may produce unexpected findings. A recent aspiration attempt may leave a bruise, alerting the radiologist to a possible hematoma.[101] The history may be quite unusual such as a horse bite to the breast

Table 2-4 **Correlative physical examination: some instances of particular benefit**

Problem	Options

Mass palpable in a dense breast	Mass present →
	     Lumpogram
	     Surgical referral
	 Mass doubtful →
	     Clinical follow-up
	     Breast ultrasound examination

Spontaneous nipple discharge	Characterize by color, location
	 If spontaneous →
	     Surgical consult
	     +/− galactogram
	 If nonspontaneous →
	     Clinical follow-up
	     Reduce caffeine

Pain and redness	Differential diagnosis:
	     Thrombophlebitis (Mondor's disease)
	     Mastitis or abscess
	     Inflammatory breast cancer

Rash or skin lesion	Dermatologic referral (e.g., eczema, mite infestation, candidiasis, rule out melanoma)
Draining periareolar sinuses	Squamous metaplasia of lactiferous ducts → surgical referral

or a motor vehicle accident–related shoulder restraint injury causing fat necrosis. An unrelated yet pertinent finding might include a skin rash, a mole suspicious for melanoma, or a chest wall lipoma that falls outside the field of view of the mammogram. Rarely, an unrecognized artifact may explain a mammographic finding such as a skin tattoo or an old Hickman catheter line (see Box 2-8). Some conditions are best diagnosed on physical examination because they leave little or no radiographic findings. Mondor's disease and squamous metaplasia of the lactiferous ducts are two such entities (Table 2-4 and Chapters 13 and 14).

Caffeine sensitivity

A significant portion of premenopausal women who are referred for a diagnostic mammogram complain of generalized breast tenderness. The severity varies from mild premenstrual tenderness to nearly continuous tenderness throughout the month. The vast majority of these women are aware that symmetric premenstrual tenderness is a reflection of cyclic hormonal activity. However, in some women the degree of discomfort is significant.

One way to quantitate the level of discomfort is to ask whether the tenderness is sufficient to wake them up at night when turning in their sleep. Many admit that this does happen and even volunteer that they choose to wear a bra to bed. These women almost invariably have a caffeine intake of more than three cups of coffee per day. Some of them admit to five to ten cups of coffee per day or an equivalent intake of tea or caffeinated sodas. Our experience has been that many such women with breast discomfort are motivated to reduce their caffeine load. We encourage them to titrate their caffeine need against their breast tenderness, warning them that a dull headache or lethargy may result if they dramatically lower their caffeine levels.

Table 2-5 **Problem-solving mammographic views**

Special mammographic views	Problems to be solved
Repeat the same projection after marking skin lesion, cleansing of deodorant or adhesive tape, reevaluating position	Artifacts suspected[96,99,100,102]
Use focal coned compression over area (a) with slight alteration of angulation (5 to 10 degrees), (b) roll breast slightly clockwise or counterclockwise, or (c) obtain a true lateral projection[115]	Pseudomass suspected from telescoping of normal parenchyma[111,113,116,119]
Cleavage view to demonstrate tissue closest to chest in medial breast	Deep medial lesion questioned[109]
True lateral projection with film closest to area of interest	Confirm milk of calcium condition Soft-tissue density evaluation (e.g., density on craniocaudal view but obscured on oblique view)[115]
Tangential view (with skin marker)	Palpable lump obscured by dense tissue or prosthesis Nipple not in profile[119] Clustered calcification—? skin location[118]
Magnification with focal spot compression	To characterize margins of a mass or size, number, and shape of microcalcifications
Modified (Eklund) views[114] with implant displaced	To better demonstrate breast parenchyma in patient with augmentation mammoplasty
Lateromedial oblique views (from lower-outer to upper-inner breast)	In case of severe thoracokyphosis, pectus excavatum, recent median sternotomy
Exaggerated craniocaudal view	Palpable or occult lesion seen in tail on oblique but not on craniocaudal view[109]
Series of views with increasing angulations	To track lesion through tissue in order to triangulate location
Coat hanger view (a lumpogram variant)	Traps palpable mass to keep in field of view[119]
Caudocranial view	Small-breasted or kyphotic woman Helpful in a man

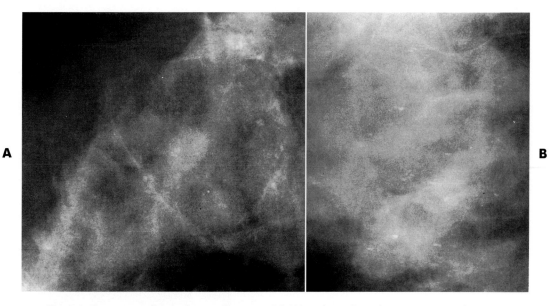

Fig. 2-3 Extensive milk of calcium. Craniocaudal **(A)** and true lateral projections **(B)** demonstrate layering of calcium in small cystic spaces.

There is no strong correlation between caffeine use and breast texture, breast cancer risk, or the presence or absence of cysts in the breast.[105,107] Nevertheless, women with a clinical fibrocystic condition are often advised to lower caffeine intake.[104,108] The benefit of lowering caffeine intake can be considerable in reducing premenstrual breast tenderness. After 4 months of abstention from methylxanthines, 80% of patients may report resolution of pain and tenderness.[106] We have experienced on more than one occasion women who have had excellent results after assiduously avoiding caffeinated beverages return to our center complaining of recurrent breast tenderness despite great care to avoid caffeine in the diet. In most cases the source of the caffeine is found to be chocolate, a dietary oversight by the patient herself. In conclusion, for mastodynia we recommend a good supporting bra, a low caffeine diet, reassurance, and analgesics as needed. Mammography is more comfortable for women with mastodynia 7 to 10 days after the beginning of the menstrual cycle.

Diagnostic mammography technique

Diagnostic or problem-solving mammography consists of routine oblique and craniocaudal projections supplemented as needed with additional views at the direction of the supervising radiologist. In some centers it is routine to augment the mediolateral oblique and craniocaudal views with a true lateral view of each breast, particularly if either a palpable or occult mass is present. The

---

BOX 2-9 MAGNIFICATION VIEWS[110,123,125]

Evaluate isolated clustered microcalcifications; confirm questionable fine microcalcifications[115,121]

Assess lesion margins on "well-defined" mass to bring out any spiculation[115,122]

Assess extent of suspicious microcalcifications before biopsy[120]

Specimen radiography (optional)[120]

After biopsy to verify removal of all suspicious microcalcifications[120]

Use selectively status postlumpectomy and radiation therapy[117]

---

true lateral projection makes triangulation of the lesion on a three-dimensional coordinate system more accurate. The lateral view is particularly useful before performing a wire localization procedure.

Many additional views are used for problem-solving situations to increase sensitivity and specificity of mammography (Table 2-5).[115,124] Frequently used supplementary projections are the exaggerated craniocaudal view for the axillary tail area or medial breast and the true lateral projection to confirm milk of calcium (Fig. 2-3) and to triangulate lesions. Magnification views (Box 2-9)

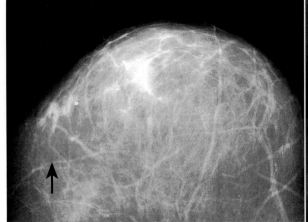

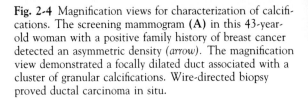

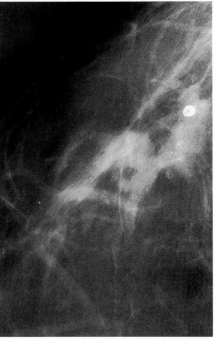

Fig. 2-4 Magnification views for characterization of calcifications. The screening mammogram **(A)** in this 43-year-old woman with a positive family history of breast cancer detected an asymmetric density *(arrow)*. The magnification view demonstrated a focally dilated duct associated with a cluster of granular calcifications. Wire-directed biopsy proved ductal carcinoma in situ.

and tangential views are frequently used for problem solving. The value of magnification mammography to characterize further a mass or grouping of calcifications cannot be underestimated (Fig. 2-4). It is necessary in preoperative and postlumpectomy assessment of suspicious calcifications. Mammographic follow-up of women treated with lumpectomy and radiation therapy may also require use of magnification mammography to assess fat necrosis versus recurrent cancer in the lumpectomy site.[117] Additional references concerning mammographic evaluation of breasts treated by lumpectomy and radiation therapy are provided at the end of this chapter. Each radiologist will develop his or her preferred combinations. It is wise to save on radiation exposure by combining approaches, such as requesting a coned-down focal compression magnification view in a true lateral projection to confirm milk of calcium layering (Fig. 2-5).[122] Additional ancillary problem-solving examinations include breast ultrasound examination and galactography, which are discussed in Chapter 3.

Artifact versus real lesion. Several artifacts have been described in mammography (see Box 2-8). Many of these artifacts will be obvious to the most casual observer. Others require some detective work and imagination to explain. The most significant artifacts may simulate a breast lesion. For example, an unrecognized skin lesion such as a skin tag or mole may appear to be a mass within the breast itself (Fig. 2-6). Direct inspection and

a tangential view of the elevated dermal lesion will solve this problem. It cannot be overemphasized to the technologists to document such skin lesions. We have been asked to consult as a second opinion on a "breast lesion" that was a nevus. The outside study even included a magnification view over the mole! How could the technologist have failed to recognize the significance of the skin lesion?

Perhaps more significant are those artifacts that simulate suspicious calcifications within the breast. It is not uncommon for antiperspirant over the tail of the breast to mimic calcification of comedocarcinoma (Fig. 2-7). We have seen residual adhesive on the skin from a chest tube bandage simulate suspicious calcifications. Repeating the view after cleansing of the skin is the best way to confirm that these radiographic changes are due to the artifact. In fact, we now provide individual packaged moist wipes for the patient to wipe her breasts before any images are obtained.

Pseudomass versus real lesion. Superimposition of normal structures may simulate a mass lesion, thus producing a "pseudomass." This is one of the more common reasons for recall in a screening population.[71,87] With experience, it is possible to recognize that a band of tissue seen in one view is producing the pseudomass observed on the other view and recall is not necessary (Fig. 2-8). Sometimes, however, special views are required to determine if the density is a real lesion or a pseudomass. It is best to change the angle slightly

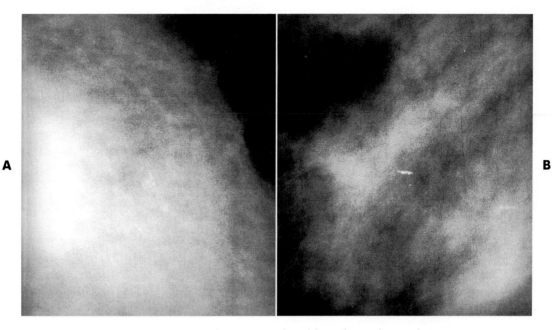

Fig. 2-5 Milk of calcium in a single cyst is confirmed by orthogonal magnification views, craniocaudal **(A)**, and true lateral **(B)**.

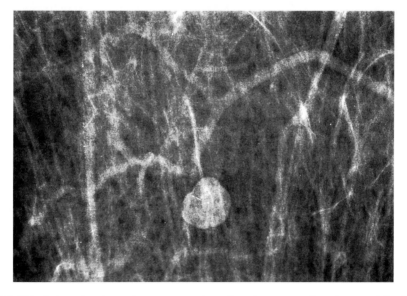

Fig. 2-6 Skin lesion: An elevated nevus traps air against the compression plate, resulting in a halo effect around the margins of the lesion.

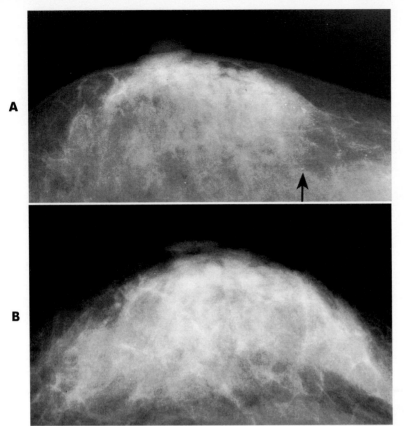

Fig. 2-7 Antiperspirant artifact: Initial image showed question of calcifications *(arrow)* on one view only **(A).** Repeat radiograph **(B)** obtained after wiping the skin with alcohol confirmed the densities to be an artifact from antiperspirant.

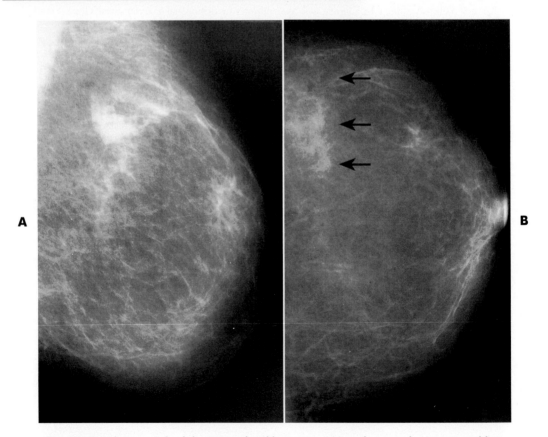

Fig. 2-8 Pseudomass: A focal density on the oblique view **(A)** in the upper breast is caused by the "telescoping" of a band of normal tissue *(arrows)* in the lateral breast on the craniocaudal view **(B).**

(5 to 10 degrees) rather than to repeat the same projection. Adding focal coned compression over the area of concern permits optimal separation of the glandular elements. Rolling the breast tissue clockwise or counterclockwise will also change the projection slightly and is very helpful to resolve a pseudomass (Fig. 2-9). A pseudomass will be resolved into normal tissues, whereas a real lesion will persist.[111-113] Magnification may be added to focal spot compression when appropriate.[122] We prefer to alter the projection angle slightly when the area in question is most likely a pseudomass. A true lateral view may be too much of a change in projection for assessing a pseudomass.

Triangulation of a real lesion seen in one view only. There are several approaches to triangulate a real lesion that is initially seen only on one view. Assuming the lesion is seen on the craniocaudal view and not on the oblique view, the simplest and most direct approach is to obtain a true lateral projection. The film should be placed against the skin surface closest to the lesion. Line draw-

ings may be helpful to approximate a lesion's location when it can be seen on two of three standard views.[124] If the location is still uncertain, the breast can be rolled clockwise from the craniocaudal position. A lesion in the upper left breast will move laterally on the resulting craniocaudal view, and a lesion in the inferior breast will move medially. Progressive angulation of the receptor 10 to 20 degrees can also be used to track a lesion from a craniocaudal projection to a lateral projection. Innovative projections may throw the lesion free of overlapping dense tissues.

If a lesion is seen on the oblique view only, one must modify the craniocaudal projection to determine if the mass is lateral or medial. The first place to search is the lateral breast, an area easily imaged by the mediolateral oblique view but incompletely surveyed on a routine craniocaudal projection. The additional view should be a laterally exaggerated craniocaudal view with 5 to 10 degrees of angulation to clear the head of the humerus. If the lesion is not confirmed in the lateral

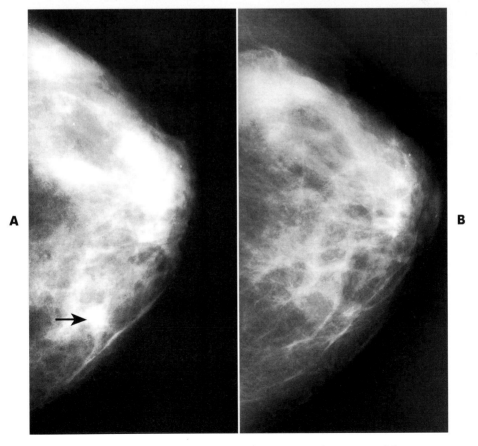

Fig. 2-9 Pseudomass: A density *(arrow)* in the medial breast on the craniocaudal view **(A)** was demonstrated to be caused by overlapping normal tissue on a repeat craniocaudal view obtained with the breast rotated counterclockwise **(B).**

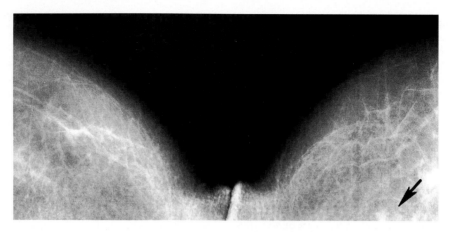

Fig. 2-10 Cleavage view: This cleavage view was used to triangulate a small mass with calcifications (*arrow*) that had been identified close to the chest wall on an oblique projection.

breast, it may be close to the chest wall in a more medial position. The cleavage view can be used to image the deep medial tissues with the breasts off-centered slightly to cover the phototimer (Fig. 2-10).

Mass obscured by dense tissue. In a dense breast it may be necessary to project a palpable mass into profile against the subcutaneous fat. This approach is often called a lumpogram (see Fig. 2-2). Drs. Logan-Young and Janus reported the "coat hanger" view for masses that tend to slide away from a focal compression cone.[119] Tangential views are also useful in the subareolar area to throw the nipple in profile and are essential to assess calcifications of dermal origin.[118] Before the modified views for augmentation mammoplasty were developed, tangential views were used to assess palpable masses in the presence of a prosthesis.

Modified views for augmented breasts (implant displaced). Prostheses can be placed in a retropectoral or retromammary position for augmentation. In the presence of such a prosthesis, the technologist should obtain the routine views and include two additional views of each breast with the implant displaced in order to optimize imaging of the breast parenchyma (Fig. 2-11). This technique, reported by Eklund in 1988, is easy to learn and teach.[114] It does not increase the woman's discomfort during imaging but does result in a study that is more accurate for detection and diagnosis of breast disease. Because these views take extra time to position, we prefer to schedule these women for a problem-solving or diagnostic rather than a screening mammographic examination.

Reporting

A problem-solving mammogram, like many other radiographic consultations, is not complete until an interpretation and recommendation have been made to the referring physician. Women who go to a diagnostic mammography practice are usually more anxious than those who go to a screening practice, making a timely report to the patient and/or physician mandatory. In general the report should indicate the level of concern, if any, for malignancy and a plan for the next step in the work-up. These recommendations may include a repeat diagnostic mammogram in 4 to 6 months, ultrasonography, or surgical consultation for possible cyst aspiration, fine-needle aspiration cytology, or excisional biopsy with or without a preoperative wire localization procedure. Some radiologists communicate directly with the patient, with the acquiescence of her referring physician. Others prefer to report directly to the referring physician, who then communicates the result to his or her patient. In our own practice we prefer the former approach. Speaking directly to the patient gives us the opportunity to decompress her anxiety as soon as possible. Women who have a personal history of breast cancer particularly appreciate this approach. We can also emphasize the importance of clinical and mammographic follow-up in her total plan for personal breast health. Since we are reporting in real time, it is also convenient to send a brief handwritten early report with the patient back to the clinic appointment, which frequently follows the mammogram appointment. We emphasize in our reports that any palpable mass requires further evaluation, usually a surgical referral.

Quality assurance

Technical and professional quality assurance for diagnostic mammography is as important as for screening mammography. Correlation of the imaging studies with surgical pathology and cytology

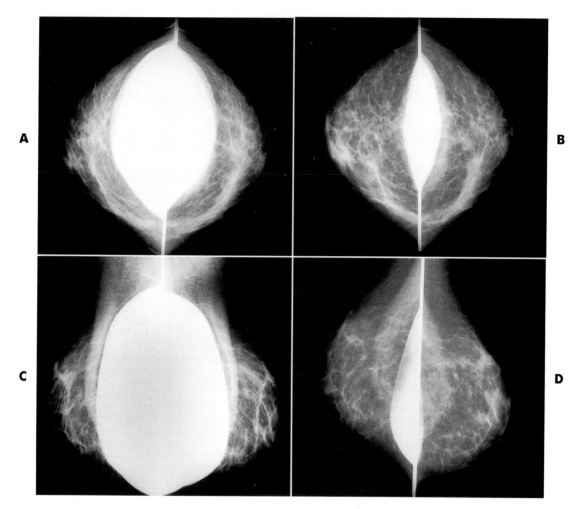

Fig. 2-11 Modified technique for augmented breasts: A complete study (eight films) includes craniocaudal and oblique projections of both breasts with the routine position (**A** and **C**) and with the implant displaced toward the chest wall (**B** and **D**).

results is invaluable for the radiologist to improve accuracy in diagnosing breast diseases, benign and malignant.

REFERENCES
Screening mammography

Definition and guidelines

1. Baker LH: Breast cancer detection demonstration project: five-year summary report, *CA* 32:194, 1982.
2. Kopans DB, Swann CA: Opinion: observations on mammographic screening and false-positive mammograms, *AJR Am J Roentgenol* 150:785, 1988.
3. Mammography 1982: a statement of the American Cancer Society, *CA* 32:226, 1982.
4. Mammography guidelines 1983: background statement and update of cancer-related checkup guidelines for breast cancer detection in asymptomatic women age 40 to 49, *CA* 33:255, 1983.
5. Mammography screening urged, *ACR Bulletin* 45:1, 1989.
6. Moskowitz M, Gartside PS: Evidence of breast cancer mortality reduction: aggressive screening in women under age 50, *AJR Am J Roentgenol* 138:911, 1982.
7. Moskowitz M: Breast cancer: age-specific growth rates and screening strategies, *Radiology* 161:37, 1986.

Risk factors

8. Anderson DE, Badzioch MD: Risk of familial breast cancer, *Cancer* 56:383, 1985.
9. Anderson DE, Badzioch MD: Bilaterality in familial breast cancer patients, *Cancer* 56:2092, 1985.
10. Dupont WD, Page DL: Menopausal estrogen replacement therapy and breast cancer, *Arch Intern Med* 151:67, 1991.
11. Henderson BE: Endogenous and exogenous endocrine factors, *Hematol Oncol Clin North Am* 3:577, 1989.
12. Knudson AG Jr: Hereditary cancers: clues to mechanisms of carcinogenesis, *Br J Cancer* 59:661, 1989.
13. Lavey RS, Eby NL, Prosnitz LR: Impact of radiation therapy and/or chemotherapy on the risk for a second malignancy after breast cancer, *Cancer* 66:874, 1990.
14. Lynch HT, Conway T, Watson P, et al: Extremely early

onset hereditary breast cancer (HBC): surveillance/management implications, *Nebr Med J* 73:97, 1988.

15. Mehta D, Khatib R, Patel S: Carcinoma of the breast and meningioma, *Cancer* 51:1937, 1983.

16. Mills PK, Beeson WL, Phillips RL, et al: Prospective study of exogenous hormone use and breast cancer in Seventh-day Adventists, *Cancer* 64:591, 1989.

17. Moskowitz M: Breast cancer: how can we reduce mortality? *Consultant* September:47, 1979.

18. Page DL, Dupont WD, Rogers LW, et al: Atypical hyperplastic lesions of the female breast: a long-term follow-up study, *Cancer* 55:2698, 1985.

19. Sadowsky NL, Kalisher L, White G, et al: Radiologic detection of breast cancer, *N Engl J Med* 294:370, 1976.

20. The Cancer and Steroid Hormone Study of the Centers for Disease Control and the National Institute of Child Health and Development: Oral-contraceptives use and the risk of breast cancer, *N Engl J Med* 315:405, 1986.

Screening mammography technique

21. Andersson I, Hildell J, Mühlow A, et al: Number of projections in mammography: influence on detection of breast disease, *AJR Am J Roentgenol* 130:349, 1978.

22. Bassett LW, Gold RH: Breast radiography using the oblique projection, *Radiology* 149:585, 1983.

23. Bassett LW, Bunnell DH, Jahanshahi R, et al: Breast cancer detection: one versus two views, *Radiology* 165:95, 1987.

24. Conway BJ, McCrohan JL, Rueter FG, et al: Mammography in the eighties, *Radiology* 177:335, 1990.

25. Haus AG: Technologic improvements in screen-film mammography, *Radiology* 174:628, 1990.

26. Ikeda DM, Sickles EA: Second-screening mammography: one versus two views per breast, *Radiology* 168:651, 1988.

27. Jackson VP, Lex AM, Smith DJ: Patient discomfort during screen-film mammography, *Radiology* 168:421, 1988.

28. Kimme-Smith C, Bassett LW, Gold RL, et al: New mammography screen/film combinations: imaging characteristics and radiation dose, *AJR Am J Roentgenol* 154:713, 1990.

29. Lundgren B: Positioning for oblique projection in mammography, *AJR Am J Roentgenol* 132:858, 1979.

30. Lundgren B, Jakobsson S: Single-view mammography screening: three-year follow-up of interval cancer cases, *Radiology* 130:109, 1979.

31. Moskowitz M: Breast cancer screening: all's well that ends well, or much ado about nothing? *AJR Am J Roentgenol* 151:659, 1988.

32. Muir BB, Kirkpatrick AE, Roberts MM, et al: Oblique-view mammography: adequacy for screening, *Radiology* 151:39, 1984.

33. Pennes DR, Homer MJ: Disappearing breast masses caused by compression during mammography, *Radiology* 165:327, 1987.

34. Sickles EA, Weber WN, Galvin HB, et al: Baseline screening mammography: one versus two views per breast, *AJR Am J Roentgenol* 147:1149, 1986.

35. Skubic SE, Yagan R, Oravee D, et al: Value of increasing film processing time to reduce radiation dose during mammography, *AJR Am J Roentgenol* 155:1189, 1990.

36. Tabar L, Haus AG: Processing of mammographic films: technical and clinical considerations, *Radiology* 173:65, 1989.

Quality assurance

37. Bird RE: Professional quality assurance for mammography screening programs, *Radiology* 177:587, 1990.

38. Brenner RJ: Medicolegal aspects of screening mammography, *AJR Am J Roentgenol* 153:53, 1989.

39. Brenner RJ: Reply, *AJR Am J Roentgenol* 154:420, 1990.

40. Galkin BM, Feig SA, Muir HD: The technical quality of mammography in centers participating in a regional breast cancer awareness program, *RadioGraphics* 8:133, 1988.

41. Golinger RC, Gur D, Fisher B, et al: The significance of concordance in mammographic interpretations, *Cancer* 44:1252, 1979.

42. Hendrick RE: Standardization of image quality and radiation dose in mammography, *Radiology* 174:648, 1990.

43. Kalisher L: Factors influencing false negative rates in xeromammography, *Radiology* 133:297, 1979.

44. Martin JE, Moskowitz M, Milbrath JR: Breast cancer missed by mammography, *AJR Am J Roentgenol* 132:737, 1979.

45. Moskowitz M: Predictive value, sensitivity and specificity in breast cancer screening, *Radiology* 167:576, 1988.

46. Moskowitz M: Screening for breast cancer: how effective are our tests: a critical review, *CA* 33:26, 1983.

47. Moskowitz M: Nonpalpable breast lesions: accuracy of prebiopsy mammographic diagnosis, reply, *Radiology* 167:285, 1988.

48. Murphy WA Jr, Destouet JM, Monsees BS: Professional quality assurance for mammography screening programs, *Radiology* 175:319, 1990.

49. Schmidt RA, Metz CE: Sensitivity of mammography, *AJR Am J Roentgenol* 154:419, 1990.

50. Sickles EA, Ominsky SH, Sollitto RA, et al: Medical audit of a rapid-throughput mammography screening practice: methodology and results of 27,114 examinations, *Radiology* 175:323, 1990.

Self-referral screening mammography

51. Bassett LW, Fox SA, Pennington E, et al: Mammographic screening in Southern California: 2½ -year longitudinal survey of fees, *Radiology* 173:61, 1989.

52. Eklund GW, Brenner RJ: The self-referred patient: a challenge to breast imaging practices, *Admin Radiol* IX:133, 1990.

53. Harper P: Self-referred breast patients pose dilemma for radiologists, *Diagnostic Imaging* September:85, 1988.

54. Monsees B, Destouet JM, Evens RG: The self-referred mammography patients: a new responsibility for radiologists, *Radiology* 166:69, 1988.

55. Sickles EA: Mammography screening and the self-referred woman, *Radiology* 166:271, 1988.

High-volume, low-cost screening mammography

56. Baron M, Strange D: The purchase of specialized mammography software: evaluating the program, *Admin Radiol* IX:137, 1990.

57. Baron M, Strange D: The purchase of specialized radiologic software: estimation of investment, *Admin Radiol* IX:53, 1990.

58. Bird RE: A successful effort to lower costs in screening mammography, *Cancer* 60:1684, 1987.

59. Bird RE, McLelland R: How to initiate and operate a low cost screening mammography center, *Radiology* 161:43, 1986.

60. Bird RE: Low-cost screening mammography: report on finances and review of 21,716 consecutive cases, *Radiology* 171:87, 1989.

61. Evens RG: Mammographic screening: how to operate successfully at low cost, *Radiology* 161:850, 1986.

62. Haug PJ, Tocino IM, Clayton DD, et al: Automated management of screening and diagnostic mammography, *Radiology* 164:747, 1986.

63. Kemp KI, Jackson GL: A simple classification system for mammographic reporting, *Radiology* 165:319, 1987.

64. Monticciolo DL, Sickles EA: Computerized follow-up of

abnormalities detected at mammography screening, *AJR Am J Roentgenol* 155:751, 1990.

65. Moskowitz M: Mammography to screen asymptomatic women for breast cancer, *AJR Am J Roentgenol* 143:457, 1984.
66. Sickles EA: Commentary: reduced-price mammography screening, *AJR Am J Roentgenol* 149:1153, 1987.
67. Sickles EA, Weber WN, Galvin HB, et al: Mammographic screening: how to operate successfully at low cost, *Radiology* 160:95, 1986.
68. Sickles EA: The usefulness of computers in managing the operation of a mammography screening practice, *AJR Am J Roentgenol* 155:755, 1990.
69. Stelling CB: Affordable screening mammography: current status, *Appl Radiol* 17:37, 1988.
70. Study recommends Medicare pay $60 for breast screening in rural areas, *ACR Bulletin* 45:11, 1989.

Recall and compliance

71. Andersson I, Andren L, Hildell J, et al: Breast cancer screening with mammography, *Radiology* 132:273, 1979.
72. Baines CJ, To T, Wall C: Women's attitudes to screening after participation in the National Breast Screening Study: a questionnaire survey, *Cancer* 65:1663, 1990.
73. Bassett LW, Bunnell DH, Cerny JA, et al: Screening mammography: referral practices of Los Angeles physicians, *AJR Am J Roentgenol* 147:689, 1986.
74. Cyrlak D: Induced costs of low-cost screening mammography, *Radiology* 168:661, 1988.
75. Feig SA: Commentary: the importance of supplementary mammographic views to diagnostic accuracy, *AJR Am J Roentgenol* 151:40, 1988.
76. Fox SA, Baum JK, Klos DS, et al: Breast cancer screening: the underuse of mammography, *Radiology* 156:607, 1985.
77. Fox SA, Klos DS, Tsou CV: Underuse of screening mammography by family physicians, *Radiology* 166:431, 1988.
78. Fox SA, Klos DS, Worthen NJ, et al: Improving the adherence of urban women to mammography guidelines: strategies for radiologists, *Radiology* 174:203, 1990.
79. Fox SA, Murata PJ, Stein JA: The impact of physician compliance on screening mammography for older women, *Arch Intern Med* 151:50, 1991.
80. Gold RH, Bassett LW, Fox SA: Mammography screening: successes and problems in implementing widespread use in the United States, *Radiol Clin North Am* 25:1039, 1987.
81. Howard J: Using mammography for cancer control: an unrealized potential, *CA* 37:33, 1987.
82. Jackson VP: The role of US in breast imaging, *Radiology* 177:305, 1990.
83. Kopans DB, Swann CA, White G, et al: Asymmetric breast tissue, *Radiology* 171:639, 1989.
84. Mann LC, Hawes DR, Ghods M, et al: Utilization of screening mammography: comparison of different physician specialties, *Radiology* 164:121, 1987.
85. Monsees B, Destouet JM, Evens RG: Communication problems after mammographic screening, *Radiology* 175:877, 1990.
86. Moskowitz M: Screening is not diagnosis, *Radiology* 133:265, 1979.
87. Pamilo M, Anttinen I, Soiva M, et al: Mammography screening: reasons for recall and the influence of experience on recall in the Finnish system, *Clin Radiol* 41:384, 1990.
88. Pisano ED, McClelland R: Strategies for more effective delivery of mammography screening services, *Curr Opin Radiol* 2:726, 1990.
89. Rimer BK, Kasper Keintz M, Kessler HB, et al: Why women resist screening mammography: patient-related barriers, *Radiology* 172:243, 1989.

90. Robertson CL, Kopans DB: Communication problems after mammographic screening, *Radiology* 172:443, 1989.
91. Sickles EA: Imaging insights: the breast lesion seen in only one view, *RSNA Today Video* 4(2), 1990.
92. Tabar L, Gad A: Screening for breast cancer: the Swedish trial. *Radiology* 138:219, 1981.
93. Williams JC: Breast cancer screening: the underuse of mammography, *Radiology* 159:566, 1986.

Problem-solving diagnostic mammography

Definition and indications

94. Council adopts definition of screening and diagnostic mammography. *ACR Bulletin* 48(10):27, 1992.

Correlative physical examination

95. Beyer GA, Thorsen MK, Shaffer KA, et al: Mammographic appearance of the retained Dacron cuff of a Hickman catheter, *AJR Am J Roentgenol* 155:1203, 1990.
96. Britton CA, Baratz AB, Harris KM: Carcinoma mimicked by the sternal insertion of the pectoral muscle, *AJR Am J Roentgenol* 153:955, 1989.
97. Brown RC, Zuehlke RL, Ehrhardt JC, et al: Tatoos simulating calcifications on xeroradiographs of the breast. *Radiology* 138:583, 1981.
98. Gilula LA, Destouet JM, Monsees B: Nipple simulating a breast mass on mammogram. *Radiology* 170:272, 1989.
99. Jackson FI, Woods JA: Letters: simulators of a breast mass on a mammogram, *Radiology* 171:877, 1989.
100. Jackson FI: Letters: breast mass simulation on a mammogram, *AJR Am J Roentgenol* 154:900, 1990.
101. Klein DL, Sickles EA: Effects of needle aspiration on the mammographic appearance of the breast: a guide to the proper timing of the mammography examination, *Radiology* 145:44, 1982.
102. Meyer JE, Stomper PC, Lee RR: Pectoralis muscle simulating a breast mass, *AJR Am J Roentgenol* 152:481, 1989.
103. Stigers KB, King JG, Davey DD, et al: Pictorial essay: abnormalities of breast caused by biopsy: spectrum of mammographic findings. *AJR Am J Roentgenol* 156:287, 1991.

Caffeine sensitivity

104. Ernster VL, Mason L, Goodson WH, et al: Effects of caffeine-free diet on benign breast disease: a randomized trial, *Surgery* 91:3, 263, 1982.
105. Lubin F, Ron E: Review letter: consumption of methylxanthine-containing beverages and the risk of breast cancer, *Cancer Lett* 53:81, 1990.
106. Minton JP, Abou-Issa H: Nonendocrine theories of the etiology of benign breast disease, *World J Surg* 13:680, 1989.
107. Parazzinni F, LaVecchia C, Riundi R, et al: Methylxanthine, alcohol-free diet and fibrocystic breast disease: a factorial clinical study, *Surgery* 90:576, 1986.
108. Russell LC: Caffeine restriction as initial treatment for breast pain, *Nurse Pract* 14:36, 1989.

Diagnostic mammography technique

109. Bassett LW, Axelrod S: A modification of the craniocaudal view in mammography, *Radiology* 132:222, 1979.
110. Bassett LW, Arnold BA, Borger D, et al: Reduced-dose magnification mammography, *Radiology* 141:665, 1981.
111. Berkowitz JE, Gatewood OMB, Gayler BW: Equivocal mammographic findings: evaluation with spot compression, *Radiology* 171:369, 1989.
112. Buchanan JB, Jager RM: Contact spot xeromammography in the early diagnosis of breast cancer, *AJR Am J Roentgenol* 130:1159, 1978.

113. Eklund GW: Technical note: innovations in mammographic compression, *AJR Am J Roentgenol* 150:791, 1988.

114. Eklund GW, Busby RC, Miller SH, et al: Improved imaging of the augmented breast, *AJR Am J Roentgenol* 151:469, 1988.

115. Feig SA: The importance of supplementary mammographic views to diagnostic accuracy, *AJR Am J Roentgenol* 151:40, 1988.

116. Hall FM, Berenberg AL: Selective use of the oblique projection in mammography, *AJR Am J Roentgenol* 131:465, 1978.

117. Hassell PR, Olivotto IA, Mueller HA, et al: Early breast cancer: detection of recurrence after conservative surgery and radiation therapy, *Radiology* 176:731, 1990.

118. Kopans DB, Meyer JE, Homer MJ, et al: Dermal deposits mistaken for breast calcifications, *Radiology* 149:592, 1983.

119. Logan WW, Janus J: Use of special mammographic views to maximize radiographic information, *Radiol Clin North Am* 25:953, 1987.

120. Schnitt SJ, Silen W, Sadowsky NL, et al: Current concepts: ductal carcinoma in situ (intraductal carcinoma) of the breast, *N Engl J Med* 318:14, 1988.

121. Sickles EA: Further experience with microfocal spot magnification mammography in the assessment of clustered breast microcalcifications, *Radiology* 137:9, 1980.

122. Sickles EA: Letters to the editor: combining spot-compression and other special views to maximize mammographic information, *Radiology* 173:571, 1989.

123. Sickles EA: Microfocal spot magnification mammography using xeroradiographic and screen-film recording systems, *Radiology* 131:599, 1979.

124. Sickles EA: Practical solutions to common mammographic problems: tailoring the examination, *AJR Am J Roentgenol* 151:31, 1988.

125. Sickles EA, Doi K, Genant HK: Magnification film mammography: image quality and clinical studies, *Radiology* 125:69, 1977.

SUGGESTED READINGS
Technique

Fabrikan JI: The BEIR-III report: origin of the controversy, *AJR Am J Roentgenol* 136:209, 1981.

Faulk RM, Sickles EA: Efficacy of spot compression-magnification and tangential views in mammographic evaluation of palpable breast masses, *Radiology* 185:87, 1992.

Feig SA, Ehrlich SM: Estimation of radiation risk from screening mammography: recent trends and comparison with expected benefits, *Radiology* 174:638, 1990.

Huda W, Sourkes AM, Bews JA, et al: Radiation doses due to breast imaging in Manitoba: 1978–1988, *Radiology* 177:813, 1990.

Kimme-Smith C, Rothschild PA, Bassett LW, et al: Mammographic film-processor temperature, development time, and chemistry: effect on dose, contrast, and noise, *AJR Am J Roentgenol* 152:35, 1989.

Moskowitz M: Screening is not diagnosis, *Radiology* 133:265, 1979.

Rothenberg LN: Patient dose in mammography, *RadioGraphics* 10:739, 1990.

Schueler BA, Gray JE, Grisvold JJ: A comparison of mammography screen-film combinations, *Radiology* 184:629, 1992.

General screening mammography

Alcorn FS: Value of mammographic screening: assessment of studies and opinion, *RadioGraphics* 10:1133, 1990.

Bailar JC: Mammography: a contrary view, *Ann Intern Med* 84:77, 1976.

Baines CJ, Miller AB, Kopans DB, et al: Canadian National Breast Screening Study: assessment of technical quality by external review, *AJR Am J Roentgenol* 155:743, 1990.

Bird RE, Wallace TW, Yankaskas BC: Analysis of cancers missed at screening mammography. *Radiology* 184:613, 1992.

Brenner RJ: Medicolegal aspects of breast imaging: Variable standards of care relating to different types of practice. *AJR Am J Roentgenol* 156:719, 1991.

Burhenne LJW, Hislop TG, Burhenne HJ: The British Columbia mammography screening program: evaluation of the first 15 months. *AJR Am J Roentgenol* 158:45, 1992.

Clark RA: Economic issues in screening mammography. *AJR Am J Roentgenol* 158:527, 1992.

Costanza ME, D'Orsi CJ, Greene HL, et al: Feasibility of universal screening mammography, lessons from a community intervention. *Arch Intern Med* 151:1851, 1991.

Dershaw DD, Liberman L, Lippin BS: Mobile mammographic screening of self-referred women: Results of 22,540 screenings. *Radiology* 184:415, 1992.

Dodd GD: Is screening mammography routinely indicated for women between 40 and 50 years of age? *J Fam Pract* 27:313, 1988.

Fajardo LL, Saint-Germain M, Meakem TJ III, et al: Factors influencing women to undergo screening mammography. *Radiology* 184:59, 1992.

Forrest APM: Screening for breast cancer: the UK scene, *Br J Radiol* 62:695, 1989.

Hall FM: Sounding board: screening mammography—potential problems on the horizon, *N Engl J Med* 314:53, 1986.

Hall FM: Opinion: the coming of age of radiologic imaging screening, *Radiology* 168:579, 1988.

Harris RP, Fletcher SW, Gonzalez JJ, et al: Mammography and age: are we targeting the wrong women? A community survey of women and physicians. *Cancer* 67:2010, 1991.

Ikeda DM, Andersson I, Wattsgard C, et al: Interval carcinomas in the Malmo mammographic screening trial: radiographic appearance and prognostic considerations. *AJR Am J Roentgenol* 159:287, 1992.

Kessler HB, Rimer BK, Devine PJ, et al: Corporate-sponsored breast cancer screening at the work site: results of a statewide program. *Radiology* 179:107, 1991.

Kopans DB: The Canadian screening program: a different perspective, *AJR Am J Roentgenol* 155:748, 1990.

McLelland R, Hendrick RE, Zinninger MD, Wilcox PA: The American College of Radiology accreditation program. *AJR Am J Roentgenol* 157:473, 1991.

American College of Radiology accreditation program. *AJR Am J Roentgenol* 157:473, 1991.

Monsees BS: Screening mammography: Who will meet the need? *Radiology* 184:30, 1992.

Mootz AR, Glazer-Waldman H, Evans WP, et al: Mammography in a mobile setting: remaining barriers. *Radiology* 180:161, 1991.

Moskowitz M: Mammographic screening: significance of minimal breast cancers: *AJR Am J Roentgenol* 136:735, 1981.

Moskowitz M: Mammography to screen asymptomatic women for breast cancer, *AJR Am J Roentgenol* 143:457, 1984.

Moskowitz M: Breast cancer: age-specific growth rates and screening strategies, *Radiology* 157:852, 1986.

Moskowitz M: Costs of screening for breast cancer, *Radiol Clin North Am* 25:1031, 1987.

Moskowitz M: Early detection of breast cancer by mammography screening, *Curr Opin Radiol* 1:193, 1989.

Moskowitz M: Impact of a priori medical decisions on screening for breast cancer, *Radiology* 171:605, 1989.

Moskowitz M, Fox SH: Opinion: cost analysis of aggressive breast cancer screening, *Radiology* 130:253, 1979.

Moskowitz M, Gartside PS: Evidence of breast cancer mortality reduction: aggressive screening in women under age 50, *AJR Am J Roentgenol* 138:911, 1982.

Peeters PHM, Verbeek ALM, Hendriks JHCL, et al: The occurrence of interval cancers in the Nijmegen screening programme, *Br J Cancer* 59:929, 1989.

Reynolds HE, Jackson VP: Self-referred mammography patients: analysis of patients' characteristics. *AJR Am J Roentgenol* 157:481, 1991.

Seago K: Mammographic screening: the pressures for reimbursement, *Medicenter Management* September 1986, p 19.

Shaw de Paredes E, Frazier AB, Hartwell GD, et al: Development and implementation of a quality assurance program for mammography, *Radiology* 163:83, 1987.

Shapiro S, Venet W, Venet L, et al: Ten-to-fourteen-year effect of screening on breast cancer mortality, *J Natl Cancer Inst* 69:349, 1982.

Sickles EA, Weber WN, Galvin HB, et al: Mammographic screening: how to operate successfully at low cost: reply, *Radiology* 161:851, 1986.

Tabar L: Control of breast cancer through screening mammography, *Radiology* 174:655, 1990.

Tabar L, Faberberg CJG, Gad A, et al: Reduction in mortality from breast cancer after mass screening with mammography, *Lancet* 1:829, 1985.

Taplin S: An opposing view, *J Fam Pract* 27:316, 1988.

U.S. Preventive Services Task Force: Screening for breast cancer, *Am Fam Physician* 39:89, 1989.

Mammographic evaluation of breasts treated by lumpectomy and radiation therapy

Dershaw DD, McCormick B, Cox L, et al: Differentiation of benign and malignant local tumor recurrence after lumpectomy, *AJR Am J Roentgenol* 155:35, 1990.

Dershaw DD, McCormick B, Osborne MP: Detection of local recurrence after conservative therapy for breast carcinoma, *Cancer* 70:493, 1992.

Dershaw DD, Shank B, Reisinger S: Mammographic findings after breast cancer treatment with local excision and definitive irradiation, *Radiology* 164:455, 1987.

Gefter WB, Friedman AK, Goodman RL: The role of mammography in evaluating patients with early carcinoma of the breast for tylectomy and radiation therapy, *Radiology* 142:77, 1982.

Hall FM: Letters to the editor: breast microcalcifications after lumpectomy and radiation therapy, *Radiology* 172:577, 1989.

Harris KM, Costa-Greco MA, Baratz AB, et al: The mammographic features of the postlumpectomy postirradiation breast, *RadioGraphics* 9:253, 1989.

Homer MJ, Schmidt-Ullrich R, Safaii H, et al: Residual breast carcinoma after biopsy: role of mammography in evaluation, *Radiology* 170:75, 1989.

Libshitz HI, Montague ED, Paulus DD Jr: Skin thickness in the therapeutically irradiated breast, *AJR Am J Roentgenol* 130:345, 1978.

Libshitz HI, Montague ED, Paulus DD: Calcifications and the therapeutically irradiated breast, *AJR Am J Roentgenol* 128:1021, 1977.

Orel SG, Troupin RH, Patterson EA, et al: Breast cancer recurrence after lumpectomy and irradiation: role of mammography in detection. *Radiology* 183:201, 1992.

Rebner M, Pennes DR, Adler DD, et al: Breast microcalcifications after lumpectomy and radiation therapy, *Radiology* 170:691, 1989.

Ryoo MC, Kagan AR, Wollin M, et al: Prognostic factors for recurrence and cosmesis in 393 patients after radiation therapy for early mammary carcinoma, *Radiology* 172:555, 1989.

Sadowsky NL, Semine A: Good mammography finds postop cancer recurrence, *Diagnostic Imaging* October 1990, p 100.

Stomper PC, Recht A, Berenberg AL, et al: Mammographic detection of recurrent cancer in the irradiated breast, *AJR Am J Roentgenol* 148:39, 1987.

Sickles EA: Low-cost mass screening for breast cancer with mammography. *AJR Am J Roentgenol* 158:55, 1992.

Wolk RB: Hidden costs of mobile mammography: is subsidization necessary? *AJR Am J Roentgenol* 158:1243, 1992.

CHAPTER
3 Ancillary Breast Imaging Modalities

Karen S. Baker

Ultrasonography
    Technique
    Indications
    Limitations and inappropriate uses
    Interpretation
    Associated procedures
Galactography
    Technique
    Indications
    Limitations
    Interpretation
    Associated procedures
Computed tomography
    Technique
    Indications
    Limitations
    Interpretation
    Associated procedures
Pneumocystography

Thermography
Transillumination
Angiography
Digital mammography
Nuclear imaging
    Immunodetection
    Positron emission tomography imaging
    Scintigraphy
Magnetic resonance imaging
    Technique
    Indications
    Limitations and inappropriate uses
    Interpretation
    Associated procedures

Standard mammography is currently the diagnostic modality of choice for breast evaluation. However, several ancillary imaging modalities have been used to evaluate the breasts. The purpose of this chapter is to discuss the technique of, indications for, limitations of, and interpretation of these modalities and to give insight as to how they fit into the spectrum of modern breast imaging.

Ultrasonography, galactography, computed tomography, and pneumocystography are modalities currently used in selected patients with clinical or mammographic breast abnormalities. Thermography and transillumination will require even further research to establish what, if any, role they may play in modern breast imaging. Angiography is mainly of historical interest and is not currently used to evaluate breast disease. The future directions in breast imaging research include digital mammography, nuclear imaging, and magnetic resonance imaging (MRI) (Table 3-1).

ULTRASONOGRAPHY
Technique

Ultrasonography of the breast was first described in 1952 by Wild and Reid[81] using A-mode contact imaging of palpable breast masses. In the late 1970s, the technique was further developed using gray-scale B-mode 5-MHz techniques[48,78] for palpable breast masses. Jellins, Kossoff, and Reeve[43] performed whole breast ultrasonography with the patient prone and the breasts immersed in a water bath. Automated whole breast ultrasonography units were developed in anticipation of a possible role in breast cancer screening.[12,13,22,23,32,57,78] This role was never achieved. Because of higher expense and longer examination time for whole breast automated scans (Boxes 3-1, 3-2), most centers now use high-resolution, high-frequency (7.5 to 10 MHz), hand-held real-time ultrasonography for problem solving in the breast.[38] Real-time ultrasound machines already available in the

46

Table 3-1 **Ancillary Breast Imaging Modalities**

Modality	Screening	Diagnostic	Research
Ultrasonography	−	+ +	+ (Doppler)
Galactography	−	+ +	−
Computed tomography	−	+	−
Pneumocystography	−	±	−
Thermography	−	−	+
Transillumination	−	−	+
Angiography	−	−	−
Digital mammography	+	+	+ +
Nuclear imaging	−	+	+ +
MRI	−	±	+ +

Note: − = not used; ± = seldom used; + = occasionally used; + + = often used.

BOX 3-1 HAND-HELD BREAST ULTRASOUND EQUIPMENT

Advantages

Readily available in most departments
Rapid determination of cystic versus solid mass
Little additional training needed
Assessment of effects of compression and motion
Biopsy and aspiration guidance
Better visualization of subareolar lesions than with automated equipment
Palpation allowed during examination

Disadvantages

Small field of view
Less reproducible examinations than with automated equipment
Difficult orientation
Difficult examination of some nonpalpable lesions
Usually performed by physician

From Jackson VP: New instrumentation in breast sonography, *Appl Radiol* November: 58, 1988.

BOX 3-2 AUTOMATED BREAST ULTRASOUND EQUIPMENT

Advantages

Large field of view
Easier orientation than with hand-held equipment
Reproducible examinations
Systematic recording of image data
Accurate performance by technologist
High-quality image with high-frequency transducers
Large areas of breast easy to cover
Multiple lesions easy to assess

Disadvantages

Expensive equipment
Longer examination time than with hand-held equipment
Need for training in technique and interpretation
Few other applications of machine
Obscuring of retroareolar lesions by nipple shadowing

From Jackson VP: New instrumentation in breast sonography, *Appl Radiol* November: 58, 1988.

radiology department may be used for breast examinations provided high-frequency probes are available (usually 7.5 to 10 MHz for sector scanners or 5 MHz for linear array scanners). Such high-frequency transducers are necessary to visualize small structures in the breast.[38] Higher frequency transducers (7.5 MHz) for whole breast automated ultrasonography units were also developed and showed improved image quality compared with 4-MHz transducers.[41]

A standoff pad or fluid-filled offset between the breast and transducer should be used for superficial lesions in order to place the lesion in the focal zone of the transducer. Some transducers have a built-in fluid offset.[1,47] For hand-held ultrasonography, the patient may be examined in the sitting or supine position or a combination of both. The orientation of the breast structures is quite different when the breast is out of the mammographic compression device. This change is most accentuated when the patient is examined by ultrasonography in a supine position. Therefore, some centers prefer to examine the patient sitting with the breast resting on a table or other firm surface while scanning. This position approximates the craniocaudal mammographic projection as much as possible without actually putting the patient's breast into the mammographic unit for sonography. Two centers use the mammographic compression device to hold the breast for ultrasonography to ensure that the lesion seen with ultrasonography correlates to the mammographic lesion.[6,18] This approach is used when the mass is not palpable.

Indications

During the evolution of breast ultrasonography as an imaging modality for breast disease, many listings of appropriate indications have been published. These indications vary depending on the reporting institution. The earliest papers on breast sonography reported on imaging of women with palpable breast masses. Most radiologists now reserve breast sonography for the following:

1. Cystic or solid differentiation of nonpalpable benign-appearing masses seen by mammography. If cystic, provide routine follow-up; if solid, either perform biopsy or provide clinical and mammographic follow-up depending on mammographic level of suspicion*
2. Palpable masses (suspected to be cysts) if needle aspiration has been attempted and has failed to yield cyst fluid[49,54,59,70]
3. Palpable mass in a young woman with dense breasts who is younger than 30 years or a pregnant woman[†]
4. Evaluation of a possible abscess; if abscess is present, then drainage is necessary[40,45,67]
5. Evaluation of a palpable mass that cannot be fully evaluated with mammography because of extreme breast density or location of the mass or because there is corresponding equivocal asymmetric density on the mammogram[‡]
6. Evaluation of lymph node status in a woman with breast cancer[7,40,64,72]
7. Guidance for interventional procedures such as cyst aspiration, preoperative needle/wire localization, fine-needle aspiration cytology, or needle core biopsy§

8. *Occasionally* for patients with prostheses or postlumpectomy patients*

Limitations and inappropriate uses

Ultrasound examination of the breast was originally investigated with the expectation that it might be used as a screening modality for breast cancer.[12] However, because of its high false-negative rate for cancer detection (owing to inability to visualize microcalcifications or small occult cancers in fatty breasts), ultrasound examination is not currently recommended as a screening tool.[†] It is more appropriately used as an adjunct to mammography, where it functions as a valuable problem-solving modality.[3] Ultrasonography is also somewhat limited for mammographically detected masses that are small (less than 0.8 to 1.0 cm) or deep within a large breast.[36] Posterior enhanced through transmission may be minimal in a very small or very deep cyst.[3] Ultrasonography also has a high-false positive rate when asymptomatic women are examined.[35] Normal structures (parenchyma, fat lobules) in the breast may simulate masses.[34,36] Therefore, only areas of the breast that are abnormal on physical examination or on mammography should be studied by adjunct sonography.

The primary use of breast ultrasonography is cystic and solid differentiation of mammographically benign-appearing, well-circumscribed masses where a simple cyst is in the differential diagnosis.[40] Ultrasonography should not be considered if the differential diagnosis does not include a cyst.[40] If the mass is solid, ultrasonography cannot reliably differentiate benign from malignant solid masses, and evaluation should be based on clinical and mammographic findings.[2,40,79]

Also, ultrasonography should not be used to *screen* the asymptomatic radiographically dense breast,[40,49] for evaluation of a *nonpalpable* asymmetric density seen at mammography[40] or for *routine* evaluation of patients after augmentation or lumpectomy and radiation therapy.[40] Ultrasonography is not recommended for evaluation of a palpable mass thought to be a cyst because needle aspiration can be accomplished quickly and at low cost.[49] The official policy statement of the ACR[65] published in 1984 states that breast ultrasonography should not be used for breast cancer screening.

Interpretation

The normal anatomy of the breast seen with ultrasonography has been previously de-

---

*References 11,20,35,39,40,43,49,67,70.
†References 4,20,31,32,39,40,44,67,82.
‡References 20,31,39,40,59,67.
§References 11,21,40,49,54,55,60,67.

---

*References 9,16,20,39,40,56,59.
†References 2,3,24,34,35,36,50,58,75.

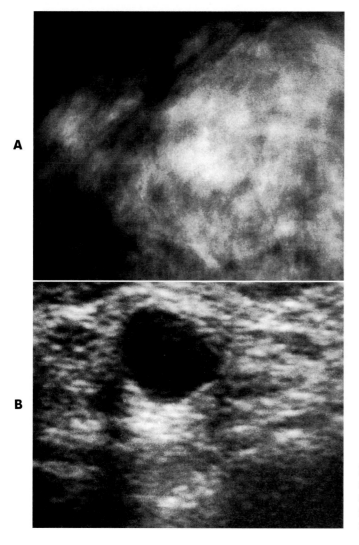

Fig. 3-1 A, Craniocaudal mammogram showing 1.5-cm mass; margins of mass are obscured by overlapping dense breast parenchyma. **B,** Ultrasonography of the mass shows a simple cyst.

scribed.[1,35,36,57,67] The skin is seen as a band of uniform echogenicity bordered on both sides by thin echogenic lines (0.5 to 2.0 mm thick). Fascial planes and Cooper's ligaments are thin, highly echogenic lines. The subareolar ducts are hypoechoic, tubular structures. Fat lobules are hypoechoic compared to the echogenic parenchyma and connective tissue. The retromammary fat is seen as a lucent zone behind the parenchyma. The pectoralis muscle demonstrates uniform, low-level echoes demarcated by surrounding bright echogenic fascial lines. Ribs are seen as oval or round structures that produce shadowing. The nipple may produce an acoustic shadow behind it. This shadow was more of a problem with whole breast scanners than hand-held scanners.

Several papers have shown that breast sonography is extremely reliable in diagnosing simple breast cysts. Sensitivities range from 96% to 100%.[22,24,35,43,76] However, one must adhere to strict criteria to make the diagnosis of a simple cyst. The mass must be round or oval, have well-circumscribed margins, and have enhanced through transmission. Most important, the mass must not contain any internal echoes (Fig. 3-1).[3] At real-time ultrasonography, simple cysts may be flattened with compression.[36] It is possible to create echoes in a cyst because of reverberation artifact. These are usually in the anterior portion of the cyst and can usually be recognized as an artifact. These echoes increase as the gain or power is increased.

Well-circumscribed (usually medullary) carcinoma may look anechoic, and this is usually caused by improperly low gain settings.[59] Once the diagnosis of a cyst has been made, the cyst must be thoroughly examined to evaluate all the cyst walls while looking for irregularity or mural nodules (Figs. 3-2 and 3-3). If wall abnormalities are found, surgical biopsy is indicated.[35,36,66] Compli-

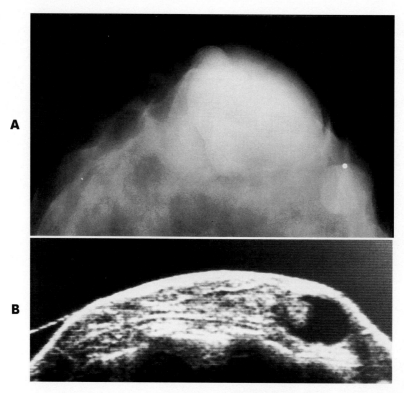

Fig. 3-2 **A,** Craniocaudal mammogram showing a 5.0-cm circumscribed mass behind the nipple. A second smaller mass is seen laterally. **B,** Ultrasonography of the 5.0-cm subareolar mass shows a cyst containing a mass along a portion of the cyst wall. Biopsy revealed intracystic papilloma.

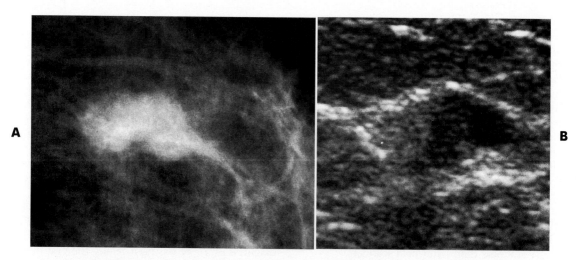

Fig. 3-3 **A,** True lateral mammogram showing ill-defined mass with a "comet-tail" anteriorly. **B,** Ultrasonography shows a complex mass with cystic and solid components. Biopsy revealed infiltrating carcinoma with an intracystic papillary component.

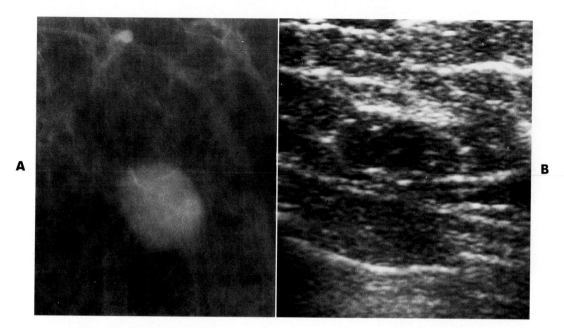

Fig. 3-4 A, Mammogram showing a 1.5-cm well-defined mass. **B,** Ultrasonography shows a well-defined solid mass. Biopsy revealed fibroadenoma.

cated cysts (bleeding, infection) or cysts containing viscous fluid usually do not meet strict criteria because they will exhibit internal echoes. Blood or debris within a cyst may be seen to layer in the dependent portion of the cyst.[2] Cysts that contain echogenic material (cellular debris, blood) should be managed with aspiration or excisional biopsy.[35,36]

Fibroadenoma is the most common benign tumor of the breast and is the most common palpable breast mass in young women under 30 years of age. This tumor has been extensively studied with sonography and has been the subject of several articles. Typical ultrasonographic features of fibroadenoma include well-circumscribed margins, homogeneous internal echoes, and round or oval shape (Fig. 3-4).* However, some masses proven to be fibroadenoma may exhibit one or more atypical ultrasonographic features such as margin irregularity, inhomogeneous echo pattern, or posterior shadowing.[42] Even for masses displaying so-called typical features of fibroadenoma, the differential diagnosis includes well-circumscribed breast carcinoma because approximately 10% to 17% of malignancies are well circumscribed.[59] Therefore, all solid masses on ultrasonography need further evaluation such as fine-needle aspiration cytology, core biopsy, or surgical biopsy.[42]

Other benign breast lesions have been described

in the literature such as breast abscess,[59] juvenile papillomatosis,[46] papilloma, hematoma,[59] galactocele,[71] lymph nodes, hamartoma,[59] fat necrosis,[59,63] and duct ectasia.[59]

Cystosarcoma phyllodes (recently renamed phyllodes tumor) has also been described in the ultrasonography literature.[8,59] This rare breast neoplasm has histologic features similar to fibroadenoma but can recur locally and metastasize in approximately 3% to 12% of cases.[8,17] This tumor can usually be diagnosed clinically. Reported ultrasonographic findings include low-level internal echoes, smooth contour, and no significant posterior shadowing. Some may show posterior enhancement. An interesting ultrasonographic feature of this tumor is the frequent finding of multiple peripheral cystic areas within the tumor, which correlate well with cystic areas seen on gross pathology. Unfortunately, the benign or malignant behavior of this tumor cannot be predicted on the basis of sonography, and wide local resection or mastectomy is required treatment depending on the size of the mass.

The appearance of breast carcinoma on ultrasonography has been well described in the literature. Typically, carcinoma exhibits ill-defined margins and inhomogeneous internal echoes (Fig. 3-5). The mass may occasionally contain cystic-appearing areas secondary to tumor necrosis.[39,58] Carcinoma typically is hypoechoic and exhibits posterior acoustic shadowing[15,22,33] but occasionally may show posterior acoustic enhancement or

---

*References 3,14,28,31,33,35,36.

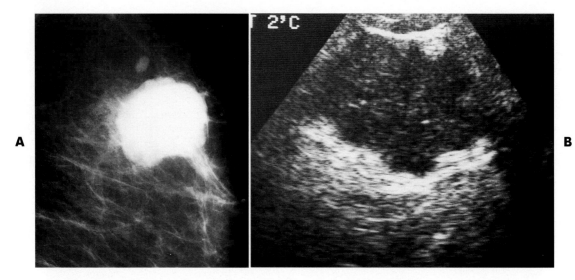

Fig. 3-5 A, Oblique mammogram showing a large 4.0-cm lobulated ill-defined mass in the upper outer quadrant. **B,** Ultrasonography shows a solid ill-defined lobulated mass with some back-wall enhancement. Biopsy revealed breast carcinoma.

have no effect.* Acoustic shadowing is most marked in carcinomas with considerable desmoplastic reaction.[59] In addition, well-circumscribed carcinoma may exhibit features similar to those of benign masses such as a homogeneous echo pattern and well-circumscribed margins. This most commonly will be ductal carcinoma, but the differential diagnosis would include special types of ductal carcinoma such as medullary, colloid (mucinous), intracystic, and solid papillary.[36,39,73] Medullary carcinoma may show little or no attenuation of sound or may show posterior acoustic enhancement.[15,39,59,62] It is this overlap of typical benign and malignant features of solid masses that makes ultrasound examination unreliable in differentiating between the two.[15,36] Secondary signs of breast malignancy such as skin thickening[51] or retraction can also be visualized with sonography.

Ultrasonography may be used to evaluate patients who have undergone lumpectomy and radiation therapy for breast carcinoma. Findings such as skin thickening, increased echogenicity of fat, poor definition of Cooper ligaments, and parenchymal distortion in the lumpectomy bed are similar to corresponding well-recognized mammographic findings.[9,30,61] However, it should be recognized that routine follow-up for these patients should be clinical breast examination and mammography with ultrasonography reserved for cases in which an abnormality is suspected.[9]

Ultrasonography has been used to evaluate women with breast implants. It is currently recommended that ultrasonography be reserved for those patients with clinical or mammographic abnormalities.[56] Ultrasonography is particularly useful in patients who are suspected of having implant-related abnormalities.[16,69] Fibrous capsule formation may manifest as a thicker, more echogenic line at the margin of the implant, and the implant itself may show a distorted shape.[16] Liebman and Kruse[56] described sonographic findings in 11 cases of breast cancer in patients with implants.

Associated procedures

More recently, ultrasound-guided fine-needle aspiration cytology, needle core biopsy and preoperative needle and wire localization procedures have become accepted techniques.[21,25,27,29,53-55] Weber and others[80] caution that mammography remains the procedure of choice for preoperative localization. Rifkin and others[68] used intraoperative ultrasonography to localize nonpalpable lesions for biopsy. Simple cysts may also be aspirated using ultrasound guidance in symptomatic patients or for masses thought to be cysts that contain internal echoes, have no acoustic enhancement, or have wall irregularity (Fig. 3-6).[21,54,60] Karstrup and others[45] reported their experience with four patients in whom breast abscesses were successfully drained percutaneously using ultrasound guidance.

Duplex Doppler ultrasonography is a technique that needs further investigation. Equipment is currently available in frequencies from 3 to 5 MHz.

---

*References 2,3,10,15,29,31,33,36,52.

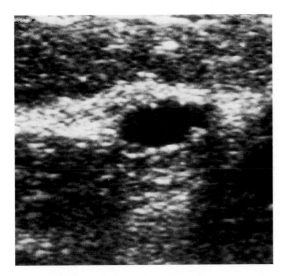

Fig. 3-6 Ultrasonogram showing a simple cyst just before ultrasound-guided needle aspiration. Needle tip is seen above the cyst.

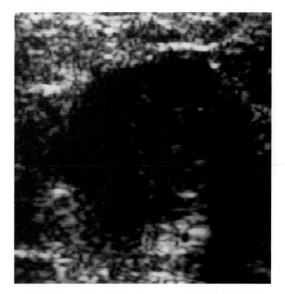

Fig. 3-7 Ultrasonogram showing a 2.2 cm solid mass that contained an abnormal signal by Doppler analysis. Proven to be ductal carcinoma at biopsy.

Sensitivity may be augmented by additional color flow capability (Fig. 3-7). Bohm-Velez and Mendelson[5] evaluated 15 solid breast masses and found that 80% of them had no identifiable vascularity by pulsed Doppler or by color flow. Cosgrove and others[19] examined 60 patients with breast masses. Of the 21 patients with breast cancer, moderate or high flow was demonstrated in 20. Their equipment operated at 3.5 to 5.0 MHz. Jackson[37] examined 54 breast lesions operating the pulsed Doppler crystal at 3.0 to 4.5 MHz. The sensitivity and specificity for diagnosis of breast carcinoma in this study were 69% and 59%, respectively. In addition, it was evident that some carcinomas did not exhibit positive Doppler signal and some benign lesions (such as fibroadenoma, fibrocystic change, and abscess) did exhibit signal. Schoenberger and colleagues[74] published 100% sensitivity in their series of 38 patients. Srivastava and others[77] also reported results showing considerable overlap in findings between benign and malignant masses.

GALACTOGRAPHY

Galactography (ductography), first described in the radiologic literature by Hicken in 1938, is mammary duct injection with water-soluble contrast material followed by mammography.[90] It is a worthwhile examination in selected patients with spontaneous nipple discharge. The patients are prescreened with clinical history, breast physical examination, and mammography. The nipple discharge can be tested for blood with a simple Hemoccult test. Cytologic examination of the discharge can be done, but most authors find this test is not highly sensitive.[88,91,94,96]

Technique

The patient is placed in a supine position on an examining table, and the discharging nipple is cleaned with alcohol. The nipple is squeezed gently until a drop of discharge is produced to localize the appropriate duct for the cannulation. The breast is then prepared with povidone-iodine (Betadine) and draped. The duct is cannulated with a small (usually 25- to 31-gauge), blunt-tipped needle or sialography cannula. Gentle straightening of the nipple may facilitate cannulation of the duct opening. A coaxial technique for cannulating the duct has also been described.[84] The needle is taped in place, with the attached syringe containing sterile water-soluble contrast material and prefilled connecting tubing. Duct injection is preferred in the supine position so that gravity can aid in the flow of contrast material and permit better filling than with the patient seated. The duct is slowly injected until the patient has a feeling of fullness or pressure in her breast. If the patient feels any sharp pain, the injection should be discontinued because this may indicate that extravasation has occurred. Usually 0.5 to 1.0 ml of contrast material is sufficient, but occasionally up to 3.0 ml can be used if the duct system is dilated. Care should be taken not to inject air bubbles so as not to confuse these artifacts with true intraluminal filling defects. The cannula can be removed or left in place for filming. The patient is then moved to the mammographic unit. The nipple may be covered with a coating of collodion to prevent leakage of contrast material from the duct. Standard craniocaudal and 90-degree true lateral views are taken using gentle compression, less than is used for routine mammography. These views may be supplemented with magnification images if needed.[96] If surgery is to be performed immediately, a mixture of methylene blue and contrast material can be injected into the duct to help pinpoint the abnormal duct system for the surgeon and pathologist.[97,98]

Indications

Appropriate indications for this examination are spontaneous, single-duct, serous, sanguineous, or serosanguineous nipple discharge in a nonlactating breast.[85,87] Bilateral, multiple-duct, nonspontaneous discharge or discharge that is milky, creamy, or green is almost always due to benign disease. Galactography is not indicated for these types of nonspontaneous nipple discharge.[93] Relative contraindications for galactography are the presence of purulent discharge or acute mastitis.[96,98]

Limitations

The patient must have expressible discharge on the day of the examination in order for the appropriate duct to be injected. Most of the time, a filling defect seen on galactography is a nonspecific finding. There is no reliable way to distinguish a benign mass such as a papilloma from ma-

lignancy, and therefore, ductal excision is usually performed.

Interpretation

The normal breast has 15 to 20 ducts emerging at the nipple. Injection of a normal ductal system shows smooth subareolar ducts with a caliber of 2 to 3 mm. The branches toward the posterior breast become progressively smaller, exhibiting a treelike pattern (Fig. 3-8). The walls of the ducts should be smooth, and the course of the ducts should be relatively straight without sudden angulation or cutoff.[88]

Excessive dilation of the ducts up to several millimeters or even 1 cm usually indicates benign duct ectasia. This benign disorder usually presents as bilateral, multiple-duct, green to black nipple discharge.

Intraluminal filling defects may be single or multiple. Although the presence of a single smooth intraluminal filling defect usually indicates a benign solitary papilloma (Fig. 3-9),[86,92] the limitation of galactography is that there is no reliable way to differentiate a benign from a malignant intraluminal mass. Therefore, intraluminal masses must be excised for pathologic diagnosis. The intranipple portion of the duct must be seen, and occasionally the cannula must be removed with repeat films in order to visualize this area.[98] Multiple small filling defects may be due to intraductal hyperplasia, papillomatosis, blood clots, or multiple papillomas. Cysts may also fill with contrast material.

Abnormal galactographic findings typically as-

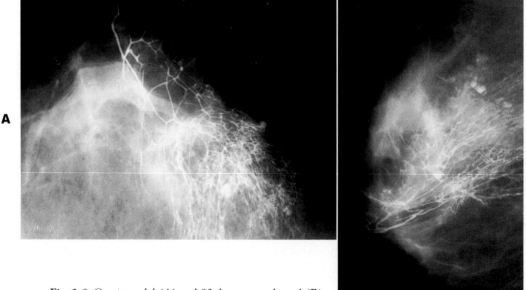

Fig. 3-8 Craniocaudal **(A)** and 90-degree true lateral **(B)** mammograms of a normal galactogram.

sociated with malignancy are irregular intraductal filling defects, invasion or displacement of the duct, or complete duct obstruction (Fig. 3-10).[83] The duct may be dilated proximal to the carcinoma. Extravasation of contrast material from the involved duct has been reported to be a possible sign of malignancy.[88] Nonfilling or distortion of part of a ductal system may also be seen.[94] Although it is possible to formulate a list of malignant and benign galactographic appearances[97] (Box 3-3), it is impossible to distinguish tissue his-tology solely on the basis of the galactogram. The galactogram should be used mainly for localization and, in fact, should not be performed if subsequent surgery is not being considered.

Associated procedures

To aid the surgeon further in localizing the abnormal area of the breast that is to be removed, methylene blue can be mixed with contrast material and injected at the time of galactography.[93,96] This is only helpful if the surgery is to be

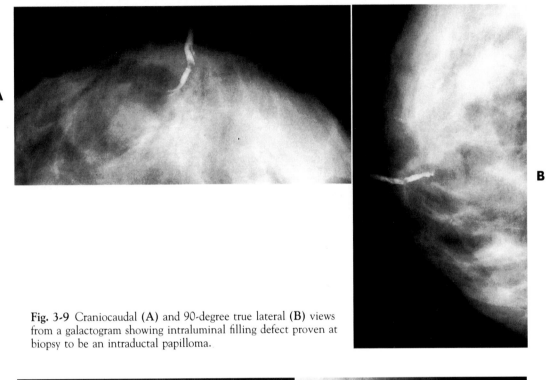

Fig. 3-9 Craniocaudal (**A**) and 90-degree true lateral (**B**) views from a galactogram showing intraluminal filling defect proven at biopsy to be an intraductal papilloma.

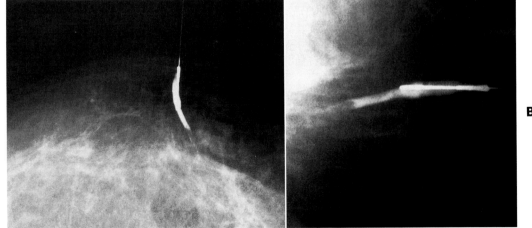

Fig. 3-10 Craniocaudal (**A**) and 90-degree true lateral (**B**) views from a galactogram showing complete duct obstruction proven at biopsy to be a ductal carcinoma.

BOX 3-3 GALACTOGRAPHIC FINDINGS OF MALIGNANCY

Complete duct obstruction
Defect or irregularity of the duct wall
Duct that ends in an ill-defined mass
Duct displacement

From Tabar L, Marton Z, Kadas I: Galactography in the examination of secretory breasts, Am J Surg 127:282, 1974.

performed immediately after injection because the blue dye tends to diffuse into the surrounding tissue. In difficult cases and depending on the surgeon's wishes, a standard needle/wire device can be placed into the breast immediately after the galactogram to localize the lesion preoperatively. Alternatively, a suture can be introduced into the duct and threaded until the suture stops at the mass within the duct in order to pinpoint the lesion for the surgeon.[89,95]

COMPUTED TOMOGRAPHY
Technique

The earliest reports of computed tomography (CT) for evaluating breast disease used a dedicated unit specifically designed for breast scanning.[99-103,106,115] The patient was placed prone on a tilting table with the breast projecting through an opening. Each breast was scanned separately while immersed in water. The scans were performed before and after rapid intravenous drip infusion of 300 ml of 30% contrast material.

In 1982, Chang and others[104] reported their experience with CT of the breast using a conventional body CT scanner. The patients were placed supine with arms above the head. Transverse images were obtained before and after rapid intravenous drip infusion of 300 ml of 30% contrast material. Muller and colleagues[110] also reported their results with conventional CT of the breast using a body scanner, but they placed their patients prone and elevated the chest from the tabletop with foam blocks so that the breasts could hang free. These investigators administered much less intravenous contrast material (60 ml) as a bolus.

Indications

Because of the need for intravenous contrast material, high cost of the examination, high radiation dose, and lengthy examination time, CT is an inappropriate breast cancer screening tool. However, CT can be used in the following situations: (1) occasionally for CT-guided preoperative wire localization when the lesion is seen in only one mammographic view,[105,107] (2) pretreatment planning before radiation therapy,[108,110-112] and (3) evaluation of postmastectomy patients for local or regional recurrence.[108,109,111-114]

Limitations

As stated, CT is not a suitable modality for breast cancer screening.[5] Microcalcifications easily seen on mammography usually are not recognized on CT (Fig. 3-11).[110] Furthermore, the scan time is relatively long and the radiation dose to the breast is considerable. Muller and colleagues[110] calculated that the radiation dose to the breast with CT may be as much as three to six times higher than with mammography.

Interpretation

The published series using CT to evaluate breast disease all were done before and after intravenous contrast administration. With this protocol, the early reports seemed to indicate that CT was much more sensitive than mammography in detecting breast cancer. The sensitivity of mammography ranged from 71% to 80%, and the sensitivity of CT ranged from 93% to 97%.[100,102-104] However, it should be pointed out that the technical limitations of film-screen mammography in the early 1980s were a significant factor in lowering the observed sensitivity of mammography. Since then, advances in film-screen combinations, positioning techniques, and equipment have dramatically improved the sensitivity of film-screen mammography. The interpretation of CT of the breast was based on the observation that malignant masses in the breast usually were enhanced with contrast administration, raising the CT number by at least 25 (50 Hounsfield units). Benign fibrocystic disease usually demonstrated precontrast CT numbers lower than or equal to those for cancer but enhanced to a lesser degree than malignant lesions. Proliferative change in some cases showed a high degree of contrast enhancement. Noncalcified fibroadenomas and breast abscesses showed a high degree of contrast enhancement, but their initial CT numbers were usually lower than for cancer.[99,100,103,104,106] These data were not clear-cut, and there was considerable overlap of response among benign and malignant lesions. Muller and colleagues[110] found no significant enhancement after injection of contrast material in five of 24 cancers and at the same time found significant enhancement in four of five benign lesions. They also reported considerable overlap between the benign and malignant groups for the initial precontrast CT numbers. These observations led these investigators to question the reliability of using enhancement as a criterion to dif-

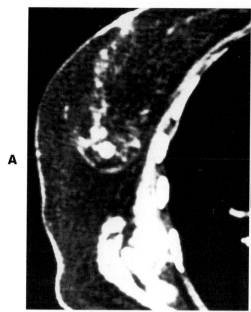

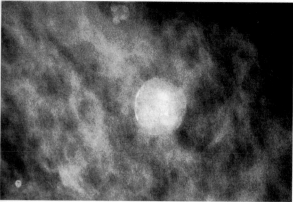

Fig. 3-11 A, Chest CT performed on this patient revealed a mass in the right breast. **B,** Mammogram of the right breast reveals a 1-cm round, well-defined mass with "eggshell" type rim calcification consistent with a simple cyst or oil cyst.

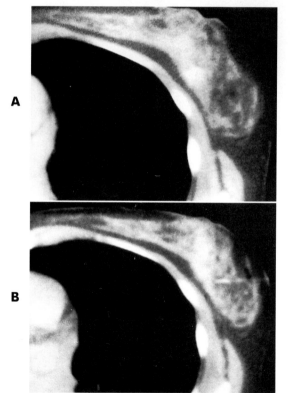

Fig. 3-12 A, CT-guided breast needle localization. CT of the chest following injection of intravenous contrast material shows a mass in the left breast. **B,** Repeat CT scan at the level of the mass showing the needle/wire localization device in place.

ferentiate benign from malignant lesions. In fact, they concluded that "although technically a whole body scanner is capable of producing good images of the breast, the number of patients in whom CT should be used instead of or in addition to mammography is limited."

Associated procedures

As stated, one of the current indications for breast CT is for preoperative wire localization of lesions that are seen on only one mammographic view (Fig. 3-12). Kopans and Meyer[107] used an N-shaped skin marker formed from surgical wire and taped it to the breast. The skin guide remained in place during the localization procedure, and the three cross sections of the marker on the CT image uniquely defined the plane of the scan. Therefore, accurate measurements could be obtained from the lesion to the skin and to the marker. Dixon[105] placed barium paste on the nipple and then defined this level as 0. Sections were then obtained through the breast to determine the distance of the lesion from the nipple cranial or caudal. Grids were superimposed on the images at the level of the nipple and at the level of the lesion to determine the distance of the lesion medial or lateral to the nipple and to determine how deep the lesion was from the skin. Although CT techniques are not used very often, they can be extremely helpful in difficult cases.

PNEUMOCYSTOGRAPHY

Pneumocystography is the insufflation of air into a previously aspirated breast cyst followed by mam-

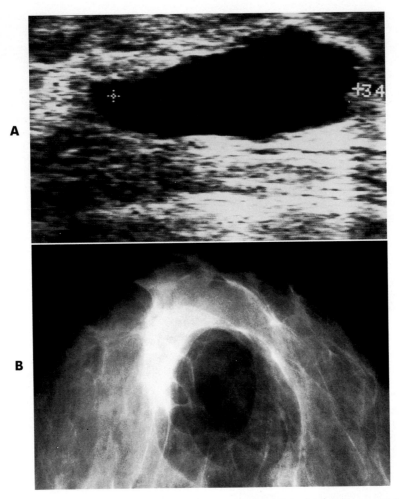

Fig. 3-13 A, Ultrasonography showing a simple cyst. **B,** Craniocaudal mammogram following pneumocystogram confirms a simple cyst with smooth borders. (Case courtesy of Dr. Judy Destouet, Baltimore, Maryland.)

mography. Usually an attempt is made to aspirate all the fluid out of the cyst before the air is injected. Room air is used in a volume about three fourths of the amount of cyst fluid obtained.[120] As the air temperature reaches body temperature, the air expands so that a lesser volume of air is used to replace the aspirated fluid.[116] Pneumocystography is used by some centers (particularly in Europe) as the diagnostic and therapeutic procedure of choice for breast cysts.[116,120-122] However, currently in North America breast ultrasonography is the modality of choice to evaluate breast cysts (see Ultrasonography section). The therapeutic benefit of air insufflation has been stressed by some and is reported to result in prevention of cyst recurrence in well over 90% of patients.[89,116,121] Ikeda and colleagues reported prevention of recurrence in 67% of patients treated with pneumocystography.[118] It is postulated that the drying effect in

the epithelium lining the cyst may prevent or delay fluid reaccumulation (Fig. 3-13).[117] The criteria for surgical biopsy include (1) intracystic mass on pneumocystography, (2) positive cytology of cyst fluid, (3) bloody cyst fluid, (4) cyst recurrence, (5) extrinsic mass compressing the cyst wall, and (6) solid mass.[116,119]

THERMOGRAPHY

Infrared thermography of the breast involves recording breast surface temperature based on infrared emission from the skin of the breast using a heat-sensitive imaging device. It is a safe test using no ionizing radiation. A variation called liquid crystal or "plate" thermography uses cholesterol esters encapsulated in a plastic film applied directly to the skin of the breast.[132] The liquid crystals change color in response to temperature changes. Thermography was initially thought to show promise as a preliminary screening test in asymptomatic women to identify those women at increased risk for breast cancer who should have subsequent mammography.[125,126,128,129] Another possible role for thermography is as a prognostic indicator in that women with breast cancer and normal thermograms had a higher survival rate than women with abnormal thermograms.[127,130] Another thermographic technique has been studied whereby microwave radiation emitted from the subcutaneous tissue is measured.[123]

Several published series indicate that thermography actually has little or no role in the detection and diagnosis of breast disease owing to unacceptably high false-positive and false-negative rates, especially for small nonpalpable stage I breast cancers.[131-133] Ulmer and colleagues[134] performed thermography on a series of 309 patients tients after lumpectomy and radiation therapy and concluded that thermography was of no value in the care and follow-up of these patients. The official policy statement of the American College of Radiology[124] says that thermography is still considered to be experimental and that "the addition of thermography to these established diagnostic examinations provides little clinically meaningful information, and substantially increases the cost of medical care."

TRANSILLUMINATION

Transillumination (Diaphanography, Light Scanning) of the breast, first described by Cutler in 1929,[137] is a noninvasive method of examining the breast using either red or infrared light. The principle of this method involves placing the light source behind the breast and recording the transmitted light. As light passes through the breast, it is reflected, scattered, and absorbed (Fig. 3-14). Solid masses in the breast absorb the light and therefore cast a dark spot in the image (Fig. 3-15). Subsequent to Cutler's first report, improvements such as development of infrared-sensitive photographic techniques[147,149-151] and computer manipulation[141,143] have enhanced the results obtained with this examination.[136,142]

Subsequent studies by several authors have shown that this examination is highly operator dependent and is not sensitive enough in the detection of early breast cancer to be a reliable screening examination.[138-140,148] The sensitivity of transillumination has been shown to be much lower than mammography for the detection of early breast cancer.[135,146] The examination is invalid in a patient with a recent biopsy or aspiration procedure, mastitis, recent trauma, or hemorrhagic cysts[147,149,150] since any hemorrhage is indistinguishable from malignancy. Microcalcifi-

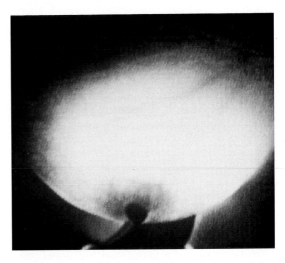

Fig. 3-14 Normal light scan of the right breast. (This is the same patient as in Fig. 3-15.) (Case courtesy of Dr. Judy Destouet, Baltimore, Maryland.)

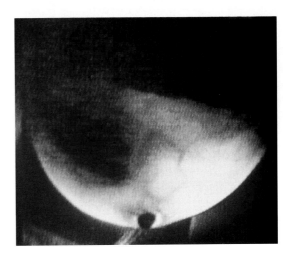

Fig. 3-15 Light scan of the left breast. Dark area corresponds to a large invasive carcinoma seen on mammogram. (This is the same patient as in Fig. 3-14.) (Case courtesy of Dr. Judy Destouet, Baltimore, Maryland.)

cations, an important mammographic finding, cannot be seen with this method.[136,138] The idea that transillumination could be used as an adjunct problem-solving examination in patients with abnormal screening mammograms has been supported by some authors[143] but discounted by others.[144-145]

The overwhelming evidence seems to support the belief that transillumination should not be used as a screening method for breast cancer and should be considered an experimental technique with no proven clinical usefulness.

ANGIOGRAPHY

Angiography of the breast was first reported in 1967.[153] However, the technique required cannulation of a major vessel, the radiation dose was high, examination time was long, and only large lesions were examined. Digital subtraction angiography of the breast is of historical interest in that several reports from one institution were published in the mid-1980s presenting data showing its potential in the evaluation of patients with abnormal mammograms and/or physical examination.[152,155,156] The goal was to determine if this examination would prove useful to distinguish benign from malignant breast disease and help to decrease unnecessary breast biopsies.

The vasculature of the breast was demonstrated by intravenous injection of a small amount of contrast material (30 ml). The patient was placed prone with the breast positioned in an immobilization device. Abnormal findings included abnormal retention of contrast material ("blush") or abnormal vessel characteristics. Although the initial results from a small group of patients seemed to be promising, this examination is relatively invasive and expensive, has a high radiation dose, and therefore is not currently used. Harrington and others[154] reported three patients in whom transcatheter embolization was necessary and life-saving for profuse bleeding from metastatic breast cancer.

DIGITAL MAMMOGRAPHY

Digital mammography has recently been considered as a possible future direction in breast imaging.[159] Three methods have been described. The first method involves digitization of conventional film mammograms.[163,164] Smathers and others[163] evaluated one such system in which they scanned conventional mammograms of a phantom with a laser scanner and then displayed the resultant images on cathode-ray tube monitors. They compared the accuracy of detection of microcalcifications by evaluating the phantom model with xeromammography, conventional film-screen mammography, and digital film-screen mammography. Their preliminary data indicated that microcalcifications were better seen on the digitized mammograms as compared with conventional mammograms. Electronic filtering enhanced the visibility of structures in the original images. Chan's work[158] suggests that microcalcification detection could be improved by using unsharp-mask filtering to enhance the digitized images.

The second method involves digitization using a photostimulable phosphor as a receptor. The image detector (imaging plate) is coated with crystals of the phosphor. The plate is exposed by conventional mammographic equipment and then introduced into a special processing system.[157,160,165] The potential advantages are better delineation of abnormal areas and production of better images with conventional mammographic equipment. Oestmann and others[161] compared conventional mammography to storage phosphor-based digital radiography with respect to detectability of malignant microcalcifications. Their data indicated that the detectability of malignant microcalcifications with the digital images was equivalent to that with conventional mammography. However, the digital images were unable to resolve the calcifications as well, probably because of lower spatial resolution.

The third method involves direct acquisition of digital mammograms using equipment with solid-state detectors.[166] The advantage may be lower dose imaging without degrading resolution. Digital mammography requires more investigation to determine if it will be as accurate as conventional mammography. If this can be achieved, digital mammography can also be linked to teleradiology systems for rapid consultation.[162] Fajardo and colleagues have begun to experiment with a charge-coupled device (CCD)–based mammography.[89]

NUCLEAR IMAGING
Immunodetection

Preliminary work has been reported using indium-111 or radioiodine-labeled human monoclonal antibodies to detect primary or metastatic sites of breast carcinoma, including the axillary lymph nodes.[175,176,179-181] This method was successful for imaging known sites of metastatic disease in a small group of 10 patients.[179] However, these techniques are strictly experimental and may have a place in the future for managing and staging breast cancer patients but as yet do not have a role in breast cancer detection.

Positron emission tomography imaging

Positron emission tomography (PET) imaging of patients with breast cancer is a new modality that may have promise in the future. Mintun and others[178] used PET imaging after intravenous injection of a radiolabeled estrogen compound (16 α [F-18] fluoroestradiol-17β) in 13 patients with breast masses. The study was interpreted as abnormal in all 12 of the patients with cancer and normal in the remaining patient with a benign mass. The results were quite promising, but more investigation is needed. Three other studies have been published using injection of [^{18}F] fluorodeoxyglucose (FDG).[177,182,183] It appears that possible uses for PET imaging may be to help confirm the diagnosis of primary and metastatic breast carcinoma. More important, in vivo PET imaging may become a more reliable indicator of estrogen receptor status than the currently used in vitro method.[178]

Scintigraphy

Breast scintigraphy has been suggested as an imaging method to be used in cases where mammography shows an abnormality that is favored to be benign.[168] However, with current diagnostic procedures such as ultrasonography and fine-needle aspiration biopsy coupled with excellent mammographic quality, breast scintigraphy does not have a place in the detection or characterization of breast abnormalities. More recently, lymphoscintigraphy has been advocated as an imaging modality to evaluate the status of internal mammary and axillary lymph nodes in patients with known breast carcinoma.[167,169-174]

MAGNETIC RESONANCE IMAGING

Research in breast magnetic resonance imaging (MRI) sequences and clinical trials has advanced significantly since the early 1980s. Several centers have acquired experience with several hundred volunteers. The data indicate a potential clinical use of gadolinium-enhanced breast MRI for selected patients.[189]

Technique

Breast MRI requires a dedicated-surface breast coil for imaging. Prototype coils obtained from equipment manufacturers may be single or double breast coils. Technical designs have included both send-receive and receive-only coils.

Pulse sequence imaging usually includes a T1-weighted spin-echo sequence for demonstration of anatomy. This sequence is most often acquired in an axial slice orientation for a double breast coil, demonstrating both breasts. This may be followed by a sagittal-orientation, high-resolution T1-weighted image. These T1-weighted scans are re-

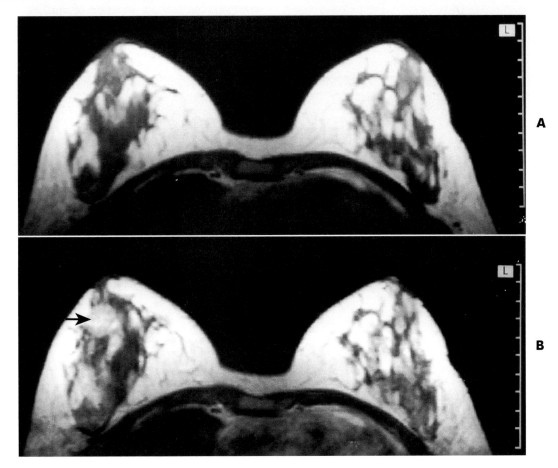

Fig. 3-16 Axial T1-weighted spin-echo images of both breasts **(A)** before and **(B)** after Gd-DTPA injection. A 1.5-cm cancer enhances after injection of contrast material (*arrow*).

peated after intravenous injection of gadolinium contrast material. Lesions are observed for pattern, intensity, and rate of enhancement (Figs. 3-16 and 3-17).

Gadolinium contrast agents have been studied to improve tissue characterization and differentiation of cancer from benign breast lesions. Some centers evaluated relative signal intensity of the breast tissues before administration of contrast material and 10 to 15 minutes after gadolinium contrast enhancement.[184] Other investigators have used the early time intervals (1 to 8 minutes after bolus injection) to create a dynamic contrast enhancement of breast tissues.[186] Preliminary data indicate an early dynamic enhancement curve during the first 4 minutes for cancer in contrast to other breast lesions.[186,188] In our center we have used T1-weighted Turboflash to track contrast enhancement of breast tissue at 3- to 6-second intervals after the bolus injection of 0.1 mmol/kg of Gd-DTPA (Figs. 3-18 and 3-19). Region of interest (ROI) intensity is graphed versus time.

A T2-weighted imaging sequence may be used to evaluate possible breast cysts. Simple cysts as small as 5 mm are easily demonstrated. Because of the cost of MRI, breast ultrasonography remains the preferred modality for confirming nonpalpable breast cysts (see Sonography section).

In addition, fat suppression techniques have potential in breast MRI to improve conspicuity of contrast-enhanced masses in breast tissues containing both fat and dense glandular parenchyma.

Indications

Breast MRI is currently a research technique in the stage of clinical feasibility testing.[187] Investigators are acquiring experience with cancers, focal and multicentric, as well as benign lesions, such as fibroadenomas, fat necrosis, radial scars, and proliferative fibrocystic disease. The data are not yet available to assess the ability of breast MRI to identify atypical ductal or atypical lobular hyperplasia and in situ carcinomas.

Potential clinical indications in those centers that have acquired experience with breast MRI are listed in Box 3-4 on p. 65. Areas of possible future potential such as detection of small cancers in dense breasts of high-risk women must await further technical advances and larger clinical tri-

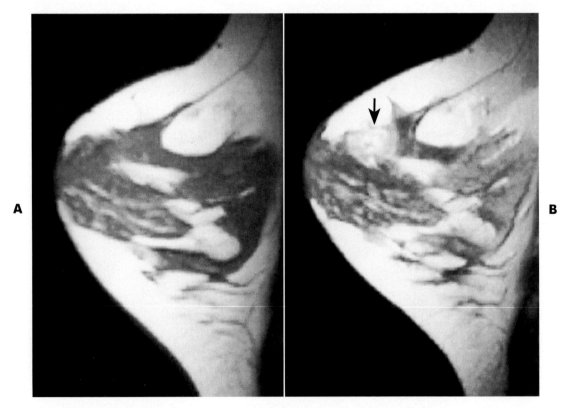

Fig. 3-17 High-resolution sagittal T1-weighted spin-echo images **(A)** before and **(B)** after Gd-DTPA injection. The cancer has a dense central area of enhancement. (This is the same patient as in Fig. 3-16.)

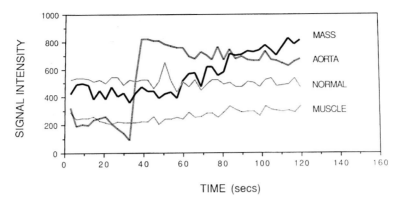

Fig. 3-18 Gd-DTPA (0.1 mmol/kg) enhancement curve of a 1-cm stellate lesion helped to differentiate this recurrent breast cancer from a scar in the lumpectomy site of a patient 7 years after conservative treatment with no interval mammographic examinations.

als to provide experience with small lesions and borderline histologic findings.

Limitations and inappropriate uses

Breast MRI has significant limitations for breast imaging. The microcalcifications easily detected by mammography are not imaged by MRI. It is uncertain whether breast MRI has the capability to detect in situ carcinoma on the order of 5 to 10 mm in size. Although incidental reports of imaging small cancers by MRI have been published, the ability of MRI to survey a breast for gadolinium-enhanced cancers has yet to be explored.

Additional limitations of the MRI technique may apply to individual patients. As for any patient having an MRI, contraindications include pacemakers, neurostimulator devices, aneurysm clips, and some heart valves. Relative contraindications include claustrophobia, obesity greater than 200 lb, and severe arthritis. The patient must be able to lie prone for approximately 45 minutes for a breast MRI using current pulse sequences with gadolinium enhancement. Women with chronic back pain or shoulder-related musculoskeletal discomfort may not be able to complete the examination.

Interpretation

The ability of in vivo breast MRI to demonstrate a lesion is dependent not only on the relative T1 and T2 values of the lesion but also on the type of surrounding breast tissue. Surrounding homogeneous fat gives good tissue contrast on T1-weighted scans with lesions that are at least 0.5 to 1.0 cm in size. The same is true in x-ray mammography. Surrounding fat permits easy identification of small water-density masses in some women that would not be visible if the surrounding tissue were inhomogeneous and contained areas of water-tissue density. On T2-weighted scans, lesions with long T2 values such as cysts will appear intense and are easily contrasted with the low signal intensity of surrounding fibrous or glandular tissues.

Calcium is not imaged by either T1- or T2-weighted spin-echo scans. Areas of heavy calcification, as in bones or coarsely calcified fibroadenomas, have no signal from the calcified areas. This produces a black area. Importantly, microcalcifications seen by mammography cannot be demonstrated by MRI techniques. Therefore, at this time MRI of the breast seems to have minimal potential as a breast cancer screening technique.

Normal breast. Fat gives a high signal intensity on both T1- and T2-weighted images. In general, fibroglandular tissue gives a low signal intensity on both images. An occasional normal premenopausal woman demonstrates symmetric areas of "blushing" on the T2-weighted scans in the central cone of the breast tissue. Normal breast parenchyma, fatty tissue, and pectoral muscle show no significant increase in ROI signal intensity measurements after enhancement. Postoperative scars over 1 year of age reportedly show no significant contrast enhancement.[185]

Cysts. On T1-weighted images, cysts are localized, smooth, rounded areas of low signal intensity surrounded by areas of moderate signal intensity (fibroglandular tissue) or high signal intensity (fat). On T2-weighted images, cysts exhibit an increased signal intensity of the cyst contents equal to or greater than the intensity of surrounding fat. Blood products may produce fluid/fluid levels in cysts by MRI.

Fibroadenomas. In the T1-weighted scans, fi-

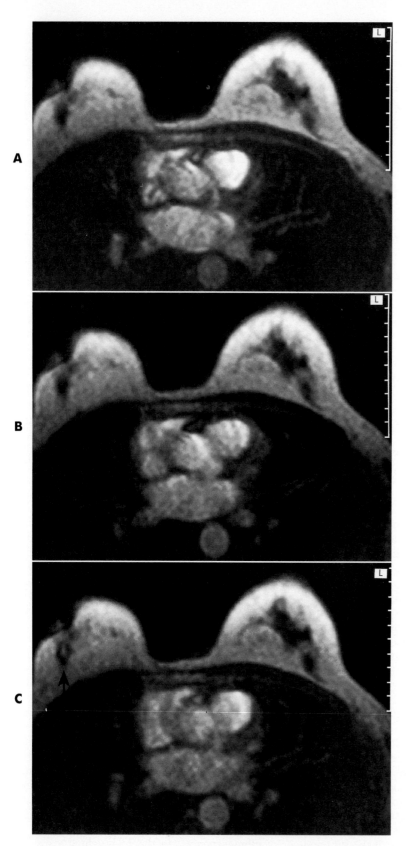

Fig. 3-19 Repeated single-slice TurboFLASH after bolus injection of 0.1 mmol/kg of Gd-DTPA demonstrates enhancement of recurrent breast cancer (*arrow*). Images were obtained at (**A**) 36 seconds, (**B**) 51 seconds, and (**C**) 117 seconds after beginning of TurboFLASH sequence. ROI of this subject is graphed in Fig. 3-18.

BOX 3-4 POTENTIAL INDICATIONS FOR BREAST MRI

Differentiation of cancer from scar tissue
Imaging of structures close to chest wall
Imaging of prostheses
Evaluation of extent of cancer for pretreatment planning (e.g., focal, multifocal, multicentric)

broadenomas have an intensity similar to normal fibroglandular tissue sometimes with areas of inhomogeneity. Fibroadenomas have been shown to enhance more slowly over time than carcinomas. On T2-weighted scans, fibroadenomas have been shown to vary from low- to high-signal intensity.[190] Preliminary data suggest that dynamic enhancement curves in the first 1 to 2 minutes after contrast injection may improve the ability of MRI to discriminate cancer from fibroadenomas.

Cancer. The morphologic appearance of breast cancer visualized on film-screen mammography is duplicated on T1-weighted MR images. Spiculated or irregular masses are visualized on both film-screen and nonenhanced MRI when surrounded by contrasting fat. On T1-weighted scans the fat signal is high intensity, and the tumor mass, including desmoplasia, is of low to intermediate signal intensity. Cancers enhance to greater than 100% of preenhancement signal levels following intravenous injection of Gd-DTPA (0.1 mmol/kg) (see Fig. 3-17). This increase in signal intensity is best evaluated by ROI measurements rather than by visualization of the relative "whiteness" of the lesion on the cathode-ray tube or on hard-copy films.

Because breast cancer is difficult for mammography to image in the dense fibroglandular breast, the capability of MRI to evaluate breast lesions in diffusely dense fibroglandular breasts is of particular interest. T1 and T2 values measured from MRI in vivo images indicate an overlap of T1 and T2 values of cancer with fibroglandular tissue. The cellularity of a tumor relative to the surrounding breast stroma is an obvious variable among cancers. Many articles on in vivo MRI have not quantitated the cellularity of cancers in relation to the cellularity of the surrounding breast stroma. This would be of particular interest for cancers in dense breasts.

The MR image provides an excellent assessment of cancer size and extent in some women. The enhanced carcinoma may become more discernible from surrounding dense fibroglandular tissues on MRI than on film-screen mammography. In women with fatty breasts, the MR image adds little more to the preoperative assessment than an excellent film-screen mammogram can provide concerning size and extent of the cancer.

Implants. Silicone implants can be imaged by MRI to assess possible rupture, herniation, and surrounding breast parenchyma. In symptomatic women MRI may be more sensitive to detect intracapsular rupture than mammography or breast ultrasonography. (See suggested readings listed at the end of this chapter.)

Associated procedures

Currently, women who have undergone MRI of the breast are part of a research protocol. Most will have a lesion requiring a pathologic diagnosis by fine-needle aspiration cytology, wire-directed biopsy, or excisional biopsy. Long-term clinical follow-up will also be essential in clinical studies to evaluate any potential false-negative diagnoses (missed cancers) by MRI of the breast.

REFERENCES
Ultrasonography

1. Bassett LW, Kimme-Smith C: Breast sonography: technique, equipment, and normal anatomy, *Semin Ultrasound CT MR* 10:82, 1989.
2. Bassett LW, Kimme-Smith C: Breast sonography, *AJR Am J Roentgenol* 156:449, 1991.
3. Bassett LW, Kimme-Smith C, Sutherland LK, et al: Automated and hand-held breast US: Effect on patient management, *Radiology* 165:103, 1987.
4. Bassett LW, Ysrael M, Gold RH: Usefulness of mammography and sonography in women less than 35 years of age, *Radiology* 180:831, 1991.
5. Bohm-Velez M, Mendelson EB: Computed tomography, duplex Doppler ultrasound, and magnetic resonance imaging in evaluating the breast, *Semin Ultrasound CT MR* 10:171, 1989.
6. Brem RF, Gatewood OMB: Template-guided breast US. *Radiology* 184:872, 1992.
7. Bruneton JN, Caramella E, Héry M, et al: Axillary lymph node metastases in breast cancer: preoperative detection with US, *Radiology* 158:325, 1986.
8. Buchberger W, Strasser K, Heim K, et al: Phylloides tumor: findings on mammography, sonography, and aspiration cytology in 10 cases, *AJR Am J Roentgenol* 157:715, 1991.
9. Calkins AR, Jackson VP, Morphis JG, et al: The sonographic appearance of the irradiated breast, *JCU* 16:409, 1988.
10. Cole-Beuglet C: Sonographic manifestations of malignant breast disease, *Semin Ultrasound* 3:51, 1982.
11. Cole-Beuglet C, Kurtz AB, Rubin CS, et al: Ultrasound mammography, *Radiol Clin North Am* 18:133, 1980.
12. Cole-Beuglet C, Goldberg BB, Kurtz AB, et al: Ultrasound mammography: a comparison with radiographic mammography, *Radiology* 139:693, 1981.
13. Cole-Beuglet C, Goldberg BB, Kurtz AB, et al: Clinical experience with a prototype real-time dedicated breast scanner, *AJR Am J Roentgenol* 139:905, 1982.

14. Cole-Beuglet C, Soriano RZ, Kurtz AB, et al: Fibroadenoma of the breast: sonomammography correlated with pathology in 122 patients, AJR Am J Roentgenol 140:369, 1983.
15. Cole-Beuglet C, Soriano RZ, Kurtz AB, et al: Ultrasound analysis of 104 primary breast carcinomas classified according to histopathologic type, Radiology 147:191, 1983.
16. Cole-Beuglet C, Schwartz G, Kurtz AB, et al: Ultrasound mammography for the augmented breast, Radiology 146:737, 1983.
17. Cole-Beuglet C, Soriano R, Kurtz AB, et al: Ultrasound, x-ray mammography, and histopathology of cystosarcoma phyllodes, Radiology 146:481, 1983.
18. Conway WF, Hayes CW, Brewer WH: Occult breast masses: use of a mammographic localizing grid for US evaluation, Radiology 181:143, 1991.
19. Cosgrove DO, Bamber JC, Davey JB, et al: Color Doppler signals from breast tumors: work in progress, Radiology 176:175, 1990.
20. Dempsey PJ: The value of ultrasound examination in diagnosing breast disease, Curr Opin Radiol 1:188, 1989.
21. D'Orsi CJ, Mendelson EB: Interventional breast ultrasonography, Semin Ultrasound CT MR 10:132, 1989.
22. Egan RL, Egan KL: Automated water-path full-breast sonography: correlation with histology of 176 solid lesions, AJR Am J Roentgenol 143:499, 1984.
23. Egan RL, Egan KL: Detection of breast carcinoma: comparison of automated water-path whole-breast sonography, mammography, and physical examination, AJR Am J Roentgenol 143:493, 1984.
24. Fleischer AC, Muhletaler CA, Reynolds VH, et al: Palpable breast masses: evaluation by high frequency, hand-held real-time sonography and xeromammography, Radiology 148:813, 1983.
25. Fornage BD: Fine-needle aspiration biopsy with a vacuum test tube, Radiology 169:553, 1988.
26. Fornage BD, Coan JD, David CL. Ultrasound-guided needle biopsy of the breast and other interventional procedures. RCNA 30(1):167, 1992.
27. Fornage BD, Faroux MJ, Simatos A: Breast masses: US-guided fine-needle aspiration biopsy, Radiology 162:409, 1987.
28. Fornage BD, Lorigan JG, Andry E: Fibroadenoma of the breast: sonographic appearance, Radiology 172:671, 1989.
29. Fornage BD, Sneige N, Faroux MJ, et al: Sonographic appearance and ultrasound-guided fine-needle aspiration biopsy of breast carcinomas smaller than 1 cm³, J Ultrasound Med 9:559, 1990.
30. Grant EG, Richardson JD, Cigtay OS, et al: Sonography of the breast: findings following conservative surgery and irradiation for early carcinoma, Radiology 147:535, 1983.
31. Harper AP, Kelly-Fry E: Ultrasound visualization of the breast in symptomatic patients, Radiology 137:465, 1980.
32. Harper AP, Kelly-Fry E, Noe JS: Ultrasound breast imaging—the method of choice for examining the young patient, Ultrasound Med Biol 7:231, 1981.
33. Harper AP, Kelly-Fry E, Noe JS: Ultrasound in the evaluation of solid breast masses, Radiology 146:731, 1983.
34. Heywang SH, Dunner DS, Lipsit ER, et al: Advantages and pitfalls of ultrasound in the diagnosis of breast cancer, JCU 13:525, 1985.
35. Hilton SV, Leopold GR, Olson LK, et al: Real-time breast sonography: application in 300 consecutive patients, AJR Am J Roentgenol 147:479, 1986.
36. Ikeda DM, Adler DD, Helvie MA: Breast ultrasound, Appl Radiol February:19, 1991.
37. Jackson VP: Duplex sonography of the breast, Ultrasound Med Biol 14:131, 1988.
38. Jackson VP: New instrumentation in breast sonography, Appl Radiol November:54, 1988.
39. Jackson VP: Sonography of malignant breast disease, Semin Ultrasound CT MR 10:119, 1989.
40. Jackson VP: The role of US in breast imaging, Radiology 177:305, 1990.
41. Jackson VP, Kelly-Fry E, Rothschild and others: Automated breast sonography using a 7.5-MHz PVDF transducer: preliminary clinical evaluation, Radiology 159:679, 1986.
42. Jackson VP, Rothschild PA, Kreipke DL, et al: The spectrum of sonographic findings of fibroadenoma of the breast, Invest Radiol 21:34, 1986.
43. Jellins J, Kossoff G, Reeve TS: Detection and classification of liquid-filled masses in the breast by gray scale echography, Radiology 125:205, 1977.
44. Jellins J, Reeve TS, Croll J, et al: Results of breast echographic examinations in Sydney, Australia. 1972–1979, Semin Ultrasound 3:58, 1982.
45. Karstrup S, Nolse C, Brabrand K, et al: Ultrasonically guided percutaneous drainage of breast abscesses, Acta Radiol 31:157, 1990.
46. Kersschot EA, Hermans ME, Paywels C, et al: Juvenile papillomatosis of the breast: sonographic appearance, Radiology 169:631, 1988.
47. Kimme-Smith C, Bassett LW, Gold RH: High frequency breast ultrasound hand-held versus automated units; examination for palpable mass versus screening, J Ultrasound Med 7:77, 1988.
48. Kobayashi T: Gray-scale echography for breast cancer, Radiology 122:207, 1977.
49. Kopans DB: What is a useful adjunct to mammography? (Editorial), Radiology 161:560, 1986.
50. Kopans DB, Meyer JE, Lindfors KK: Whole-breast US imaging: four-year follow-up, Radiology 157:505, 1985.
51. Kopans DB, Meyer JE, Proppe KH: The double line of skin thickening on sonograms of the breast, Radiology 141:485, 1981.
52. Kopans DB, Meyer JE, Steinbock RT: Breast cancer: the appearance as delineated by whole breast water-path ultrasound scanning, JCU 10:313, 1982.
53. Kopans DB, Swann CA: Preoperative imaging-guided needle placement and localization of clinically occult breast lesions, AJR Am J Roentgenol 152:1, 1989.
54. Kopans DB, Meyer JE, Lindfors KK, et al: Breast sonography to guide cyst aspiration and wire localization of occult solid lesions, AJR Am J Roentgenol 143:489, 1984.
55. Laing FC, Jeffrey RB, Minagi H: Ultrasound localization of occult breast lesions, Radiology 151:795, 1984.
56. Leibman AJ, Kruse B: Breast cancer: mammographic and sonographic findings after augmentation mammoplasty, Radiology 174:195, 1990.
57. Maturo VG, Zusmer NR, Gilson AJ, et al: Ultrasound of the whole breast utilizing a dedicated automated breast scanner, Radiology 137:457, 1980.
58. Maturo VG, Zusmer NR, Gilson AJ, et al: Ultrasonic appearance of mammary carcinoma with a dedicated whole-breast scanner, Radiology 142:713, 1982.
59. McSweeney MB, Murphy CH: Whole-breast sonography, Radiol Clin North Am 23:157, 1985.
60. Meyer JE, Greenes RA, Sonnenfeld MR: Breast immobilization for occult mass aspiration, Radiology 169:266, 1988.
61. Meyer JE, Kopans DB: The appearance of the therapeutically irradiated breast on whole-breast water-path ultrasonography, J Ultrasound Med 2:211, 1983.
62. Meyer JE, Amin E, Lindfors KK, et al: Medullary carcinoma of the breast: mammographic and US appearance, Radiology 170:79, 1989.
63. Morgan CL, Trought WS, Peete W: Xeromammographic

and ultrasonic diagnosis of a traumatic oil cyst, *AJR Am J Roentgenol* 130:1189, 1978.

64. Pamilo M, Soiva M, Lavast EM: Real-time ultrasound, axillary mammography, and clinical examination in the detection of axillary lymph node metastases in breast cancer patients, *J Ultrasound Med* 8:115, 1989.

65. Policy statement: On sonography for the detection and diagnosis of breast disease, ACR 1984.

66. Reuter K, D'Orsi CJ, Reale F: Intracystic carcinoma of the breast: the role of ultrasonography, *Radiology* 153:233, 1984.

67. Reynolds HE, Jackson VP: The role of ultrasound in breast imaging. *Appl Radiol* 11:55, 1991.

68. Rifkin MD, Schwartz GF, Pasto ME, et al: Ultrasound for guidance of breast mass removal, *J Ultrasound Med* 7:261, 1988.

69. Rosculet KA, Ikeda DM, Forrest ME, et al: Ruptured gel-filled silicone breast implants: sonographic findings in 19 cases, *AJR Am J Roentgenol* 159:711, 1992.

70. Rubin E, Miller VE, Berland LL, et al: Hand-held real-time breast sonography, *AJR Am J Roentgenol* 144:623, 1985.

71. Salvador R, Salvador M, Jimenez JA, et al: Galactocele of the breast: radiologic and ultrasonographic findings, *Br J Radiol* 63:140, 1990.

72. Scatarige JC, Hamper VM, Sheth S, et al: Parasternal sonography of the internal mammary vessels: technique, normal anatomy, and lymphadenopathy, *Radiology* 172:453, 1989.

73. Schneider JA: Invasive papillary breast carcinoma: mammographic and sonographic appearance, *Radiology* 171:377, 1989.

74. Schoenberger SG, Sutherland CM, Robinson AE: Breast neoplasms: duplex sonographic imaging as an adjunct in diagnosis, *Radiology* 168:665, 1988.

75. Sickles EA, Filly RA, Callen PW: Breast cancer detection with sonography and mammography: comparison using state-of-the-art equipment, *AJR Am J Roentgenol* 140:843, 1983.

76. Sickles EA, Filly RA, Callen PW: Benign breast lesions: ultrasound detection and diagnosis, *Radiology* 151:467, 1984.

77. Srivastava A, Webster DJ, Woodtock JP, et al: Role of Doppler ultrasound flowmetry in the diagnosis of breast lumps, *Br J Surg* 75:851, 1988.

78. Teixidor HS, Kazam E: Combined mammographic-sonographic evaluation of breast masses, *AJR Am J Roentgenol* 128:409, 1977.

79. Vilaro MM, Kurtz AB, Needleman L, et al: Hand-held and automated sonomammography: clinical role relative to x-ray mammography, *J Ultrasound Med* 8:95, 1989.

80. Weber WN, Sickles EA, Calun PW, et al: Nonpalpable breast lesion localization: limited efficacy of sonography, *Radiology* 155:783, 1985.

81. Wild JJ, Reid JM: Further pilot echographic studies of the histologic structure of tumors of the living intact human breast, *Am J Pathol* 28:839, 1952.

82. Williams SM, Kaplan PA, Peterson JC, et al: Mammography in women under age 30: is there clinical benefit? *Radiology* 161:49, 1986.

Galactography

83. Alberti GP, Troiso A: Secreting breast: the role of galactography, *Eur J Gynaecol Oncol* 3:96, 1982.

84. Berna JD, Guirao J, Garcia V: A coaxial technique for performing galactography, *AJR Am J Roentgenol* 153:273, 1989.

85. Berni D, De Giuli E: The value of ductogalactography in the diagnosis of intraductal papilloma, *Tumori* 69:539, 1983.

86. Bjorn-Hansen R: Contrast mammography, *Br J Radiol* 38:947, 1965.

87. Ciatto S, Bravetti P, Berni D, et al: The role of galactography in the detection of breast cancer, *Tumori* 74:177, 1988.

88. Diner WC: Galactography: mammary duct contrast examination, *AJR Am J Roentgenol* 137:853, 1981.

89. Fajardo LL, Jackson VP, Hunter TB: Interventional Procedures in Diseases of the Breast: Needle biopsy, Pneumocystography, and Galactography, *AJR Am J Roentgenol* 158:1231, 1992.

90. Hicken NF, Best RR, Hunt HB, et al: The roentgen visualization and diagnosis of breast lesions by means of contrast media, *AJR Am J Roentgenol* 39:321, 1938.

91. Kindermann G, Rummel W, Bischoff J, et al: Early detection of ductal breast cancer: the diagnostic procedure for pathological regional discharge from the nipple, *Tumori* 65:555, 1979.

92. Nunnerley HB, Field S: Mammary duct injection in patients with nipple discharge, *Br J Radiol* 45:717, 1972.

93. Osborne J: Galactography with contrast and dye—a two stage radiological/surgical approach to serous or bloody nipple discharge, *Australas Radiol* 33:266, 1989.

94. Ouimet-Oliva D, Hebert G: Galactography: a method of detection of unsuspected cancers, *AJR Am J Roentgenol* 120:55, 1974.

95. Sadowsky N: Personal communication, March 1992.

96. Tabar L, Dean PB, Pentek Z: Galactography: the diagnostic procedure of choice for nipple discharge, *Radiology* 149:31, 1983.

97. Tabar L, Marton Z, Kadas I: Galactography in the examination of secretory breasts, *Am J Surg* 127:282, 1974.

98. Threatt B, Appelman HD: Mammary duct injection, *Radiology* 108:71, 1973.

Computed tomography

99. Chang CH, Sibala JL, Gallagher JH, et al: Computed tomography of the breast: a preliminary report, *Radiology* 124:827, 1977.

100. Chang CHJ, Sibala JL, Fritz SL, et al: Computed tomographic evaluation of the breast, *AJR Am J Roentgenol* 131:459, 1978.

101. Chang CH, Sibala JL, Lin F, et al: Preoperative diagnosis of potentially precancerous breast lesions by computed tomography breast scanner: preliminary study, *Radiology* 129:209, 1978.

102. Chang CHJ, Sibala JL, Fritz SL, et al: Specific value of computed tomographic breast scanner (CT/M) in diagnosis of breast diseases, *Radiology* 132:647, 1979.

103. Chang CH, Sibala JL, Fritz SL, et al: Computed tomography in detection and diagnosis of breast cancer, *Cancer* 46:939, 1980.

104. Chang CH, Nesbit DE, Fisher DR, et al: Computed tomographic mammography using a conventional body scanner, *AJR Am J Roentgenol* 138:553, 1982.

105. Dixon GD: Preoperative computed-tomographic localization of breast calcifications, *Radiology* 146:836, 1983.

106. Gisvold JJ, Reese DF, Karsell PR: Computed tomographic mammography (CTM), *AJR Am J Roentgenol* 133:1143, 1979.

107. Kopans DB, Meyer JE: Computed tomography guided localization of clinically occult breast carcinoma—the "N" skin guide, *Radiology* 145:211, 1982.

108. Lindfors KK, Meyer JE, Busse PM, et al: CT evaluation of local and regional breast cancer recurrence, *AJR Am J Roentgenol* 145:833, 1985.

109. Meyer JE, Munzenreider JE: Computed tomographic demonstration of internal mammary lymph node metastasis in patients with locally recurrent breast carcinoma, *Radiology* 139:661, 1981.

110. Muller JWT, Van Waes PFGM, Koehler PR: Computed tomography of breast lesions: comparison with x-ray mammography, *J Comput Assist Tomogr* 7:650, 1983.

111. Scatarige JC, Boxen I, Smathers RL: Internal mammary lymphadenopathy: imaging of a vital lymphatic pathway in breast cancer, *Radiographics* 10:857, 1990.

112. Scatarige JC, Fishman EK, Zinreich ES, et al: Internal mammary lymphadenopathy in breast carcinoma: CT appraisal of anatomic distribution, *Radiology* 167:89, 1988.

113. Shea WJ Jr, de Geer G, Webb WR: Chest wall after mastectomy Part I. CT appearance of normal postoperative anatomy, postirradiation changes, and optimal scanning techniques, *Radiology* 162:157, 1987.

114. Shea WJ Jr, de Geer G, Webb WR: Chest wall after mastectomy Part II. CT appearance of tumor recurrence, *Radiology* 162:162, 1987.

115. Sibala JL, Chang CH, Lin F, et al: Computed tomographic mammography: diagnosis of mammographically and clinically occult carcinoma of the breast, *Arch Surg* 116:114, 1981.

Pneumocystography

116. Dyreborg U, Blichert-Toft M, Boegh L, et al: Needle puncture followed by pneumocystography of palpable breast cysts, *Acta Radiol* 26:277, 1985.

117. Hoeffken W, Lanyi M: Mammography: *technique, diagnosis, differential diagnosis, results*, Philadelphia, 1977, WB Saunders.

118. Ikeda DM, Helvie MA, Adler DD, et al: The role of fine-needle aspiration and pneumocystography in the treatment of impalpable breast cysts, *AJR Am J Roentgenol* 158:1239, 1992.

119. Sanders TJ, Morris DM, Cederbom G et al: Pneumocystography as an aid in the diagnosis of cystic lesions of the breast, *J Surg Oncol* 31:210, 1986.

120. Tabar L, Pentek Z: Pneumocystography of benign and malignant intracystic growths of the female breast, *Acta Radiol* 17:829, 1976.

121. Tabar L, Pentek Z, Dean PB: The diagnostic and therapeutic value of breast cyst puncture and pneumocystography, *Radiology* 141:659, 1981.

122. Tabar L, Kadas I, Marton Z, et al: The significance of mammography, galactography and pneumocystography in detecting occult carcinomas of the breast, *Surg Gynecol Obstet* 137:965, 1973.

Thermography

123. Barrett AH, Myers PC, Sadowsky NL: Microwave thermography in the detection of breast cancer, *AJR Am J Roentgenol* 134:365, 1980.

124. College policy reviews use of thermography: *ACR Bulletin* January 1984, p 13.

125. Feig SA, Shaber GS, Schwartz GF, et al: Thermography, mammography, and clinical examination in breast cancer screening, *Radiology* 122:123, 1977.

126. Gautherie M, Gros CM: Breast thermography and cancer risk prediction, *Cancer* 45:51, 1980.

127. Isard HJ, Sweitzer CJ, Edelstein GR: Breast thermography: a prognostic indicator for breast cancer survival, *Cancer* 62:484, 1988.

128. Isard HJ, Becker W, Shilo R, et al: Breast thermography after four years and 10,000 studies, *AJR Am J Roentgenol* 115:811, 1972.

129. Jones CH, Greening WP, Davey JB, et al: Thermography of the female breast: a five-year study in relation to the detection and prognosis of cancer, *Br J Radiol* 48:532, 1975.

130. Libshitz HI: Thermography of the breast: current status and future expectations, *JAMA* 238:1953, 1977.

131. Moskowitz M, Milbrath J, Gartside P: Lack of efficacy of thermography as a screening tool for minimal and stage I breast cancer, *N Engl J Med* 295:249, 1976.

132. Moskowitz M, Fox SH, Brun del Re R, et al: The potential value of liquid-crystal thermography in detecting significant mastopathy, *Radiology* 140:659, 1981.

133. Sterns EE, Curtis AC, Miller S, et al: Thermography in breast diagnosis, *Cancer* 50:323, 1982.

134. Ulmer HU, Brinkmann M, Frischbier HJ: Thermography in the follow-up of breast cancer patients after breast-conserving treatment by tumorectomy and radiation therapy, *Cancer* 65:2676, 1990.

Transillumination

135. Alveryd A, Andersson I, Aspegren K, et al: Lightscanning versus mammography of the detection of breast cancer in screening and clinical practice, *Cancer* 65:1671, 1990.

136. Bartrum RJ Jr, Crow HC: Transillumination lightscanning to diagnose breast cancer: a feasibility study, *AJR Am J Roentgenol* 142:409, 1984.

137. Cutler M: Transillumination as an aid in the diagnosis of breast lesions, *Surg Gynecol Obstet* 48:721, 1929.

138. Drexler B, Davis JL, Schofield G: Diaphanography in the diagnosis of breast cancer, *Radiology* 157:41, 1985.

139. Geslien GE, Fisher JR, DeLaney C: Transillumination in breast cancer detection: screening failures and potential, *AJR Am J Roentgenol* 144:619, 1985.

140. Gisvold JJ, Brown LR, Swec RG, et al: Comparison of mammography and transillumination light scanning in the detection of breast lesions, *AJR Am J Roentgenol* 147:191, 1986.

141. Greene FL, Hicks C, Eddy V, et al: Mammography, sonomammography, and diaphanography (lightscanning): a prospective, comparative study with histologic correlation, *Am Surg* 51:58, 1985.

142. Marshall V, Williams DC, Smith KD: Diaphanography as a means of detecting breast cancer, *Radiology* 150:339, 1984.

143. Merritt CRB, Sullivan MA, Segaloff A, et al: Real-time transillumination light scanning of the breast, *Radiographics* 4:989, 1984.

144. Monsees B, Destouet JM, Gersell D: Light scan evaluation of nonpalpable breast lesions, *Radiology* 163:467, 1987.

145. Monsees B, Destouet JM, Gersell D: Light scanning of nonpalpable breast lesions: reevaluation, *Radiology* 167:352, 1988.

146. Monsees B, Destouet JM, Totty WG: Light scanning versus mammography in breast cancer detection, *Radiology* 163:463, 1987.

147. Ohlsson B, Gundersen J, Nilsson D-M: Diaphanography: a method for evaluation of the female breast, *World J Surg* 4:701, 1980.

148. Sickles EA: Breast cancer detection with transillumination and mammography, *AJR Am J Roentgenol* 142:841, 1984.

149. Wallberg H: Diaphanography in various breast disorders: clinical and experimental observations, *Acta Radiol* 26:271, 1985.

150. Wallberg H, Alveryd A, Bergvall UK et al: Diaphanography in breast carcinoma, *Acta Radiol* 26:33, 1985.

151. Wallberg H, Alveryd A, Nasiell K et al: Diaphanography in benign breast disorders, *Acta Radiol* 26:129, 1985.

Angiography

152. Ackerman LV, Watt AC, Shetty P, et al: Breast lesions examined by digital angiography: work in progress, *Radiology* 155:65, 1985.

153. Feldman F, Habif DV, Fleming RJ, et al: Arteriography of the breast, *Radiology* 89:1053, 1967.

154. Harrington DP, Barth KH, Baker RR et al: Therapeutic

embolization for hemorrhage from locally recurrent cancer of the breast, *Radiology* 129:307, 1979.

155. Watt AC, Ackermann LV, Shetty PC et al: Differentiation between benign and malignant disease of the breast using digital subtraction angiography of the breast, *Cancer* 56:1287, 1985.

156. Watt AC, Ackerman LV, Windham JP, et al: Breast lesions: differential diagnosis using digital subtraction angiography, *Radiology* 159:39, 1986.

Digital mammography

157. Asaga T, Chiyasu S, Mastuda S, et al: Breast imaging: dual-energy projection radiography with digital radiography, *Radiology* 164:869, 1987.

158. Chan HP, Vyborny CJ, MacMahon H, et al: Digital mammography ROC studies of the effects of pixel size and unsharp-mask filtering on the detection of subtle microcalcifications, *Invest Radiol* 22:581, 1987.

159. Kimme-Smith C: Mammographic image receptors and image processing, *Current Opinion in Radiology* 2:719, 1990.

160. Kimme-Smith C, Bassett LW, Gold RH, et al: Digital mammography: a comparison of two digitization methods, *Invest Radiol* 24:869, 1989.

161. Oestmann JW, Kopans D, Hall DA, et al: A comparison of digitized storage phosphors and conventional mammography in the detection of malignant microcalcifications, *Invest Radiol* 23:725, 1988.

162. Shtern F: Digital mammography and related technologies: A perspective from the National Cancer Institute, *Radiology* 183:629, 1992.

163. Smathers RL, Bush E, Drace J, et al: Mammographic microcalcifications: detection with xerography, screen-film, and digitized film display, *Radiology* 159:673, 1986.

164. Sommer FG, Smathers RL, Wheat RL, et al: Digital processing of film radiographs, *AJR Am J Roentgenol* 144:191, 1985.

165. Sonoda M, Takano M, Miyahara J, et al: Computed radiography utilizing scanning laser stimulated luminescence, *Radiology* 148:833, 1983.

166. Tesic MM, Sones RA, Morgan DR: Single-slit digital radiography: some practical considerations, *AJR Am J Roentgenol* 142:697, 1984.

Nuclear imaging

167. Bourgeois P, Fruhling J, Henry J: Postoperative axillary lymphoscintigraphy in the management of breast cancer, *Int J Radiat Oncol Biol Phys* 9:29, 1983.

168. Cancroft E, Goldfarb CR: Breast scintigraphy as an imaging modality in the diagnosis of breast masses, *Semin Nucl Med* 11:289, 1981.

169. Collier BD, Palmer DW, Wilson JF, et al: Internal mammary lymphoscintigraphy in patients with breast cancer, *Radiology* 147:845, 1983.

170. Ege GN: Internal mammary lymphoscintigraphy: the rationale, technique, interpretation, and clinical application—a review based on 848 cases, *Radiology* 118:101, 1976.

171. Ege GN: Radiocolloid lymphoscintigraphy in the management of breast carcinoma, *Contemp Surg* 20:1982.

172. Ege GN: Lymphoscintigraphy: techniques and applications in the management of breast carcinoma, *Semin Nucl Med* 13:26, 1983.

173. Ege GN, Clark RM: Internal mammary lymphoscintigraphy in the conservative management of breast carcinoma: an update and recommendations for a new TNM staging, *Clin Radiol* 36:469, 1985.

174. Ege GN, Elhakim T: The relevance of internal mammary lymphoscintigraphy in the management of breast carcinoma, *J Clin Oncol* 2:774, 1984.

175. Khaw BA, Strauss HW, Cahill SL, et al: Sequential imaging of indium-111-labeled monoclonal antibody in human mammary tumors hosted in nude mice, *J Nucl Med* 25:592, 1984.

176. Khaw BA, Bailes JS, Scheider SL, et al: Human breast tumor imaging using ^{111}In labeled monoclonal antibody: athymic mouse model, *Eur J Nucl Med* 14:362, 1988.

177. Kubota K, Matsuzang T, Amemiya A et al: Imaging of breast cancer with [18F]Fluorodeoxyglucose and positron emission tomography, *J Comput Assist Tomogr* 13:1097, 1989.

178. Mintun MA, Welch MJ, Siegel BA, et al: Breast cancer: PET imaging of estrogen receptors, *Radiology* 169:45, 1988.

179. Ryan KP, Dillman RO, DeNardo ST, et al: Breast cancer imaging with In-111 human IgM monoclonal antibodies: preliminary studies, *Radiology* 167:71, 1988.

180. Stacker SA, Thompson C, Riglar C, et al: A new breast carcinoma antigen defined by a monoclonal antibody, *J Natl Cancer Inst* 75:801, 1985.

181. Thompson CH, Lichtenstein M, Stacker SA, et al: Immunoscintigraphy for detection of lymph node metastases from breast cancer, *Lancet* 2:1245, 1984.

182. Wahl RL, Cody RL, Hutchins GD, et al: Primary and metastatic breast carcinoma: initial clinical evaluation with PET with the radiolabeled glucose analogue 2-[F-18]-fluoro-2-deoxy-D-glucose, *Radiology* 179:765, 1991.

183. Wahl RL, Henry CA, Ethier SP: Serum glucose: Effects on tumor and normal tissue accumulation of 2-[F-18]-Fluoro-2-deoxy-D-glucose in rodents with mammary carcinoma, *Radiology* 183:643, 1992.

Magnetic resonance imaging

184. Heywang SH, Wolf A, Pruss E, et al: MR imaging of the breast with Gd-DTPA: use and limitations, *Radiology* 171:95, 1989.

185. Kaiser WA: Dynamic magnetic resonance breast imaging using a double breast coil: an important step towards routine examination of the breast, *Frontiers in European Radiology* 7:39, 1990.

186. Kaiser WA, Zeitler E: MR imaging of the breast: fast imaging sequences with and without Gd-DTPA, *Radiology* 170:681, 1989.

187. Moskowitz M, Feig SA, Cole-Beuglet C, et al: Evaluation of new imaging procedures for breast cancer: proper process, *AJR Am J Roentgenol* 140:591, 1983.

188. Stack JP, Redmond OM, Codd MB et al: Breast disease: tissue characterization with Gd-DTPA enhancement profiles, *Radiology* 174:491, 1990.

189. Stelling CB: Magnetic resonance imaging and spectroscopy of the breast, *Curr Opin Radiol* 2:746, 1990.

190. Stelling CB, Powell DE, Mattingly SS: Fibroadenomas: histopathologic and MR imaging features, *Radiology* 162:399, 1987.

SUGGESTED READINGS
Ultrasonography

Evans WP: Fine needle aspiration cytology and core biopsy of nonpalpable breast lesions, *Curr Opin Radiol* 4:1301, 1992.

Feig SA: Breast masses: mammographic and sonographic evaluation, *RCNA* 30(1):67, 1992.

Heywang-Kobrunner SH: Nonmammographic breast imaging techniques, *Curr Opin Radiol* 4:146, 1992.

Piccoli CW: Current utilization and future techniques of breast ultrasound, *Curr Opin Radiol* 4:139, 1992.

Magnetic resonance imaging

Gorczyca DP, Sinha S, Ahn CY, et al: Silicone breast implants in vivo: MR imaging. *Radiology* 185:407, 1992.

Harms SE, Pierce WB, Flamig DP, et al: New pulse sequence for improved resolution, fat suppressed 3D imaging of the breast. Works in Progress Abstract, Society of Magnetic Resonance in Medicine, Tenth Annual scientific meeting and exhibition. August 10-16, 1991, San Francisco, California, USA.

Lewis-Jones HG, Whitehouse GH, Leinster SJ: The role of magnetic resonance imaging in the assessment of local recurrent breast carcinoma, *Clin Radiol* 43:197, 1991.

Pierce WB, Harms SE, Flamig DP, et al: Three-dimensional gadolonium-enhanced MR imaging of the breast: pulse sequence with fat suppression and magnetization transfer contrast work in progress, *Radiology* 181:757, 1991.

Steinbach BG, Hiskes SK, Fitzsimmons JR, et al: Phantom evaluation of imaging modalities for silicone breast implants. *Invest Radiol* 27:841, 1992.

Breast Self-Examination and Clinician Breast Examination

Daniel E. Kenady

BREAST SELF-EXAMINATION
Guidelines and technique

Breast self-examination (BSE) has been advocated as a potentially very important factor in the early diagnosis of breast cancer.[2] Estimates indicate that 65% of all breast nodules are discovered by this type of examination.[1] Nevertheless, a Gallup Poll initiated in 1973 indicated that only 23% of women routinely examined their own breasts.[9] Patient education is an important issue in increasing compliance. Examination of the breasts by either patient, nurse practitioner, or physician is of obvious importance, because a painless nodule is by far the most common presentation of breast carcinoma.[1] Pain is a symptom of breast cancer in only 15% to 24% of patients. Other presenting symptoms, such as breast enlargement, nipple discharge, retraction or contour changes, ulceration, erythema, axillary mass, and back and bone pain, are relatively infrequent presenting symptoms. Most attention, therefore, has appropriately been directed toward self-examination in an attempt to downstage tumors at their presentation.

It is recommended that all women examine their breasts monthly starting at menarche. Because two thirds of women have fibrocystic breasts, the examination should be timed to occur at the same part of the menstrual cycle on subsequent examinations. This will minimize the confusion caused by normal cyclic changes in the breasts. We normally recommend examination on day 4 or 5 of the menstrual cycle, because engorgement is minimized and the breasts are normally less tender at this time. BSE on a monthly basis is recommended so that the patient detects change at the earliest possible time. Women who practice monthly BSE frequently detect very minimal changes. Examining the breasts more frequently than monthly is usually counterproductive, because monthly cyclic changes can be so confusing that the patient has no idea whether a significant change has actually occurred.

Some studies indicate that the importance of BSE is minimized if the patient is not carefully instructed in proper technique.[5] The first phase of BSE should always involve inspection while the patient is standing in front of a mirror. The patient should be informed about what skin retraction or dimpling looks like and what it implies. The patient also should look for nipple flattening or retraction. The patient must realize that the upper outer quadrant is commonly more nodular and contains more breast tissue than the other quadrants. Inspection should address symmetry, skin ulceration, erythema, and nipple retraction or changes. The patient should be instructed to raise her hands over her head for initial inspection and then to press them into her waist and tense the pectoral muscles (Fig. 4-1).

The next step in the self-examination involves palpation. The patient should be thoroughly instructed in the techniques used in this portion of the examination. Palpation should be performed with the patient in three different positions: seated, standing in the shower, and supine with a small pillow under the shoulder (Fig. 4-2). The fingers of the opposite hand are used to examine the entire breast in a systematic manner either transversely, vertically, radially, or circularly, depending on the method with which the patient feels most comfortable (Fig. 4-3). All four methods should result in complete coverage of breast tissue. One study indicated that the vertical strip

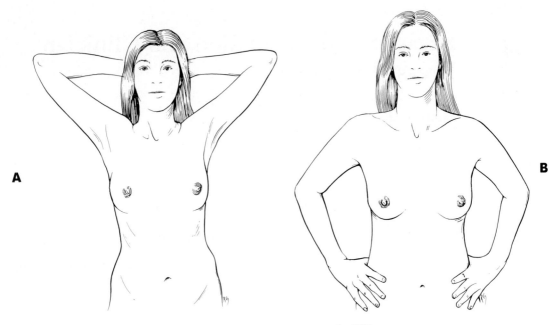

Fig. 4-1 Inspection positions for BSE.

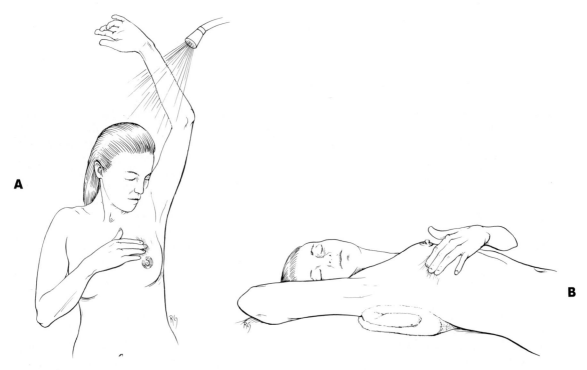

Fig. 4-2 Palpation positions for BSE.

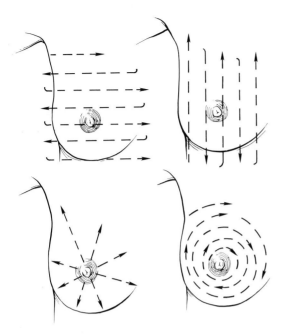

Fig. 4-3 Methods of palpation during BSE or CBE.

method may result in a more thorough coverage of total breast tissue than concentric circles or radial methods.[7] Physicians and nurse clinicians should teach the method with which they believe the patient will be most compliant. The axilla should also be examined during the palpation portion of the examination. Covering the breast with soap, cold cream, or talcum powder may increase the sensitivity of the examination.[6]

Impact on early detection

Nearly all women (90% to 99%) are aware of BSE. Far fewer (15% to 40%) perform BSE on a monthly basis.[5] Older women perform BSE less frequently than do younger women. This is of concern because older women are at a higher risk for developing breast cancers. Women with high incomes and educational attainment practice BSE more frequently[5] than do other women.

Considerable controversy remains as to whether self-examination of the breast is beneficial in terms of detecting early breast cancers. Hill and colleagues reported a meta-analysis of 12 studies involving 8118 patients with breast cancer. This review related the practice of BSE both to regional histologic lymph node status and to the diameter of the primary tumor at diagnosis.[3] These authors divided the data into two subsets. The first six studies compared nodal status and tumor size in patients who had practiced BSE at least once prior to treatment and in patients who had never practiced BSE. This analysis revealed that only 39%

of patients who had practiced BSE had metastases to axillary nodes, as compared to 50% of those who had never practiced BSE (odds ratio 0.66). Disturbingly, however, 56% of the patients who had practiced BSE had tumors of 2 cm or larger, as compared to 66% of those who had never practiced BSE (odds ratio 0.56).

The second subset of data analyzed by Hill and colleagues was taken from six additional studies in which the data were presented differently; that is, the comparison was between patients who had discovered their cancer during BSE and those who had discovered it accidentally. This analysis revealed that, in the group that found the tumor during BSE, 42% of patients had metastatic axillary nodes, compared to 46% of those who found the tumor accidentally. Only two of these six studies reported data on the size of tumors discovered by the two methods. Neither indicated a difference in size by method. Hill and colleagues made the point that accidental discovery does not preclude BSE practice and hypothesized that, even though they might discover a tumor accidentally, patients who practice BSE might be more likely to discover it at a smaller size. The authors concluded that their second analysis was not as important as looking at the overall practice of BSE. The conclusion of this meta-analysis was that the six studies investigating prediagnostic BSE practice are the most beneficial and have established BSE as helpful in detecting small cancers as well as in decreasing the incidence of nodal metastases.

Senie and associates[8] reported data indicating that one cannot determine what effect regular BSE has on the size of tumors when they are detected unless one controls for annual physical examination. Unfortunately, all of our data on BSE benefits result from descriptive studies with questionable methods. There have been no long-term prospective controlled trials.

A more recent study[4] reports interviews of 209 patients with advanced-stage breast cancers and a random sample of 433 women from the same population without advanced-stage breast cancer. The interviews indicated that the frequency of BSE did not differ between women with advanced-stage breast cancer and control subjects. However, it should be pointed out that self-described "proficiency in BSE" was low for both groups. A small percentage of these women described a more thorough BSE technique. These women demonstrated a 35% decrease in the occurrence of advanced-stage breast cancer as compared with women who did not perform BSE. Because it is difficult to quantify proficiency in BSE, it is very difficult to evaluate these studies.

Certainly, the fact that at least 70% of women discover their own breast cancers highlights the need for emphasizing BSE.[6] Although one third of patients state that they have practiced BSE, most are probably inadequately trained. At present, it cannot be determined whether BSE as a single modality is of benefit in the early detection of breast cancer.

CLINICIAN BREAST EXAMINATION
Guidelines and technique

The American Cancer Society guidelines recommend that all women older than 40 years of age have an annual clinician breast examination (CBE) and that those younger than 40 years of age (starting at menarche) have examinations every 3 years. This schedule assumes the absence of family or personal history of breast pathology other than fibrocystic change. Most women have fibrocystic changes in the breast that make physical examination somewhat more difficult. Any woman who has had a breast biopsy should have a CBE at least annually. A woman with a mother or sister who has had breast cancer should have annual examinations starting at least 10 years before the age of diagnosis of the affected relative. If the patient's mother was premenopausal at the time of diagnosis, annual examination should start at menarche.

Women are routinely examined in the sitting and supine positions. The supraclavicular and axillary areas are examined by a bimanual method performed with the patient in a seated position. The patient is then placed in the supine position and the examination of each breast is repeated. The chances of detection may be increased by also examining patients in the right and left semilateral decubitus positions to conform to mammographic positions. As is true with self-examination, it is important to conduct both inspection and palpation while the patient is in the sitting and supine positions. Inspection should assess shape, size, symmetry, presence of edema, erythema, nipple inversion or change, and skin retraction. Palpation should include the axillary, cervical, supraclavicular, and infraclavicular nodal areas. Just as with the patient's own examination, any of the four standard techniques is acceptable, as long as the entire breast tissue is examined.

Impact of clinician breast examination

Physical examination of the breast by physicians or nurse clinicians has proved effective in detecting breast cancers. The Health Insurance Plan of Greater New York (HIP) study[10] indicated that clinician and radiologic examinations were independent of each other in terms of effectiveness and that clinician examination particularly was effective at all ages (unlike mammography, which was shown to have its greatest effect in women 50 years of age and over). In the HIP study, 45% of the cancers were detected by clinician examination alone. In patients who are on regular follow-up schedules, it is often helpful to plan physical examination immediately after consultative mammograms. Mammographic findings can be helpful in targeting physical examinations to areas of concern revealed by radiograph. Equally important, negative mammograms should never delay biopsy of clinically dominant lesions. Certainly, physical examination and mammography are complementary; maximum use of each modality should be the goal in treating patients.

As previously referenced, Senie and associates[8] have presented data indicating that controlling for annual CBE may remove any possible benefit of patient BSE on tumor size at detection. When patients were examined yearly and divided into groups of those who did and did not perform BSE, the percentage of tumors less than 2 cm was only 6% greater in those women practicing BSE (47% versus 53%). In those women who underwent yearly examination (60% in this series), the mean size of cancer diagnosed was 2.3 cm. This contrasted with those who had not had examinations within the past 10 years. In this latter group, the mean size of the cancer was 3.4 cm. In patients who had a yearly CBE, 51% of tumors were smaller than 2 cm, contrasting with 21% of the tumors in women who had never had a physician examination. Nodal status was also affected: 63% of women who underwent yearly CBE had normal axillary nodes free of metastatic disease as compared with only 44% of those who never had a CBE. A major conclusion of these data is that patients found it difficult to detect tumors smaller than 2 cm. Only 38% of these tumors were first detected by the patient, compared with 62% of tumors that were larger than 2 cm.

Certainly the final verdict is not yet available on BSE in those patients who have a yearly CBE. Most would agree that BSE sensitizes the patient to a more compulsive follow-up schedule with a clinician and thus should not be deemphasized.

Postbiopsy examination

Close follow-up by physical examination is extremely important for patients who have undergone breast biopsies. An ipsilateral mammogram is normally obtained 3 months after biopsy to reestablish a baseline that can be correlated with physical examination. Often a depression resulting from breast biopsy can result in a "shelf," which may raise concern that an area of fibrocystic change is dominant. If there is any question of a new dominant mass after biopsy, a repeat fine-needle aspirate or excisional biopsy is scheduled. Biannual examination is preferred in patients who have histologic confirmation of atypical hyperplasia of ductal or lobular origin or lobular or ductal carcinoma in situ that is not treated with total mastectomy. Patients who have been diagnosed with invasive breast cancer and treated conservatively are examined every 3 months for the first 4 years, every 6 months during years four through eight, and then annually. If the patient has had a mastectomy, careful examination of both the upper and lower flap areas must be performed in addition to examination of nodal areas. If the patient has had a breast-conserving procedure, particular attention is paid to the area under the incision and to the quadrant of the lumpectomy.

In summary, BSE and CBE are important adjuncts to mammography in the detection of breast cancer and as part of follow-up in the patient who has had breast cancer. Patient and physician education concerning appropriate techniques and their scheduling will increase the benefit of these modalities.

REFERENCES
Breast self-examination

1. Haagensen CD: *Diseases of the breast,* Philadelphia, 1986, WB Saunders, pp 502, 505, 574.
2. Haagensen CD, Bodian C, Haagensen DE Jr: *Breast carcinoma: risk and detection,* Philadelphia, 1981, WB Saunders, p 461.
3. Hill D, White V, Jolley D, Mapperson K: Self-examination of the breast: is it beneficial? Meta-analysis of studies investigating breast self examination and extent of disease in patients with breast cancer, *BMJ* 297:271, 1988.
4. Newcomb PA, Weiss NS, Storer BE, and others: Breast self-examination in relation to the occurrence of advanced breast cancer, *J Natl Cancer Inst* 83:260, 1991.
5. O'Malley MS, Fletcher SW: Screening for breast cancer with breast self-examination. A critical review, *JAMA* 257:2196, 1987.
6. Rosato FE, Rosenberg AL: Examination techniques: role of the physician and patient in evaluating breast diseases. In Bland KI, Copeland EM III, editors: *The breast: comprehensive management of benign and malignant diseases,* Philadelphia, 1991, WB Saunders, pp 409–418.
7. Saunders KJ, Pilgrim CA, Pennypacker HS: Increased proficiency of search in breast self-examination. *Cancer* 58:2531, 1986.
8. Senie RT, Rosen PP, Lesser ML, Kinne DW: Breast self-examination and medical examination related to breast cancer stage, *Am J Public Health,* 71:583, 1981.
9. *Women's attitudes regarding breast cancer: The Gallup Poll.* Princeton, NJ, 1973, Gallup Organization.

Clinician breast examination

10. Venet L, Strax P, Venet W, Shapiro S: Adequacies and inadequacies of breast examinations by physicians in mass screening, *Cancer* 28:1546, 1971.

CHAPTER 5

The Role of the Surgeon in Breast Disease Diagnosis

Patrick C. McGrath

INTRODUCTION

The surgeon's position at the center of the multidisciplinary approach to the diagnosis and treatment of breast disease is unique. In most instances patients will either be seen by or referred to the surgeon early in the evaluation of a breast lesion. Thus, the surgeon must not only be familiar with the various disease entities of the breast but also be able to coordinate the workup and treatment of patients effectively. As will be pointed out in the following discussion, cooperation among the surgeon, the radiologist, and the pathologist is extremely important to ensure the proper treatment of the patient with breast disease.

CLINICAL EVALUATION

When a patient presents for evaluation of a palpable breast mass, critical information can be obtained from a thorough history and physical examination. This information can ensure that the subsequent workup is carried out in an orderly fashion. The majority of palpable breast lesions are discovered by the patient, often accidentally. Self-detected lesions are the most common presentation for carcinoma of the breast[1] (Table 5-1). Duration, rapidity of onset, and fluctuation in the size of the mass are all factors that may help in determining the nature of the lesion. All need to be interpreted with some caution because no absolutes exist in distinguishing between benign and malignant disease.

Pain as a presenting symptom is often underemphasized and misinterpreted. Although some studies note that only 5% of patients with breast cancer present with pain,[1,4] others have reported an incidence of pain in up to 24%.[2,3] The pain associated with cancer has no specific characteristics. It differs, however, from that seen with mastalgia due to fibrocystic disease in that it is unilateral, persistent, and well localized. Although pain is not a common symptom of breast cancer, its presence does not exclude the diagnosis, especially in a postmenopausal woman. In this situation, one must rule out the presence of carcinoma before establishing a diagnosis of mastalgia due to underlying fibrocystic changes.

Other symptoms that may prompt a woman to seek medical attention involve changes associated with the nipple, including discharge, retraction, crusting, erythema or itching, or changes associated with the breast, including enlargement, edema, ulceration, erythema, or skin retraction. Occasionally a patient will present with an axillary mass, and much less frequently with symptoms attributable to metastases, such as bone pain. Although these symptoms are relatively infrequent as the presenting complaint, they should alert physicians to the possibility of an underlying carcinoma. Only 10% to 20% of women who present with breast symptomatology have carcinoma, and up to 50% may have no specific breast pathology.[1] Nevertheless, each patient should undergo thorough evaluation and appropriate follow-up.

In addition to evaluating specific symptoms, the physician should take a thorough history, including factors such as menstrual and reproductive pat-

Table 5-1 **Frequency of initial symptoms of breast carcinoma reported by patients***

Author and year of report Period included in report	Harnett (1948) 1938-1939	Donegan (1967) 1940-1958	Yorkshire Group† (1983) 1976-1981	Haagensen‡ (1983) 1943-1980
Lump	77.4%	66.5%	76%	65.3%
Pain	10.0%	11.0%	5%	5.4%
Enlargement of the breast		1.0%		1.0%
Skin of breast retraction			1%	3.1%
Nipple flattening or retraction	2.0%	3.0%	4.0%	2.1%
Skin of breast ulceration				0.2%
Edema of breast		1.0%		0.0%
Redness of skin of breast		1.0%		0.8%
Nipple discharge	2.2%	9.0%	2.0%	1.8%
Nipple itching				0.4%
Redness and thickening of the epithelium of the nipple				0.1%
Nipple crusting and erosion	2.7%	2.0%		1.1%
Axillary tumor	0.8%		1.0%	2.0%
No symptoms— carcinoma found by previous examiner	1.6%			14.1%
Number of patients	2529	774	1205	2198

*From Haagensen CD: *Diseases of the breast,* Philadelphia: WB Saunders, 1968, p. 502.
†The Yorkshire report did not include patients with Paget's carcinoma.
‡During the last 13 years carcinoma was found by mammograms in 10 patients who had not had any symptoms of breast disease.

terns, previous use of exogenous hormones, gynecologic surgery, breast biopsies, exposure to radiation, or a family history of breast cancer. The combination of a thorough history and physical examination, in conjunction with the appropriate use of mammography, will allow differentiation between benign and malignant disease in the majority of women. However, confirmation of the diagnosis can be made only by microscopic examination of the tissue involved. Thus it is essential to decide which of these patients should have a biopsy and by what technique it should be performed.

The need for a biopsy in the evaluation of a pal-pable three-dimensional mass is well accepted. The only exception might be in women younger than 25 years of age with small clinically benign lesions. These patients may be followed at appropriate intervals. However, even in these young women, if the mass increases in size to the range of 1.5 to 2 cm, most physicians would recommend biopsy. The difficulty arises in those patients who present with a questionable breast mass that is not clearly distinct from the underlying fibrous breast tissue. These patients usually have a general pattern of nodularity, in which the abnormality is diffuse and not a distinct, persistent mass. This nodularity may be localized to an area of one breast, most commonly the upper outer quadrant, or it may be present throughout both breasts. At times it can be difficult to separate this exaggerated nodularity from a discrete mass, and in many cases it is necessary to make a tissue diagnosis. This is particularly true in cases of invasive lobular carcinoma. Mammography is often not helpful in these cases because of the density of the underlying breast tissue.

BIOPSY TECHNIQUES FOR A PALPABLE BREAST MASS

Biopsy of palpable breast lesions that warrant a histologic diagnosis may be performed by one of several techniques. The type of biopsy performed will depend in part on factors such as the stage of the tumor, the treatment plan in the event that the tumor should prove to be malignant, and the expertise of the cytopathologist. Each of the biopsy techniques will be briefly reviewed from the standpoint of the surgeon.

Fine-needle aspiration biopsy

Fine-needle aspiration (FNA) biopsy of a palpable breast mass, when available, is the preferred initial technique for establishing a tissue diagnosis. FNA is fast, efficient, cost effective, relatively painless, and reliable.[5-7,9] It can be performed in the office by the surgeon or the pathologist. The technique, described in greater detail in Chapter 6, involves the aspiration of individual cells or clumps of cells through a 22-gauge needle into a 10- or 20-ml syringe, and the preparation of these cells for cytologic examination. Complications from this procedure are extremely rare. No cases have been reported in which the needle track was seeded with tumor cells after FNA. The diagnostic accuracy of this technique has been reported to be as high as 95%, and the number of false-positive interpretations is nearly zero.[5-7] Accuracy appears to be somewhat operator dependent. Ideally this procedure should be performed by the cytopathologist in the clinic. Greater accuracy, fewer false-positives, and fewer unsatisfactory samples are obtained if the cytopathologist performs the FNA, prepares the smear of the cytologic material, and makes the diagnosis.[7]

One of the limitations of FNA biopsy is the possibility of false-negative results, usually caused by sampling errors. The absence of malignant or atypical cells on FNA does not rule out the possibility of cancer. In fact, if FNA biopsy of a suspicious palpable breast mass does not yield a diagnosis of cancer, then an excisional or incisional biopsy is necessary to exclude malignancy. The practice of follow-up open surgical biopsy on all negative

FNA biopsies should preclude the possibility of missing the diagnosis of breast cancer.

An experienced cytopathologist should make a uniformly accurate diagnosis of cancer, permitting definitive treatment to be carried out without confirmation by open biopsy.[6,8,10] A review of more than 8500 FNA biopsies recorded in the literature from 1975 to 1988 confirms the high accuracy of a malignant diagnosis by this method. Only 5 (0.05%) false-positives were reported, all occurring early in the cytopathologists' experience.[6] Many cytopathologists, taking a conservative approach, require the confirmation of two other pathologists before calling a specimen malignant. Any FNA that is extremely suggestive of malignancy but not unequivocal requires frozen section confirmation before definitive treatment is carried out.

Although FNA biopsy does not allow the pathologist to perform quantitative estrogen and progesterone receptor assays, the presence of these receptors on cytologic specimens can be determined by immunocytochemical methods.[11] The cytologic sample can also be used for flow cytometry to determine DNA ploidy and S-phase fraction. FNA is also unable to differentiate between intraductal and invasive ductal carcinoma. This is discussed in greater detail in Chapter 6.

Core-needle biopsy

The core-needle biopsy, another less invasive technique that can be performed in an office setting, uses a cutting needle such as Tru-cut to obtain a core of tissue. In general, this technique involves anesthetizing the skin overlying the breast mass and nicking it with a No. 11 blade. The Tru-cut needle is then introduced into the mass, and a core of tissue approximately 1 cm in length is obtained for histologic, not cytologic, interpretation. The risks of bleeding, tissue disturbance, and tumor implantation are certainly much greater than those associated with FNA biopsy. A core-needle biopsy that reveals malignant cells is diagnostic for breast cancer, but because of the possibility of a sampling error, the absence of malignant cells in the core of tissue cannot exclude the diagnosis of cancer. Multiple FNA biopsies appear to be more likely to sample malignant cells than a single core-needle biopsy, proving FNA to be the superior technique in establishing the diagnosis of clinically suspicious palpable breast masses.[12]

Although FNA has replaced it in many centers, core-needle biopsy is still useful at those institutions where cytology is not available or the cytologist is not experienced. Core-needle biopsy may be useful in cases in which previous FNA was extremely suggestive of carcinoma but the pathologist requests frozen section confirmation. In those situations, the surgeon can perform a core-needle biopsy at the beginning of the operation to establish a definitive diagnosis, proceeding to incisional biopsy only if necessary. It is important to remember that the puncture site and the core needle track should be located so as to be easily included within the subsequent excision at the time of the definitive surgery.

Incisional biopsy

An incisional biopsy involves removal of a portion of a breast mass to provide the pathologist with tissue for histologic evaluation. The main purpose of this type of biopsy is to establish a diagnosis and provide tissue for quantitative hormone receptor assays. It is generally performed in situations in which the tumor is too large for complete excision or in which complete excision would compromise subsequent definitive procedures. It is also performed just before the definitive mastectomy in those cases in which frozen section confirmation is necessary. Incisional biopsy also proves useful in cases of inflammatory carcinoma. In this disease it is important to include a section of the overlying skin with the biopsy so that involvement of the dermal lymphatics can be documented.

Excisional biopsy

Excisional biopsy is the complete removal of a discrete mass in the breast. It should be used primarily when FNA biopsy is unsuccessful in establishing a diagnosis. In general, excisional biopsy is performed in an outpatient setting under local anesthesia. Several important factors must be taken into account when one is performing an excisional biopsy. First, the location and type of incision are extremely important both for cosmetic results and possible further surgical procedures. In general, curvilinear incisions along the skin lines (Langer's lines) directly over the tumor mass are preferable (Fig. 5-1). Curvilinear scars provide much better cosmetic results than radial scars, and they are easy to incorporate into a subsequent mastectomy if this should prove necessary. A poorly placed biopsy incision can make subsequent management of a breast cancer, whether by mastectomy or breast conservation, extremely complicated. Dissection of the tumor should not be performed by electrocautery because thermal injury to the tissue may make histologic interpretation of the margin difficult and will interfere with the hormone assays. When the excisional biopsy is per-

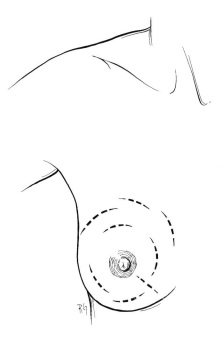

Fig. 5-1 Recommended incisions for breast biopsies. Curvilinear incisions along Langer's lines provide optimal cosmetic results. In the lower half of the breast, if skin is resected, a radial incision is preferred.

formed, it is important to include a rim of normal tissue around the tumor mass. If the lesion proves to be malignant, the biopsy could then serve as the "lumpectomy" if the patient desires breast conservation. In a "lumpectomy," the goal is to achieve gross and microscopically negative margins. To ensure that it will be possible to determine whether the margin is involved with the tumor, it is important to orient the specimen and take it fresh to the pathologist. At that point the pathologist should ink the margins and then bisect the specimen to obtain tissue for diagnosis as well as for receptor studies. If there is any concern about a gross positive margin, the pathologist can perform a frozen section to determine whether the margin is involved. If necessary, additional breast tissue corresponding to the margin of concern can then be easily removed. Rarely is it advisable to perform multiple frozen sections to determine margin involvement. All breast masses removed by excisional biopsy should be treated as though they were malignant. The appropriate initial management of a palpable breast lesion is crucial because it will determine the outcome for the patient.

One should never biopsy a mass without first attempting needle aspiration. The lesion may be a cyst that could easily be diagnosed and treated with a simple aspiration, thus avoiding an unsightly scar. When a patient experiences dense fibrocystic changes in the surrounding breast tissue, one must be very careful to remove only the mass in question. There is a temptation to remove additional fibrotic tissue because it feels abnormal, but removal of excessive tissue may cause significant cosmetic deformity. At the completion of the excision, meticulous hemostasis must be obtained, especially in densely fibrotic breast tissue. The wound should never be drained because this leads to obliteration of the dead space and an inferior cosmetic result. It has been recommended that only subcutaneous fat and skin should be closed and no attempt should be made to close the dead space.[13]

THE SURGEON'S APPROACH TO SELECTED BREAST CONDITIONS

The majority of palpable breast masses (80%) are benign. The following sections discuss the surgeon's perspective towards the management of the common benign lesions of cysts and fibroadenomas. The subject of nipple discharge is also included with guidelines for selection of patients for galactography and discussion of microdochectomy and major ductal excision. The specific entities of fibroadenomas, solitary papilloma, and fibrocystic change are discussed respectively in Chapters 9-11.

Cysts

Cysts are the most common dominant mass found in the breast. Approximately 7% of all women will develop a symptomatic breast cyst during the premenopausal period and up to 27% of women will have incidental cysts in breast cancer specimens.[16] Although most cysts rarely continue to develop in the postmenopausal years, occasionally the use of exogenous hormones will be associated with persistent cyst development. Macroscopic cysts are frequently asymptomatic, noticed by the patient only accidentally or during breast self-examination. Alternatively, sudden pain can alert the patient to the presence of a large cyst. This pain is believed to be caused by the distention of the surrounding tissue or possibly by leakage of fluid into the surrounding tissue, resulting in chemical irritation. The majority of cysts occur in the upper half of the breast, and their physical characteristics vary according to their size and depth and the character of the surrounding breast tissue.[16] The consistency of the cyst will depend on the pressure of the fluid within it. Tense, deep cysts may often feel like a solid tumor. A large cyst may dis-

place surrounding Cooper's ligaments, mimicking skin attachment or even retraction (pseudo-retraction of Haagensen).[15]

A gross cyst is significant mainly in that it is a dominant mass that requires differentiation from a malignant tumor. Differentiation is easily accomplished by needle aspiration of the mass, which in the case of a cyst is both diagnostic and therapeutic. This procedure is performed in the office or clinic with a 22-gauge needle and a syringe. The cyst is fixed in place between two fingers, and the needle is plunged directly into it (Fig. 5-2). In general, no local anesthetic is required. A cyst may contain as little as 0.5 ml of fluid or as much as 60 ml. In a benign, gross cyst, the fluid will vary from straw-colored to green or brown. The fluid may be discarded because cytologic evaluation is neither helpful nor cost effective. Cystic malignant growths of the breast are extremely uncommon (1% of all carcinomas of the breast), and all have bloody or peculiar (thick, cloudy) cyst fluid that should be sent for cytologic evaluation.[14] After the aspiration, the breast should be reexamined to make sure that the mass has completely disappeared. A persistent mass that differs from the rim of compressed breast tissue should be treated in the manner previously discussed. Recurrence of the cyst is not uncommon but occurs less frequently than might be expected. About 10% of cysts refill to form a palpable lesion. These can be easily managed by reaspiration. Some surgeons advocate excision after more than two aspirations, while others believe that recurrence may be an indication for mammography but not for excision. A carcinoma associated exclusively with refilling of a cyst without bloody fluid would be extremely unusual. The absolute indication for surgical excision is a persistent mass or bloody cyst fluid.

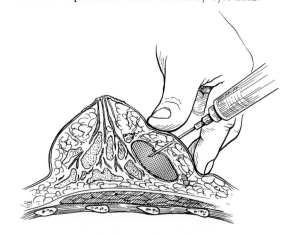

Fig. 5-2 Technique of aspirating a cyst.

Fibroadenoma

Fibroadenomas are discrete, benign tumors of the breast showing evidence of connective tissue and epithelial proliferation.[19] They are the most common benign solid tumor of the female breast and can occur anytime after puberty. Median age at diagnosis is approximately 30 years, and the highest incidence is in women between the ages of 21 and 25 years.[17] Postmenopausal women can experience fibroadenomas, but usually the tumors have developed earlier and become clinically apparent only when surrounding breast tissue is replaced by fat. Fibroadenomas are most common in the left breast and in the upper outer quadrants. These tumors are hormone dependent and may increase in size toward the end of each menstrual cycle or during pregnancy. Estrogen and progesterone receptors have been found in low concentrations in both the glands and stroma of fibroadenomas.[18]

Clinically, the fibroadenoma occurs in young women as a rubbery, firm, smooth, sometimes lobulated, very mobile mass. When left untreated it will gradually increase in diameter to 3 to 4 cm. Because of its unique clinical features, fibroadenoma can usually be diagnosed with relative certainty in young women. However, differentiating fibroadenoma from a solitary tense cyst by physical examination may be difficult, and it would be unfortunate to excise in the operating room what could easily be handled by aspiration alone. Therefore it is reasonable to attempt aspiration of these lesions to rule out the possibility of a simple cyst and avoid unnecessary surgery.

The recommended management of a fibroadenoma usually involves simple gross excision, regardless of its size or the age of patient. Some surgeons, however, prefer to observe small lesions in women younger than 25 years of age. Occasionally, fibroadenomas regress, especially in the postpartum period, but most of these tumors remain static or gradually increase in size. If an observed lesion increases in size, excision is advised. In general, most fibroadenomas are excised upon initial diagnosis to alleviate patient concern, but occasionally one can individualize treatment according to the size of the tumor, the age of the patient, and other considerations such as pregnancy.

In general, mammography does not play a role in the management of a fibroadenoma in a young woman. Not only does the density of breast tissue result in a low diagnostic yield, but also the patient is exposed to unnecessary radiation. All too often a 25-year-old woman with a clinically obvious fibroadenoma is referred for evaluation and treatment with a previously obtained mammogram in hand. It is important to remember that the role of mammography is the detection of occult disease and that all palpable masses need to be assessed regardless of the mammographic findings. Up to 10% of palpable cancers are not detected by mammography.

Nipple discharge

Nipple discharge is seen in only about 2% of patients with carcinoma (Table 5-1) and in up to 10% of patients with benign breast disease. The character of the discharge is perhaps the most important indicator of the significance of the underlying pathology. Pathologic discharge is serous, serosanguinous, or bloody; spontaneous rather than produced only by squeezing the nipples; persistent; and nonlactational. In Haagensen's series, up to 65% of pathologic nipple discharge was caused by a solitary intraductal papilloma.[22] The overall incidence of malignancy in patients with pathologic nipple discharge ranges from 5% to 20%. Most studies report about a 10% incidence.[21,22,25,26] The risk of malignancy increases with age and is much higher in postmenopausal women. Among patients presenting with only nipple discharge, the incidence of carcinoma was 3% in patients younger than 40 years of age, 10% in those between the ages of 40 and 60 years, and 32% for patients older than 60 years.[22,27] Other causes of pathologic spontaneous nipple discharge include duct ectasia, fibrocystic changes, cysts, or ductal papillomas.

Evaluation of a patient presenting with a nipple discharge requires a careful history and physical examination to determine whether she may require a biopsy to establish a diagnosis. The physician should obtain a complete review of reproductive and endocrine systems, and a history of medications and trauma. Examination should include careful, systematic palpation around the areola to determine at what point pressure will produce a discharge. In addition to the standard breast examination, one should carefully examine the segment that has been localized to feel for a palpable mass or dilated duct. The character of the discharge should be noted. If there is any question whether there is blood in the discharge, a sample can be placed on a hemoccult slide or laboratory test stick (as used for urinanalysis) and tested immediately for the presence of hemoglobin or hemoglobin breakdown products.[21] If a definite palpable mass is associated with the discharge, it should be treated as previously discussed.

Mammography is advisable for all patients with nipple discharge, with the exception of those patients under 30 in which the yield would be low. The most important mammographic finding would be microcalcifications along the duct suggesting carcinoma. The role of a galactogram in the evaluation of an abnormal nipple discharge is not well established. This technique involves the cannulation of a single duct with a small catheter and the injection of a water-soluble contrast agent and is discussed further in Chapter 3. Small papillomas or carcinomas may be identified by this technique, but debris or clot may mimic a tumor, and dilated ducts may obscure a lesion. Galactography has been reported to diagnose correctly only 79% of lesions.[20] Careful localization of the involved duct on physical examination precludes the routine use of galactography for this reason, and in general the technique is reserved for unusual or difficult cases.

The role of exfoliative cytology is also controversial. If the results are positive it may be useful, but its high false-negative rate precludes its routine use as a diagnostic tool. Studies that report a false-negative cytology in up to 16% of cases and a 4% false-positive result indicate that this technique is much less reliable than FNA.[23,24] Negative cytologic examination should be disregarded and biopsy pursued in appropriate patients.

Patients with nipple discharge and an associated palpable mass should receive treatment appropriate for the mass. Where there is no palpable mass, treatment will depend on the nature of the discharge. In patients with galactorrhea (milky discharge), mechanical stimulation, medications including hormones, or a prolactinoma should be excluded. Those patients older than 35 years of age who have a colored (creamy, green, brown, black), nonsanguinous discharge need a thorough examination and mammogram. Biopsy or ductal excision should not be performed unless an abnormality is detected on evaluation or the discharge is so profuse that the patient desires excision.

Because of the risk of cancer, those patients with serous, serosanguineous, or bloody discharge are of most concern. All patients older than 30 years of age who exhibit these symptoms need to undergo mammography. Palpation or galactography should be performed to determine the source of the discharge. If the discharge can be localized to a single duct, then the procedure of choice is a microdochectomy. In older patients, where the risk of carcinoma is much greater, and in those patients in whom the discharge cannot be localized, an excision of the major ducts is required.

A ductal excision performed under local anesthesia is commonly carried out in the outpatient operating room. A circumareolar incision no larger than 50% of the circumference of the areola is made in the region of the localized duct. The midpoint of the incision should lie at the site where palpation produces discharge. The skin of the areola is then raised with fine dissecting scissors past the entrance of the ducts into the nipple. If the dilated duct in question cannot be visually discerned, a small lacrimal duct probe may be passed through the opening in the nipple to identify the duct. When one is performing a microdochectomy, the duct of concern is dissected free from the other ducts in the nipple and dissected all the way into the dermis. This distal duct is then marked with a suture, and the remainder of the duct leading deeper into the breast is excised along with a small amount of surrounding breast tissue. Removal of 5 to 6 cm of the duct system usually removes any papilloma present, but if the duct remains dilated past this point, it should be followed into the periphery of the breast. In performing a major ductal excision, the surgeon makes no effort to dissect individually a single involved duct but rather includes all the major ducts and a core of underlying breast tissue. At the completion of the dissection, meticulous hemostasis is obtained, an absorbable purse-string suture is used to evert the nipple, and the skin is reapproximated without a drain.

EVALUATION OF A NONPALPABLE BREAST MASS

The major goal of breast imaging techniques is to detect carcinoma at an early stage, when surgical therapy can achieve its greatest positive effect. Approximately 15% of screening mammograms are abnormal,[33] and increasing numbers of women are being referred to surgeons for evaluation and treatment of abnormal mammographic findings. Although mammography can detect small abnormalities in the breast, the clinical significance of these abnormalities remains imprecise. A review of seven published studies including over 2000 patients with mammographic abnormalities that met strict criteria for biopsy yielded a positive predictive value of only 21%.[28-30,32,34-36] It is not clear what the positive predictive value for abnormal mammograms should be, but the practice of routinely performing a biopsy on every abnormality is being critically analyzed. A review of the experience at our institution over the past 4 years has revealed an increase from 19% to 33% in the positive predictive value of needle localized biopsies for nonpalpable lesions with the application of stricter criteria for biopsy. The higher rate of positive biopsies is due in part to the availability of magnification mammography and to a willingness on the part of surgeons to follow closely "indeterminate" mammographic lesions with repeat mammograms every 6 months, performing a biopsy only on those lesions that have changed. This policy has reduced the number of wire-

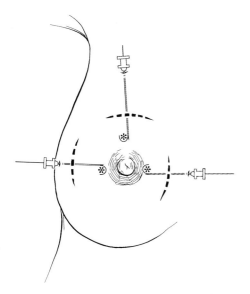

Fig. 5-3 Appropriate incisions for needle localization biopsies of nonpalpable lesions. The incision near the middle of the wire allows easier incorporation into subsequent mastectomies.

directed biopsies by 25%, with no adverse effect on patient outcome.[31] It is extremely important for the surgeon to review all abnormal mammograms with the radiologist and to combine the clinical and radiologic features to obtain a better idea of which patients require immediate biopsy and which need close follow-up. This type of approach will reduce the number of negative biopsies and improve patient management.

Excisional breast biopsy after needle localization

Once the decision is made to proceed with a biopsy of the breast tissue corresponding to the mammographic abnormality, this area should be localized to allow the surgeon to remove the appropriate tissue. A variety of localization techniques are covered in greater detail in Chapter 7. This section discusses the biopsy techniques after needle localization. In general, the procedure is performed under local anesthesia in outpatient surgery. Location of the incision is extremely important to potential further surgery, especially

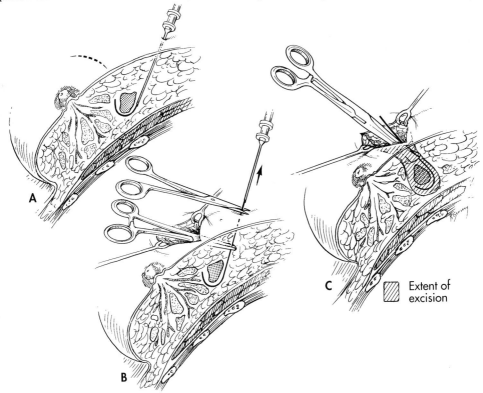

Fig. 5-4 Technique of excisional breast biopsy after needle localization. **A,** The needle lies posterior to the suspicious lesion and serves as a guide for the surgeon to remove the appropriate tissue. The incision is made near the middle of wire. **B,** Dissection is carried down the middle of wire, which is secured after the needle shaft is removed. The wire is divided at the skin. **C,** The cut edge of the wire is then brought out through the wound, enabling easy removal of the lesion with a rim of normal tissue. Specimen radiography is performed once the specimen has been oriented.

Extent of excision

when the needle enters the skin a long distance from the lesion. By careful evaluation of the location of the lesion with respect to the length of the wire, one can make an appropriate curvilinear incision near the middle of the wire (Fig. 5-3). This technique for incision placement, described by Wilhelm and Wanebo,[37] allows the surgeon to remove less tissue and makes it easier to incorporate the incision into a subsequent mastectomy if necessary (Fig. 5-4). The wire should not be pulled during the dissection lest it become dislodged. One can best avoid dislodging the wire by blocking out the area to be resected with as little manipulation of the wire as possible. As with other excisional biopsies, it is preferable to excise a margin of normal tissue around the lesion so that this procedure could serve as the "lumpectomy" if the lesion proved to be malignant. Once the specimen is removed, it is essential to orient it and take it immediately to pathology for specimen radiography to confirm the presence of the suspect lesion in the excised tissue. The specimen is then inked to determine whether the margins are involved. Frozen section analysis is not routinely performed because most of these lesions are so small that the technique of frozen section may compromise the ability to make a histologic diagnosis. However, if the lesion involved is a mass lesion, the specimen can be bisected to see if there is enough tissue for hormone assays. Significant cooperation among the surgeon, the radiologist, and the pathologist is required to ensure not only accurate processing of the tissue but also an appropriate diagnosis.

REFERENCES
Clinical evaluation

1. Haagensen CD: *Diseases of the Breast,* ed 2, Philadelphia, 1986, WB Saunders.
2. Preece PE, Baum M, Mansel RE, et al: Importance of mastalgia in operable breast cancer, *Br Med J* 284:1299, 1982.
3. Smallwood JA, Kye DA, Taylor I: Mastalgia: is this commonly associated with operable breast cancer? *Ann R Coll Surg Engl* 68:262, 1986.
4. Symptoms and signs of operable breast cancer 1976-1981, *Br J Surg* 70:350, 1983.

Biopsy techniques for a palpable breast mass
Fine needle aspiration biopsy

5. Frable WJ: Needle aspiration of the breast, *Cancer* 53:671, 1984.
6. Nicastri GR, Reed WP, Dziura BR: The accuracy of malignant diagnoses established by fine needle aspiration cytologic procedures of mammary masses, *Surg Gynecol Obstet* 172:457, 1991.
7. Palombini L, Fulciniti F, Vetrani A, et al: Fine-needle aspiration biopsies of breast masses; a critical analysis of 1956 cases in 8 years (1976-1984), *Cancer* 61:2273, 1988.
8. Sheikh FA, Tinkoff GH, Kline TS, Neal HS: Final diagnosis by fine-needle aspiration biopsy for definitive operation in breast cancer, *Am J Surg* 154:470, 1987.

9. Smith TJ, Safaii H, Foster EA, Reinhold RB: Accuracy and cost-effectiveness of fine needle aspiration biopsy, *Am J Surg* 49:540, 1985.
10. Wanebo HJ, Feldman PS, Wilhelm MC, et al: Fine needle aspiration cytology in lieu of open biopsy in management of primary breast cancer, *Ann Surg* 199:569, 1984.
11. Weintraub J, Weintraub D, Redard M, Vassilakos P: Evaluation of estrogen receptors by immunocytochemistry on fine-needle aspiration biopsy specimens from breast tumors, *Cancer* 60:1163, 1987

Core-needle biopsy

12. Shabot MM, Goldberg IM, Schick P, et al: Aspiration cytology is superior to Tru-Cut needle biopsy in establishing the diagnosis of clinically suspicious breast masses, *Ann Surg* 196:122, 1982.

Excisional biopsy

13. Margolese R, Poisson R, Shibata H, et al: The technique of segmental mastectomy (lumpectomy) and axillary dissection: a syllabus from the National Surgical Adjuvant Breast Project workshops, *Surgery* 102:828, 1987.

The surgeon's approach to selected breast conditions
Cysts

14. Devitt JE, Barr JR: The clinical recognition of cystic carcinoma of the breast. *Surg Gynecol Obstet* 159:130, 1984.
15. Haagensen CD. *Diseases of the breast,* ed 2, Philadelphia, 1986, WB Saunders, 541.
16. Hughes LE, Mansel RE, Webster DJT: *Benign disorders and diseases of the breast: concepts and clinical management,* London, 1989, Bailliere Tindall, pp. 93,94,96.

Fibroadenoma

17. Hughes LE, Mansel RE, Webster DJT: *Benign disorders and diseases of the breast: concepts and clinical management,* London, 1989, Bailliere Tindall, p. 60.
18. Nardelli GB, Lamaina V, Siliotti F: Steroid receptors in benign breast disease, gross cystic disease and fibroadenoma, *Clin Exp Obstet Gynecol* 14:10, 1987.
19. *Histological Typing of Breast Tumours,* ed 2, no 2 *International Histological Typing of Tumours,* Geneva, 1981, World Health Organization.

Nipple discharge

20. Berni D, De Giuli E: The value of ductogalactography in the diagnosis of intraductal papilloma, *Tumori* 69:539, 1983.
21. Chaudary MA, Millis RR, Davies GC, Hayward GL: The diagnostic value of testing for occult blood, *Ann Surg* 196:651, 1982.
22. Haagensen CD: *Diseases of the breast,* ed 2, Philadelphia, 1986, WB Saunders, p.504.
23. Kjellgren O: The cytologic diagnosis of cancer of the breast, *Acta Cytol* 8:216, 1964.
24. Knight DC, Lowell DM, Heimann A, Dunn E: Aspiration of the breast and nipple discharge cytology, *Surg Gynecol Obstet* 163:415, 1986.
25. Leis HP Jr, Greene FL, Cammarata A, Hilfer SE: Nipple discharge: surgical significance, *South Med J* 81:20, 1988.
26. Murad TM, Contesso G, Mouriesse H: Nipple discharge from the breast, *Ann Surg* 195:259, 1982.
27. Seltzer MH, Perloff LJ, Kelly RI, Fitts WT: The significance of age in patients with nipple discharge, *Surg Gynecol Obstet* 131:519, 1970.

Evaluation of a nonpalpable breast mass

28. Chetty U, Kirkpatrick AE, Anderson TL, et al: Localization and excision of occult breast lesions, *Br J Surg* 70:607, 1983.
29. Erickson EJ, McGreevy JM, Muskett A: Selective nonoperative management of patients referred with abnormal mammograms, *Am J Surg* 160:659, 1990.
30. Marrujo G, Jolly PC, Hall MH: Nonpalpable breast cancer: needle-localized biopsy for diagnosis and considerations for treatment, *Am J Surg* 151:599, 1986.
31. Hamby LS, McGrath PC, Stelling CB, et al. The management of indeterminate mammographic lesions. *Am Surg* 59:4, 1993.
32. Meyer JE, Kopans DB, Stomper PC, Lindfors KK: Occult breast abnormalities: percutaneous preoperative needle localization, *Radiology* 150:335, 1984.
33. Nesin N, Elliott BA, Elliott TE: Screening mammography in a primary care setting, *Minn Med* 71:209, 1988.

34. Rogers JV Jr, Powell RW: Mammographic indications for biopsy of clinically normal breasts: correlation with pathologic findings in 72 cases, *Am J Roentgenol Radium Ther Nucl Med* 115:794, 1972.
35. Symmonds RE Jr, Roberts JW: Management of nonpalpable breast abnormalities, *Ann Surg* 205:520, 1987.
36. Wilhelm MC, deParedes ES, Pope T, Wanebo HJ: The changing mammogram: a primary indication for needle localization biopsy, *Arch Surg* 121:1311, 1986.

Excisional breast biopsy after needle localization

37. Wilhelm MC, Wanebo HJ: Technique and guidelines for needle localization biopsy of nonpalpable lesions of the breast, *Surg Gynecol Obstet* 167:439, 1988.

Breast Cytology: Fine-Needle Aspiration and Other Techniques

Diane D. Davey

Fine-needle aspiration (FNA) of the breast is a technique in which an abnormality is sampled using a thin needle (usually 22 gauge or smaller) for cytologic studies. This technique should be differentiated from a cutting or Tru-Cut needle biopsy in which the sample is processed by histologic methods.

Martin, Ellis, Stewart, and other coworkers reported results of FNA procedures at Memorial Hospital in New York in the 1930s.[8,12] However, FNA did not become widely used in the United States until the 1970s. Breast FNA has been used extensively in Europe for approximately 40 years since Soderstrom, Lopes-Cardozo, Franzen, Zajicek, Lowhagen, and others popularized it.[4,6,7,11]

Breast FNA can be used to evaluate single or multiple masses and is useful in differentiating cysts from other processes. FNA, clinical examination, and mammography together are a useful triple diagnostic triage approach to decide whether a mass requires surgical excision or can be observed.[1,5] More recently, FNA has become a definitive diagnostic modality for treatment of breast cancer. FNA can be used to acquire tissue for special studies (see Chapter 8). It is valuable for evaluating recurrent breast or chest wall masses after breast surgery. Extramammary FNAs can be used to stage breast cancers.

Advantages of breast FNA are many. This is an office procedure that can be done quickly and easily with minimal patient preparation. The ability to diagnose a mass quickly provides psychological benefits to the patient. The clinician can discuss various treatment options with the patient and plan surgery and therapy more definitively. By decreasing the numbers of excisional biopsies and frozen sections, FNA can save money and operating room expenses.[3,9,10]

Significant complications of FNA are few.[2,3] The patient experiences minimal discomfort. Bleeding is usually minimal, with occasional small hematomas occurring. Local infections and pneumothorax are theoretical risks but are not reported with any frequency. Since the needle used is thin, needle tract spread has also not been documented.

Inadequate specimens and false-positive and false-negative diagnoses remain the major problems of this technique. Inadequate specimens are more numerous when this technique is used by inexperienced physicians, but they cannot be completely eliminated. Fibrotic masses may yield little or no cellular material when aspirated. Also, as smaller masses are sampled, some inadequate specimens can be expected. The problems with false-positive and false-negative diagnoses are discussed throughout this chapter, with results of large series summarized at the end. In learning this technique and evaluating results, one must differentiate false diagnoses into sampling errors and interpretive errors. Correlation of FNA specimens with histologic preparations is critical in gaining expertise.

FINE-NEEDLE ASPIRATION TECHNIQUES

The choice of aspirator

Who should perform the FNA? This question remains a subject of debate among many cytopathologists and clinicians, but this need not be so. The main objective of FNA is to provide an optimal specimen for diagnosis with minimal delay and inconvenience. An advantage of having the clinician perform the FNA is that it can be done immediately whenever an abnormality is encountered. The clinician may be more experienced in breast examination and may have observed the patient over a long period. The cytopathologist has the advantage of more experience in specimen preparation and adequacy. Knowledge of physical findings and other patient history is often essential in interpreting FNA specimens. Finally, the radiologist may choose to perform FNAs in the setting of a breast diagnostic center when abnormalities are detected by mammogram or on physical examination. As special localization techniques gain more prominence in the diagnosis of small breast lesions, radiologists will play a larger role in the FNA procedure. The most important factor in obtaining adequate specimens is experience. If the clinician or radiologist obtains the specimen, it is essential to provide the cytopathologist with good clinical information and correlation with any mammographic findings.

Materials and equipment

Materials and equipment used for the FNA procedure are listed in Box 6-1. A special FNA handle or gun (Cameco, Inrad, or others) for the syringe is often useful but not essential. A variety of needles and slides is useful, so that the procedure and specimen preparation can be tailored to the individual patient. We also believe that the issue of local anesthesia may be an individual one, depending on both the patient and the physician performing the FNA. If the patient is very anxious or if several needle passes are anticipated, we have found that local anesthesia can be useful. However, many physicians perform FNAs with excellent results using no anesthetic.

The question of immediate assessment of aspirates using a quick stain such as Diff-Quik is also

---

BOX 6-1 MATERIALS NEEDED FOR FINE-NEEDLE ASPIRATION

Syringes: 10 or 20 ml
Needles: 22, 23, and 25 gauge
Aspiration handle or gun (optional)
Slides: Frosted one-end and totally frosted
Fixative: 95% ethanol or spray fixative
Saline solution (Plasma-Lyte or similar)
Alcohol preparation pads or local disinfectant
Gauze squares
Gloves
Empty container for air-dried slides
Pencil, labels, and requisitions
Lidocaine, 3-ml syringe, small needles (optional)
Microscope and Diff-Quik (optional)

---

an individual decision. If several passes are performed and the patient can return for a repeat FNA with minimal inconvenience, rapid assessment is probably not necessary. If the patient lives a long distance away or if some immediate therapeutic decision is needed, immediate assessment may be helpful. In any case, FNA specimens should receive high priority for staining and interpretation in the cytology laboratory, so that this technique continues to be useful for rapid assessment of breast abnormalities.

The aspiration procedure

The FNA technique should be explained to the patient before the procedure is started. Often the patient is very anxious and does not know what to expect. Assembling materials and labeling slides in advance is also useful so that the procedure goes smoothly once begun. The patient should be positioned to optimally palpate and localize the mass. Cleansing the skin with an alcohol preparation pad is usually sufficient to sterilize the area. Sterile drapes are unnecessary. Although some physicians perform FNAs without gloves, we would advise their use as part of the universal precautions procedure for handling potentially infectious body fluids. With experience, masses can be palpated adequately wearing good-quality gloves.

If a local anesthetic is desired, a smaller needle is useful, 25 to 30 gauge. The anesthetic should first be injected intradermally to form a skin wheal

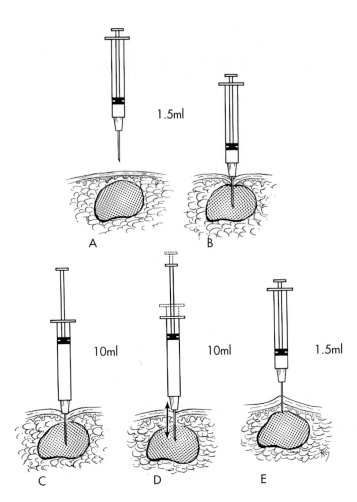

Fig. 6-1 Technique for performing FNA biopsy. **A,** Procedure is begun with 1 to 2 ml of air in syringe. **B,** While the mass is localized with one hand, needle is inserted. **C,** Suction is applied to syringe. **D,** Needle is moved back and forth within the mass. **E,** Suction is released before withdrawal of the needle from the mass, allowing plunger to return to original position.

and then injected into subcutaneous tissue. The injection should occur very slowly to minimize patient discomfort. Only small amounts of anesthetic should be used so that the mass is not obscured and the aspirate diluted by anesthetic.

Starting the procedure with 1-2 ml of air in the syringe is useful (Fig. 6-1). The air can be used to expel material onto the slide immediately after performing the aspirate. The breast mass should be localized between the fingers and thumb of one hand, while the needle is inserted into the mass using the other hand. Frequently, a change in resistance can be felt when the needle enters the mass. While applying continuous suction to the syringe, the needle is moved back and forth several times within the mass, generally staying in the same plane. If the mass is sufficiently large, the direction of the needle can be altered after partial withdrawal, but separate passes will often better sample different foci. The sampled material should remain in the lumen and hub of the needle unless the mass is cystic or hemorrhagic. Care should be exercised to stay within the mass as much as pos-

sible. Suction should be released before withdrawing the needle from the mass, allowing the syringe to return to the original volume of air. Direct pressure is applied to the area using a gauze square.

Smears are made by gently expressing a few drops of material onto the slide. A second slide is placed on top of the material, and then the two slides are gently but quickly pulled apart either sideways or lengthwise (Fig. 6-2 A to D). We prefer to make paired alcohol-fixed and air-dried slides. The alcohol-fixed slides should be immediately immersed in 95% ethanol or spray fixed to prevent air-drying artifacts. Frequently, more than one set of slides can be made with a single aspiration. Additional material can often be expressed from the needle hub by first removing the needle, aspirating air into the syringe, and then reattaching the needle.

Alternate methods exist for preparing the slides, including techniques to concentrate particles. The reference by Abele and others details several concentration techniques.[13]

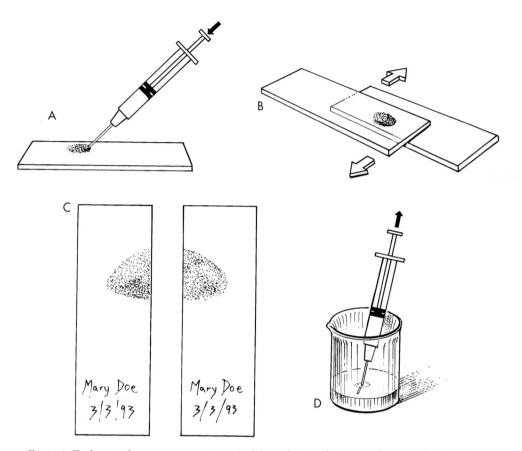

Fig. 6-2 Technique for smear preparation. **A,** Material is gently expressed onto a slide. **B,** Second slide is placed on top, and two slides are quickly but gently pulled apart. **C,** Appearance of paired smears. **D,** Needle is rinsed in saline or fixative solution.

The needle should be rinsed into a saline solution to recover the maximum amount of material. Our laboratory places aliquots of about 10 ml of Plasma-Lyte into specimen containers for this purpose. Other laboratories use fixative to rinse the needles[24] but this may limit the types of special stains to be performed later.

Some physicians sample masses using a thin needle without syringe or aspiration.[57] Holding the needle hub directly may allow a greater degree of manual control, but inadequacy rates may be higher for benign masses.[20] If a cystic mass is encountered, a syringe is attached to the needle. Attaching intravenous extension tubing between the needle and syringe accomplishes a similar degree of control.[53] An assistant can apply negative pressure to the syringe.

Most physicians perform two to six separate passes; this is often tailored to the individual circumstances and studies needed in our institution. Separate passes should ideally sample separate portions of the mass. Pennes and colleagues studied the incremental yield of additional needle passes. Three or four passes were recommended to optimize yield within practical limitations.[52]

Special situations and other helpful hints

Cysts. If a cystic mass is encountered, the cyst contents should be aspirated completely. The area should be palpated again and any residual mass reaspirated. Bloody or turbid cyst fluid should be examined cytologically.[18] Samples from patients with residual masses should also be examined. Clear or serous cyst fluids may rarely contain carcinoma.[37] Whether these should be cytologically examined may depend on clinical circumstances and suspicion of cancer.

Fatty masses and fat necrosis. Fatty material often does not adhere well to an unfrosted slide. We use one frosted slide and one unfrosted slide to spread at least one pair of slides from a fatty aspirate. The frosted slide is always alcohol fixed. Use of specially coated slides (polylysine or albumin) may also aid adherence of fatty material.

Fatty aspirates can often be grossly diagnosed because the material is yellow, semiclear, and greasy in appearance. The fatty material forms small pools after the material is smeared. An aspirate from fat necrosis is yellow-white and more opaque, but otherwise similar.

Hemorrhagic masses. If bloody material is observed within the needle hub, the needle pass should be terminated to avoid diluting the specimen with blood and causing further local trauma. Subsequent needle passes should be directed to another site within the mass. Use of a smaller gauge needle may be useful.[51] Carnoy's fixative may be useful for bloody smears.[34]

Necrotic masses. If necrotic material is aspirated, a different site within the mass should be sampled with later passes. Aspiration of the edge of the mass may be useful.

Scirrhous and rubbery masses. Masses with a large amount of fibrous stroma may yield very scanty material with aspiration. Sampling different portions of the mass or sampling the edge of the mass may be useful.[51] Varying the size of the needle with different passes may also be helpful; small needles often collect more cells.[43]

Scouting aspirates. Scouting-needle aspiration in the area of mammographic abnormality has been used to aid in detection of nonpalpable breast masses.[21] Quadrant aspirates from women with a family history of breast cancer have also been attempted to detect proliferative and atypical fibrocystic disease.[45]

Examination of nipple secretions

Intraductal lesions such as papillomas and papillary carcinomas may occasionally present with nipple discharge. Cytologic examination may aid in establishing a diagnosis, especially if the discharge is hemorrhagic or unilateral.[56] Physiologic secretions are usually bilateral and milky or serous in appearance.[32] A drop of material is obtained by gently squeezing the nipple while maintaining pressure on the areola. A plain slide is passed quickly over the drop and immediately alcohol fixed.[53]

Radiologic guidance procedures for fine-needle aspiration

Needle placement by mammographic guidance, ultrasound guidance, and stereotaxic devices has been used to obtain aspirates from small or deep nonpalpable breast abnormalities.[16,28,31,38] Most of the series of stereotaxic biopsies have been reported from European centers. The rate of insufficient specimens with stereotaxic techniques var-

ies from about 8% to 27%.[*] There is a higher rate of inadequate specimens for benign lesions. Abundant fibrosis and deviation of the needle are common causes of inadequate specimens. The sensitivity of this technique for diagnosing cancer ranges from about 80% to 100% if insufficient samples are not considered false-negatives and atypical or suspicious diagnoses are considered true-positives. The sensitivity is lower if inadequate samples are counted as true-negatives. Specificity is somewhat higher, 91% to 100%. Some of the false-positive or suspicious diagnoses reported included cases of atypical hyperplasia. This cytologic technique cannot differentiate cases of in situ carcinoma from invasive carcinoma, which may be disadvantageous for treatment decisions.

Using standard mammographic techniques for localization, most investigators have reported a higher rate of inadequate specimens, with 36% reported in two series.[30,41] However, one investigator reported an insufficient rate of only 9% using standard techniques.[50]

Radiologic guidance techniques require skill, experience, and a team approach between the radiologist, cytopathologist, and surgeon. Accuracy improves if multiple needle passes are used or if there is immediate assessment of the specimen. For these techniques to be cost effective, benign results must be accurate enough to decrease the number of open biopsies performed. Stereotaxic equipment is expensive, and such techniques are probably best used at breast centers with a high volume of patients and procedures. Breast ultrasound is a cost effective way to direct FNA of those nonpalpable lesions which can be identified sonographically.

Processing of specimens

Routine stains include the Papanicolaou stain or a hematoxylin-eosin stain for alcohol-fixed smears, and a Wright-Giemsa or May-Grunwald-Giemsa stain for air-dried smears. We prefer the simple Diff-Quik stain, a modified Wright-Giemsa stain, for air-dried smears. Cyst fluid or material present from the needle rinse can be used to make either cytospin preparations, cell blocks, or both.

Special studies in fine-needle aspiration specimens

Either unstained smears or cell block sections can be used for many special stains. For optimal re-

---

sults, material for hormone receptor studies should be placed on slides coated with polylysine and immediately processed or stored at −70° C. Edelman and Waisman found that reactivity was well preserved in most air-dried smears stored at room temperature for up to 2 weeks, however.[25] We usually reserve ample material in the needle rinse solution and prepare hormone receptor slides using the cytospin immediately after returning to the laboratory. Several studies have compared estrogen and/or progesterone receptor studies by estrogen receptor immunochemical assay (ER-ICA) methods on FNA specimens with biochemical methods and/or with frozen-section immunochemical stains.* In general, there is good but not perfect correlation between different methodologies. Sensitivity of FNA compared with that of biochemical methods on excised tissue ranges from 78% to 96% in most studies with specificities of 70% to 100%. Overall concordance figures range from 76% to 94%.[48,49] In our experience, the sensitivity is higher than the specificity; we have had false-negative FNA ER-ICA stains, but only rare false-positive results. A significant number of cells (at least 20%) with intense staining should be observed to interpret the stain as positive.

DNA analysis can be performed by both flow cytometry and image cytometry on breast FNA specimens.[14,17,22,36,55] We prefer DNA image cytometry since less specimen is required and abnormal cells can be selectively measured. Slides for DNA ploidy studies are initially air dried and then fixed in 10% neutral buffered formalin. Stains for oncogene products can also be performed on aspirate smears or cytospins. Oncogene stains for Her-2-neu show good correlation with studies on excised breast cancers.[46]

INTERPRETATION OF FINE-NEEDLE ASPIRATE SPECIMENS
Findings in normal breasts

An adequate breast FNA specimen is one that shows cells explaining the physical findings. Smears that contain only blood should be considered unsatisfactory rather than negative. Usually, smears that do not contain ductal epithelial cells are also considered unsatisfactory; the exceptions are masses consistent with lipomas and cases of fibrous mastopathy or fatty replacement in elderly women.

Cellular constituents present in normal breast FNAs include ductal cells, myoepithelial cells,

stripped or naked nuclei, breast lobules, histiocytes or foam cells, and adipose tissue. Ductal cells are cuboidal cells present in cohesive sheets with occasional papillary formations (Fig. 6-3). Nuclei are slightly larger than a red cell, chromatin is even and finely granular, and nucleoli are inconspicuous. Cytoplasm is scant and cyanophilic and cell membranes are ill defined. Normal ductal cells present on a smear serve as a convenient baseline for comparison to pathologic conditions.

Bipolar stripped (naked) nuclei have smaller, darker nuclei that are often elongated. These nuclei are thought to originate from myoepithelial cells and/or stromal cells.

Breast lobules show branching lobular structures with peripheral spindled nuclei. Lobules are most commonly identified during pregnancy or lactation (Fig. 6-4).

Histiocytes or foam cells have abundant foamy cytoplasm, and small, frequently eccentric nuclei (Fig. 6-5). Since many of these cells probably originate from ductal cells, we prefer the term *foam cells.*

Adipose tissue is frequently present in tissue fragments (Fig. 6-6A, p. 94). Fat cells have abundant clear cytoplasm, small, dark nuclei, and distinct cell membranes.

Other findings occasionally present on breast FNAs include skeletal muscle (Fig. 6-6B, p. 94) and skin constituents. Platelet clumps are frequently seen in bloody aspirates and should be distinguished from stroma. Stain precipitates and other artifacts need to be easily recognized to avoid misidentification.[51]

Benign breast lesions

Inflammatory conditions. With acute inflammation or abscesses, numerous neutrophils are seen along with cellular debris, fibrin, macrophages, and occasional atypical or reactive epithelial cells (Fig. 6-7A, p. 95). A subareolar abscess is characterized by numerous neutrophils and anucleated squamous cells (Fig. 6-7B, p. 95).[67]

Chronic mastitis shows histiocytes, plasma cells, lymphocytes, multinucleated giant cells, and granulation tissue in addition to a variable component of acute inflammation. Duct ectasia shows a creamy exudate containing debris and a predominance of histiocytes.[51] A granulomatous inflammation can be seen with tuberculosis, with fungal infections, and as a response to foreign material introduced during breast augmentation or reconstruction. After excisional biopsies, mastectomies, or lumpectomies, we are frequently asked to aspirate thickened areas under scars. Such aspirates

---

*References 27, 33, 35, 42, 44, 47-49, 54.

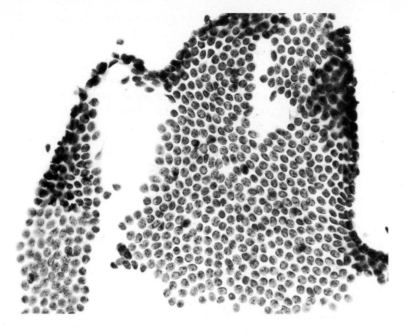

Fig. 6-3 Honeycomb sheet of benign ductal cells. Scattered bipolar stripped nuclei are visible at the edges of the groups (Papanicolaou ×100).

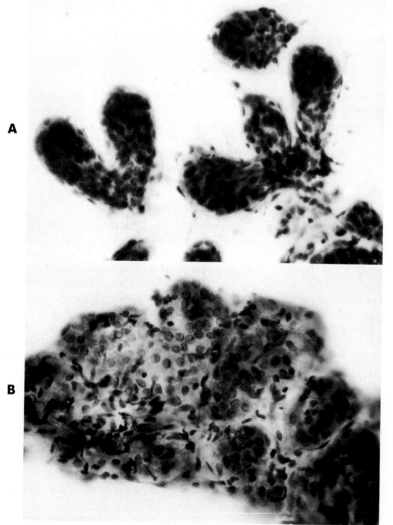

A

B

Fig. 6-4 A, Normal breast lobules showing branching clusters of cells with peripheral spindled nuclei (Papanicolaou ×100). **B,** Acinar clusters of lobular cells with small nucleoli aspirated from a vague mass in pregnancy (Papanicolaou ×100).

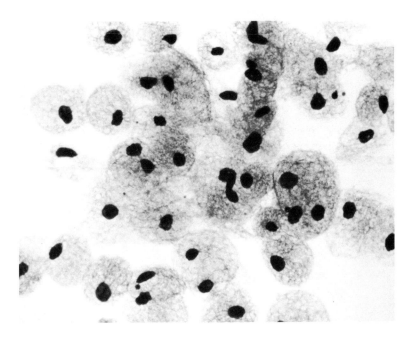

Fig. 6-5 Bilateral creamy breast discharge showing numerous foam cells (Diff-Quik ×132).

usually show chronic inflammation, granulation tissue, fat necrosis, and foreign body giant cells. Carcinoma is identified in the minority of cases.

Fat necrosis is often found after surgical procedures or trauma but may have no prior history. Because it presents as a hard mass, it may be confused with cancer. Aspirates usually yield abundant yellow-white, somewhat opaque material. Degenerating fat cells have a granular appearance, and fat globules of varying size are present (Fig. 6-8A, p. 96). Abundant cellular debris is present. The inflammatory component varies with the age of the injury. Lipid-laden histiocytes and multinucleated giant cells predominate (Fig. 6-8B, p. 96); scattered neutrophils are seen in early stages. If a component of organizing hematoma is present, hemosiderin may be prominent. Reactive fibroblasts with prominent nucleoli and occasional mitotic figures may also be observed.[6] In late stages, the lesion may become fibrotic and calcified, yielding less material with aspiration.

Depending on the clinical situation, culture and organism stains may occasionally be indicated in inflammatory processes. Ductal cells may show some atypical features in inflammatory processes but usually remain cohesive. Granulation tissue and reactive fibroblasts are often a source of concern unless one is aware of their cytologic appearance. The inflammatory background and sparse number of epithelial cells are useful criteria for avoiding false-positive diagnoses.

Fibrocystic disease. The principal cytologic

BOX 6-2 CYTOLOGIC FINDINGS IN FIBROCYSTIC DISEASE

Low cellularity, unless proliferative component
Cyst fluid with protein material and "blobs"
Foam cells
Apocrine cells
Clusters and sheets of ductal epithelial cells
Occasional bipolar nuclei and stromal fragments

---

findings in fibrocystic disease are listed in Box 6-2. The relative proportion of each element varies according to the histologic composition. Overall, aspirates from fibrocystic disease usually have low cellularity. With abundant stromal fibrosis, there is often resistance to moving the needle, and the lesion feels rubbery. The aspirate sample is usually scant. Occasional stromal fragments containing spindle-shaped fibroblasts and bipolar naked nuclei may be observed.

Cysts are often a target of the aspirate. Cyst fluid usually contains predominately proteinaceous material, foam cells, and apocrine cells. Blobs of basophilic material representing degenerated foam cells are frequently seen in the background.[94] The apocrine cells have abundant granular cytoplasm that stains a variable color with the Papanicolaou stain. The nuclei are slightly enlarged with single

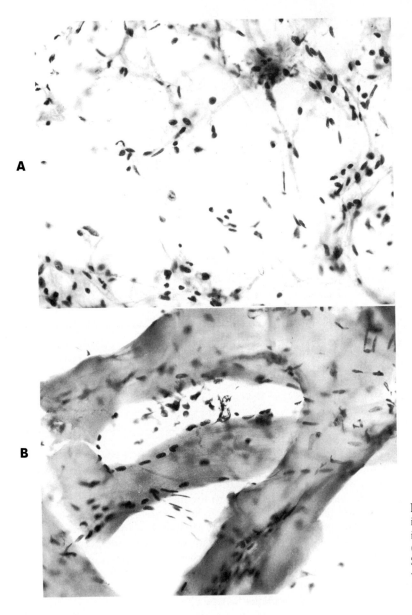

Fig. 6-6 A, Adipose tissue illustrating clear fat cells and intermixed stromal cells (Papanicolaou ×80). **B,** Skeletal muscle fibers with visible striations (Papanicolaou ×80).

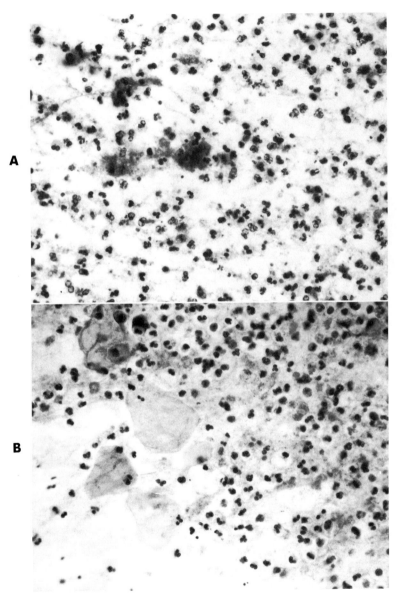

Fig. 6-7 A, Debris and numerous acute inflammatory cells from FNA of acute mastitis (Papanicolaou ×132). **B,** FNA of subareolar abscess. Note numerous inflammatory cells and anucleated squamous cells (Papanicolaou ×100).

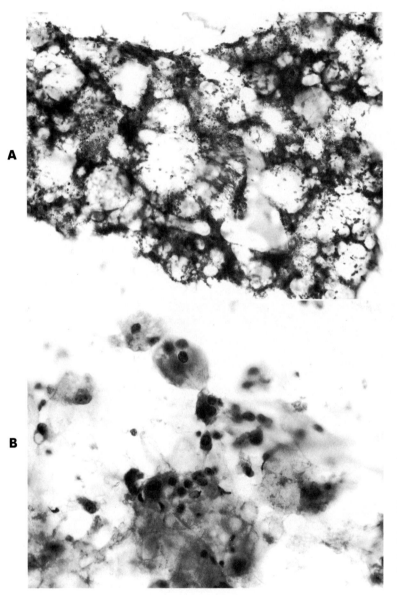

Fig. 6-8 A, Degenerated adipose cells with granular appearance in FNA from fat necrosis (Papanicolaou ×66). B, FNA from firm area under scar showing fat necrosis and foreign body reaction with numerous foamy histiocytes and chronic inflammatory cells (Papanicolaou ×100).

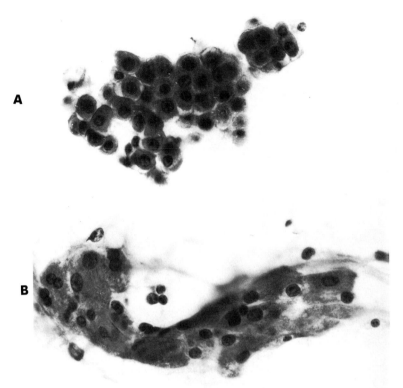

Fig. 6-9 A, Apocrine cells with granular cytoplasm and central nucleoli from an aspirate of fibrocystic disease (Papanicolaou ×132). **B,** Sheet of atypical apocrine cells showing binucleation and variation in nuclear size in a patient with fibrocystic disease (Papanicolaou ×80).

prominent central nucleoli (Fig. 6-9A). Apocrine cells may be present singly but are often present in orderly honeycomb sheets or papillary configurations. Some variation in nuclear size and other atypical features may be seen (Fig. 6-9B).[37] Caution should be exercised before diagnosing such a process as malignant, since most apocrine cells are benign. After cyst fluid is obtained, the area should be palpated, and any residual mass reaspirated.

Ductal epithelial cells usually are present in small clusters and sheets (Fig. 6-10). Ductal cells are usually uniformly spaced and have small benign nuclei with smooth borders and even fine chromatin.[82] Larger clusters of ductal cells with interspersed lacunae may be seen in patients with prominent ductal hyperplasia.[37] The presence of dark bipolar nuclei overlying the sheets of epithelial cells or in the background is helpful in diagnosing the lesion as benign.

A few studies have attempted to correlate cytologic findings in fibrocystic disease with the degree of atypia seen histologically.[50,58,59,82] In the study by Masood and others, cytologic features, including cell arrangement, cellular pleomorphism, chromatin pattern, and numbers of myoepithelial cells, were graded. Cases of atypical hyperplasia usually had scores intermediate between proliferative fibrocystic disease without atypia and carci-

noma. Image analysis techniques have also been used to evaluate atypical hyperplasia.

Other diagnostic difficulties with fibrocystic disease include fibroadenomas and well-differentiated or tubular carcinomas. (See discussion in these sections.)

Fibroadenomas. The clinical presentation of a well-circumscribed, movable mass is helpful when one is making the cytologic diagnosis of fibroadenoma. Fibroadenomas generally have a rubbery texture when aspirated, and the smears are usually very cellular. Cytologic features include large branching sheets and fronds of uniform, evenly spaced epithelial cells (Box 6-3 and Fig. 6-11A). Some describe the fronds as having an "antler horn appearance."[62] Occasionally, some loss of cell cohesion is present at the edges of the groups. Bipolar stripped nuclei are usually numerous in the background of the smears and overlying the epithelial sheets. Fragments of hypocellular stromal tissue are usually seen but are less numerous than the epithelial fragments (Fig. 6-11B). Fibroadenomas may show some overlapping features with fibrocystic disease (Fig. 6-12A, p. 100), and a minority of cases cannot be reliably distinguished by cytologic means.[37] Fibrocystic disease is more likely to show numerous apocrine cells and foam cells.[51] Using stepwise regression analysis, Bottles and others found that marked cellularity, stroma,

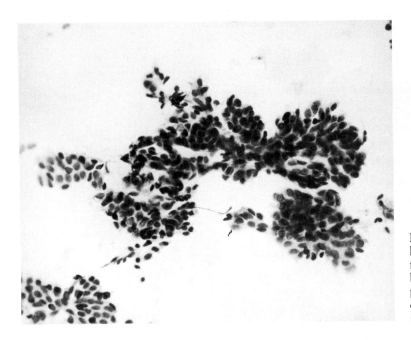

Fig. 6-10 Clusters of hyperplastic ductal cells from fibrocystic disease. Scattered bipolar stripped nuclei are present in the background and overlying the cell clusters (Papanicolaou ×100).

BOX 6-3 CYTOLOGIC FINDINGS IN FIBROADENOMAS

Moderate to high cellularity
Fronds of epithelial cells (honeycomb sheets)
Numerous bipolar stripped nuclei
Stromal fragments

---

and antler horn clusters were most useful in differentiating fibroadenomas from fibrocystic disease.[62]

Some epithelial cells in fibroadenomas may show nuclear enlargement and other atypical features (Fig. 6-11C). Fibroadenomas in pregnancy are especially likely to show epithelial atypia (Fig. 6-12B).[51] Helpful features in avoiding a diagnosis of malignancy are the general cohesion of the epithelial cells, the absence of single atypical epithelial cells, and the presence of numerous myoepithelial cells. In a study of carcinomas simulating fibroadenoma or fibrocystic change, Rogers and Lee found that nuclear hyperchromasia indicated malignancy.[85] Bottles and others identified stromal fragments, antler horn epithelial clusters, and honeycomb epithelial sheets as the best criteria to differentiate fibroadenomas from carcinomas.[62] A few fibroadenomas will require excision to differentiate them from tubular carcinomas.

Intraductal papillomas. Intraductal papillomas found in large subareolar ducts are often associated with bloody or serous nipple discharge. Occasionally, a subareolar mass is present that can be aspirated. Multiple peripheral papillomas are often found as a component of proliferative fibrocystic disease and are less often associated with nipple discharge. Cytologically, papillomas are characterized by tight papillary clusters and sheets of cells (Fig. 6-13). If the lesion is cystic, balls of epithelial cells are common.[37] Hyalinized fibrovascular stalks may appear as metachromatic globoid or cylindric structures surrounded by epithelial cells.[74] In the large solitary forms the epithelial cells have a more columnar shape compared with the proliferative ductal cells seen in fibrocystic disease. The nuclei may be slightly enlarged or hyperchromatic because of degeneration. Foam cells and apocrine cells are commonly observed, and blood and hemosiderin-laden macrophages may be seen in the background. Papillomas may be difficult to distinguish from papillary carcinomas, but isolated tall columnar cells are more frequent in carcinomas.[37]

Pregnancy and lactation. Aspirates from lactating or pregnant breast tissue are often cellular with abundant amorphous material in the background.[6,53] Cells show some loss of cohesion and have fragile vacuolated or granular cytoplasm, which is frequently stripped from the nucleus. Nuclei are enlarged and have prominent nucleoli. The hypercellularity and dyshesion mimic findings of carcinoma, but nuclei remain uniform with smooth borders and even chromatin.[53] Acinar configurations of lobular cells may also be observed (see Fig. 6-4B).[80] If a distinct mass is aspirated and

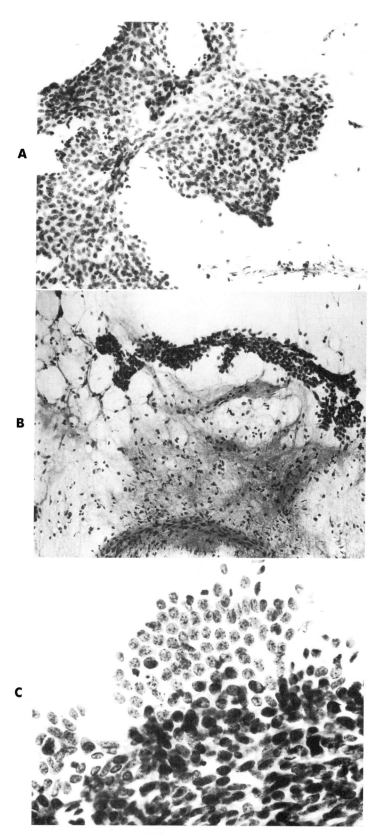

Fig. 6-11 A, FNA of fibroadenoma showing large branching sheets of epithelial cells (Papanicolaou ×50). **B,** Fronds of benign epithelium admixed with stroma in a fibroadenoma (Papanicolaou ×40). **C,** Fibroadenoma showing evenly spaced nuclei at top of illustration but nuclear overlapping and atypical features at bottom (Papanicolaou ×132).

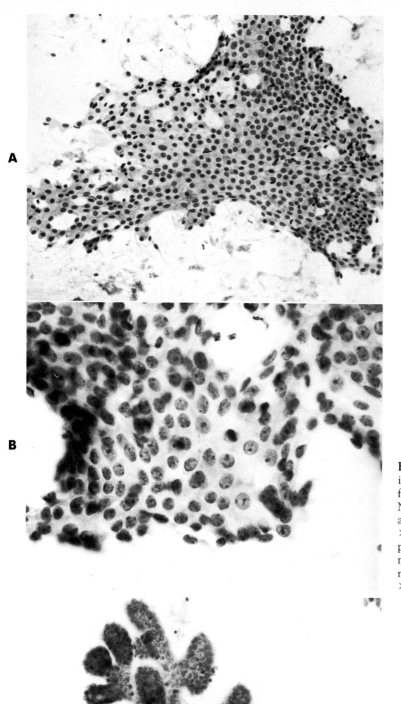

Fig. 6-12 A, Fibroadenoma illustrating slight apocrine features in the epithelial cells. Numerous bipolar nuclei are also evident (Papanicolaou ×80). B, Fibroadenoma in pregnancy showing prominent nucleoli but otherwise bland nuclear features (Papanicolaou ×132).

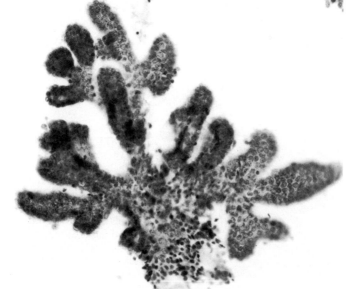

Fig. 6-13 Branching papillary cell clusters from FNA of a papilloma (Papanicolaou ×66).

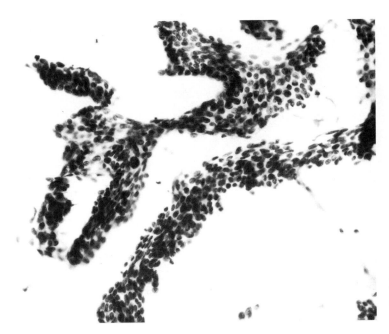

Fig. 6-14 FNA of gynecomastia showing branching sheets of cohesive epithelial cells (Papanicolaou ×66).

numerous acini or lobules identified, this is consistent with a lactating adenoma. Fibroadenomas may enlarge in pregnancy and show some loss of cohesion with nuclear enlargement and atypia.[51] Therefore, clinical history of pregnancy or lactation is essential when interpreting breast FNAs. Novotny and others have recently reviewed FNA in pregnancy.[80]

Gynecomastia. Cohesive sheets of ductal cells, naked bipolar nuclei, and occasional stromal fragments are the principal cytologic findings in gynecomastia (Fig. 6-14). These are similar to the cytologic findings in fibroadenomas, but cellularity is usually lower in gynecomastia and the epithelial groups tend to be smaller. Papillary formations, scattered loosely adherent cells, and columnar cells may also be observed.[37] The nuclei may show some atypical features, including enlargement and hyperchromasia. These atypical features may be accentuated by recent chemotherapeutic agents.[83] The overall cell cohesion and lack of numerous isolated malignant cells support a benign diagnosis. Early lesions of gynecomastia yield a more cellular aspirate and often show fragments of loose myxoid stroma.

Radiation changes. Breast aspirations are occasionally performed after lumpectomy and radiation therapy for breast carcinoma. Atypical epithelial cells in microacinar clusters may be seen in nonneoplastic breast tissue. The cytoplasm is often vacuolated, and nuclei show variation in size with occasional prominent nucleoli.[60,81] Usually bipolar naked nuclei are present. If prominent cell

dissociation or high cellularity is observed, recurrent tumor should be suspected.[66] Comparison with the previous breast cancer may be useful. Many masses aspirated after radiation therapy show changes of fat necrosis.[81]

Other benign lesions. A lipoma or fatty replacement of the breast may be suggested if one is sure that the mass has been sampled adequately and only adipose tissue is obtained. A lipoma should be soft and discrete with no needle resistance to make this diagnosis.[51]

The rare adenomas that have been aspirated have shown similar features to fibroadenomas. Lactating adenomas show acinar structures and isolated cells with vacuolated cytoplasm and nucleoli.[68] A ductal adenoma has been reported that had overlapping features with mucinous carcinoma and lactating adenoma.[92] Subareolar papillomatosis or nipple adenoma is characterized by a cellular aspirate with clustered and isolated columnar cells.[79] Clusters of squamous cells may also be seen.[37] Clinical findings are important to avoid a false-positive diagnosis of cancer.

Granular cell tumors may be confused with cancer clinically because of hardness and fixation to the skin. These neoplasms are often gritty when aspirated. The cells will occur in loose clusters or be isolated on the smears (Fig. 6-15). Cytoplasm is granular and occasional nucleoli may be observed.[78]

The reader is referred to more detailed references to obtain further information on rare neoplasms.

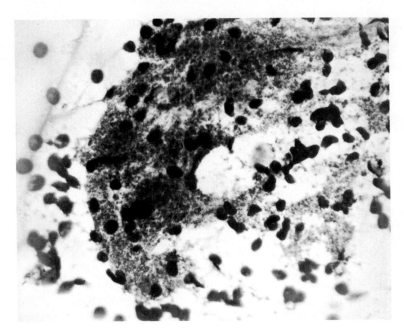

Fig. 6-15 Touch preparation of granular cell tumor (hematoxylin-eosin ×80).

Carcinomas

General findings. General features of carcinoma are shown in Box 6-4 and Fig. 6-16. Most aspirates are cellular, with scirrhous ductal cancers and some lobular cancers being exceptions. The cell groups in cancer are usually syncytial and three dimensional, in contrast to the orderly monolayered sheets of epithelial cells characteristic of most benign lesions.[6] Cancer cell groups tend to be smaller than benign groups, and bipolar naked nuclei are sparse or absent.[82] The cells within the groups are disordered and often crowded. Loss of cell cohesion is present at the edges of many groups, which often have a frayed appearance. The presence of single malignant cells is one of the most important criteria for the diagnosis of cancer.[6] Malignant nuclear criteria, including enlargement, pleomorphism, hyperchromasia, coarse and irregular chromatin distribution, irregular nuclear shapes with "bites" and indentations, and abnormal nucleoli, are present to a variable extent depending on the type of carcinoma (Fig. 6-17A). Some carcinomas have bland nuclear features but are readily diagnosed by the marked cell dispersion (Fig. 6-17B).

Nuclear grading techniques have been used successfully in breast carcinoma aspirates.[22,91]

Ductal adenocarcinoma. The aspirate cellularity of ductal carcinomas depends on the amount of stroma in the background. Most ductal carcinomas are easily aspirated, but the extremely scirrhous cancers will feel gritty and yield a scant as-

> ### BOX 6-4 GENERAL CYTOLOGIC FEATURES OF CARCINOMAS
>
> Cellular aspirate (some exceptions)
> Loss of cell cohesion
> Syncytial or three-dimensional cell clusters
> Disordered or crowded cell arrangement
> Nuclear enlargement with irregular nuclear borders
> Presence of single malignant cells

pirate. Cell groupings are also quite variable. Some will have mostly cohesive syncytial clusters of cells with few single cells (see Fig. 6-17A). Others show very loose clusters of cells or single dispersed cancer cells (see Fig. 6-17B). Nuclei are enlarged to at least twice the size of red blood cells. Comparison with benign ductal cells, red cells, or lymphocytes in the background is useful to appreciate the degree of nuclear enlargement. Malignant nuclear criteria are usually readily recognized, including hyperchromasia, nuclear membrane irregularity, irregular chromatin distribution, and prominent nucleoli. Necrotic debris and pyknotic cells may be seen in the background, especially if there is a component of comedocarcinoma.

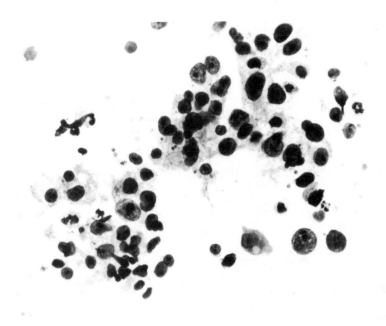

Fig. 6-16 Loose cell clusters and single ductal carcinoma cells with malignant nuclear criteria (Papanicolaou ×132).

Small cell variants of ductal carcinoma may be seen, especially in older women. Nuclei are more uniform with fewer malignant criteria. Some may show a plasmacytoid appearance (Fig. 6-17C).[87] Loss of cell cohesion is prominent with many single cells. This variant shows some cytologic overlap with lobular carcinoma but is usually more cellular (Fig. 6-17D).[87]

Intraductal carcinoma cannot usually be cytologically distinguished from infiltrating ductal carcinoma. Benign ductal cells admixed with cancer cells may suggest an intraductal process, and the presence of necrotic debris may suggest comedocarcinoma.[43,91,93] Cytologic features of specific subtypes of intraductal carcinomas have been described recently.[76,77]

Medullary carcinoma. Medullary carcinomas are relatively soft when aspirated and usually yield a very cellular specimen. The exception is medullary carcinoma with areas of cystic necrosis, which may yield relatively few cells and mimic a hemorrhagic breast cyst.[69] Loose clusters and individual malignant cells are present on smears of medullary carcinoma. The nuclei are greatly enlarged, vesicular, and irregular with prominent nucleoli (Fig. 6-18, p. 106). Cytoplasm is pale, ill defined, and delicate. Stripped and damaged nuclei are common.[72] Lymphocytes are present in variable numbers in the background.

Mucinous (colloid) carcinoma. Mucinous carcinomas are soft on aspiration, and the material has a glistening mucoid appearance. The mucin stains variably with the Papanicolaou stain but is often a pale pink. The bright purple mucin is more obvious on the Diff-Quik stain (Fig. 6-19A and B, p. 107). A mucicarmine stain may also be useful to confirm the presence of mucin.[72] Balls or clusters of monotonous epithelial cells are seen within the mucin. Since the cells are relatively small and show minimal nuclear abnormalities, a diagnosis of mucinous carcinoma may at times be difficult to make.[64] The presence of numerous cell balls, occasional isolated neoplastic cells, and a classic mucinous background are the most useful criteria. Foci of mucinous differentiation can also be seen within ordinary ductal carcinomas.

Papillary carcinoma. Papillary carcinomas may be associated with bloody or serous nipple discharge. Aspirates from papillary carcinoma are commonly blood tinged, and if the lesion is cystic, the aspirate may yield abundant hemorrhagic fluid. The smears show tight papillary cell clusters and scattered smaller loosely cohesive clusters (Fig. 6-20, p. 107). Tall columnar cells can be identified at the edges of the groups and also isolated in the smears.[71] The nuclei show only slight pleomorphism. Naked nuclei, debris, and hemosiderin-laden macrophages are common in the background. The cytologic features overlap those of papillomas and occasionally fibroadenomas. The smaller loose cell clusters, debris, and hemosiderin-laden macrophages help exclude the diagnosis of fibroadenoma. Some papillomas and papillary carcinomas can only be distinguished by excision.

Tubular carcinoma. The cells from a tubular carcinoma show more cohesion than ordinary ductal carcinoma and often only mild nuclear atypia

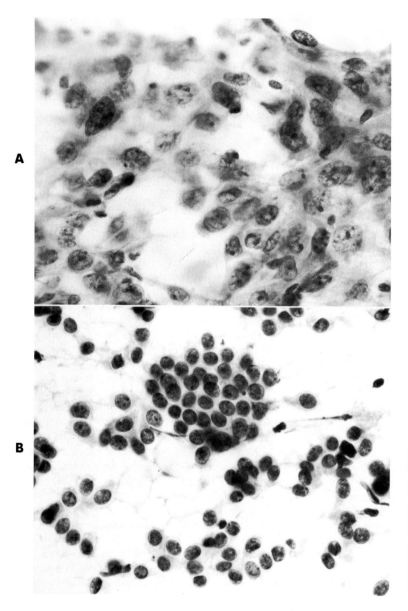

Fig. 6-17 A, Poorly differentiated ductal carcinoma showing syncytial sheets of cells with pleomorphic nuclei and frequent multiple nucleoli (Papanicolaou ×132). B, Well-differentiated ductal carcinoma showing bland nuclear features but prominent loss of cell cohesion (Papanicolaou ×160).

C

D

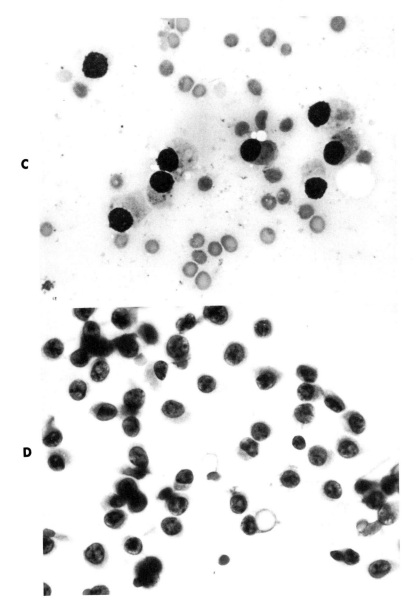

Fig. 6-17, cont'd C, Ductal carcinoma showing small dispersed cells with plasmacytoid appearance (Diff-Quik ×160). **D,** Ductal carcinoma composed of small dispersed cells with occasional signet ring forms (Papanicolaou ×200). This variant of ductal carcinoma shows overlapping features with lobular carcinoma.

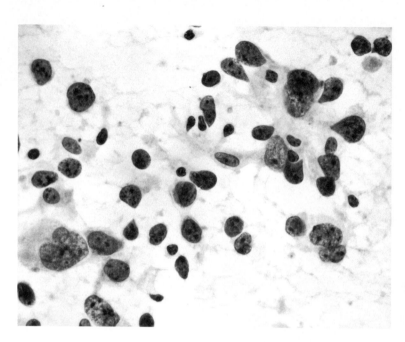

Fig. 6-18 FNA of a medullary carcinoma. Note the large pleomorphic carcinoma cells with background lymphocytes (Papanicolaou ×160).

(Fig. 6-21). Angular epithelial clusters are commonly described on aspirate smears.[61,63] Rare single atypical epithelial cells can usually be identified.[63] Although myoepithelial cells or bipolar nuclei are not seen in most cases, about 20% will show prominent myoepithelial cells.[61,63] The main differential diagnosis is fibroadenoma. The presence of angular clusters, single cells, and nuclear atypia should raise the possibility of tubular carcinoma rather than fibroadenoma. Some cases require excision for definitive diagnosis.

Lobular carcinoma. Aspirates from lobular carcinomas are generally less cellular than those from ductal carcinomas. Lobular carcinoma cells are present in small clusters, in short chains, or as single dispersed cells.[72] The cells are small and monomorphic with a cuboidal shape (Fig. 6-22). Nuclei are oval and often eccentric. The nuclei are hyperchromatic with coarse chromatin. The coarse chromatin and eccentric nuclei may cause the cells superficially to resemble plasma cells.[6] Some lobular carcinomas are characterized by many signet ring cells. Such cells have eccentric distorted nuclei and intracytoplasmic vacuoles that often contain a central condensed mucin droplet.[6]

The features of lobular carcinoma may overlap with small cell ductal carcinomas, especially when the histology shows a variant (solid or alveolar pattern) of lobular carcinoma.[75] Such distinctions may not be critical to the FNA diagnosis, however. We often make a diagnosis of "mammary carcinoma" in such cases and provide a differential

diagnosis. Of more importance is the fact that lobular carcinomas have a higher incidence of false-negative diagnoses than ductal carcinomas, probably because of the scanter cellularity and small uniform appearance of the cells.

Lobular carcinoma in situ (LCIS) is relatively difficult to diagnose by FNA. Loosely cohesive cell groups with a "dilapidated brick wall" appearance, eccentric nuclei with slight atypia, and intracytoplasmic lumina were described as the most useful criteria in a recent study.[86] Atypical lobular hyperplasia could not be distinguished from LCIS. LCIS features overlapped with findings of invasive lobular carcinoma, but invasive lesions usually had higher cellularity and more single cells.

Other breast carcinomas. Aspirates in the presence of Paget's disease show findings of ductal carcinoma. Skin scrapings or touch preparations of saline-moistened skin can also be made. Cells often show degenerative changes.[94] The cells have large pleomorphic nuclei with nucleoli as compared with benign squamous cells from the skin. Mucin can be demonstrated in the cytoplasm. Immunohistochemistry may be useful to differentiate Paget's disease from malignant melanoma.[87]

Apocrine carcinoma cytologically may show sheets of cells, syncytial groups, or isolated cells.[37] Apocrine cells have abundant granular cytoplasm, enlarged vesicular nuclei, and prominent, often multiple nucleoli. If well differentiated, this carcinoma may be difficult to distinguish from benign

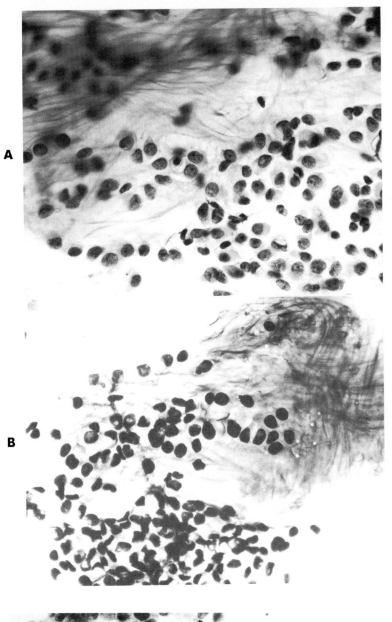

Fig. 6-19 **A** and **B,** Loosely
cohesive carcinoma cells
embedded in mucinous
material; FNA of mucinous
carcinoma (**A,** Papanicolaou
×132 and **B,** Diff-Quik ×100).

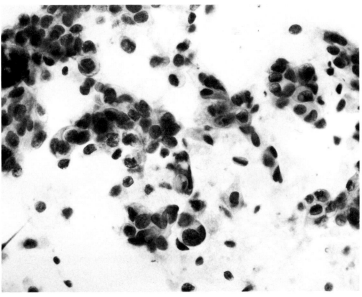

Fig. 6-20 Breast discharge of
papillary carcinoma showing
cell clusters with abnormal
nuclei. Debris and histiocytes
are present in the background
(Papanicolaou ×132).

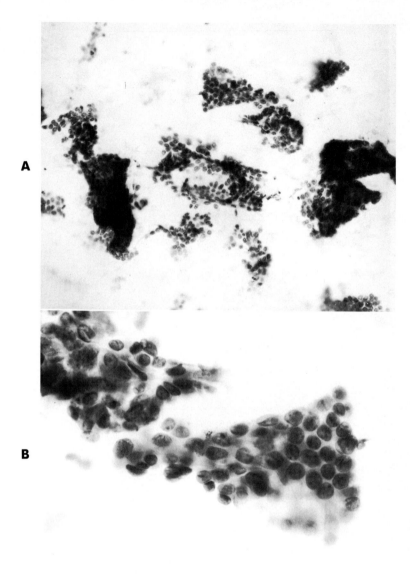

Fig. 6-21 A and **B,**
Well-differentiated tubular
carcinoma showing
characteristic angular cohesive
cell clusters. Some nuclear
membrane abnormalities are
seen at high power (**A,**
Papanicolaou ×50 and **B,**
×160).

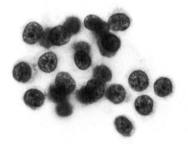

Fig. 6-22 Loose cell clusters and individual small
carcinoma cells from FNA of lobular carcinoma
(Papanicolaou ×200).

apocrine metaplasia. The clinical presentation of a solid suspicious mass rather than a cystic lesion is helpful. Most apocrine carcinomas show a predominance of pleomorphic apocrine cells with disordered or syncytial arrangement.[70]

Male breast cancer, when aspirated, usually has features similar to ductal carcinomas in women. The main differential diagnosis is gynecomastia (see previous section).

The reader is referred to other texts for discussion of other rare cancers, including metaplastic and secretory carcinoma.

Other neoplasms

Phyllodes tumor and mesenchymal neoplasms. Phyllodes tumors (cystosarcoma phyllodes) with benign behavior are cytologically very similar to fibroadenomas (Fig. 6-23). Fronds and monolayered sheets of epithelial cells are seen as well as naked nuclei.[90] Occasional crowded clusters of epithelial cells may be seen that are probably aspirated from areas of epithelial hyperplasia; these may cause diagnostic confusion with ductal carcinomas.[65,88] The stromal fragments may be more prominent and more cellular than the usual fibroadenoma.[90] Isolated fibroblasts, foam cells, and multinucleated giant cells may be seen in the background.[84] Size alone is not a useful feature in separating phyllodes tumors from fibroadenomas. Excision with ample margins is recommended in questionable cases.

Malignant phyllodes tumors show pleomorphic sarcomatoid elements on the aspirate smears.[88] If only rare epithelial elements are present, this tumor may be misdiagnosed as a sarcoma. Since the cytologic features are not specific for predicting biologic behavior, final diagnosis is best made after excision of the mass.

The reader is referred to more detailed references for discussion of other mesenchymal tumors.[37,88]

Metastatic tumors. Less than 2% of breast malignancies are metastatic tumors. Common primary sites include ovarian, lung, and genitourinary carcinomas, melanoma, leukemia (granulocytic sarcoma), and lymphoma.[37,89] Correctly diagnosing such lesions is often dependent on knowing the clinical history. Metastatic lesions usually produce cellular aspirates with cytologic characteristics of malignancy.

Lymphomas and leukemias are characterized by primarily single cells with a high nuclear to cytoplasmic ratio. These must be differentiated from stripped or naked nuclei seen in the background of benign breast aspirates and from single malignant breast carcinoma cells. Most leukemic infiltrates are from acute myelogenous leukemia. The nuclei have fine chromatin, nucleoli, and occasional nuclear irregularity. A Wright or Diff-Quik stain is useful for identifying evidence of myeloid differentiation, including cytoplasmic granules and Auer rods. Histochemical stains for peroxi-

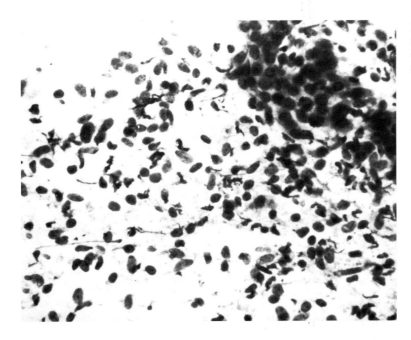

Fig. 6-23 FNA of phyllodes tumor illustrating epithelial cell clusters and numerous atypical stromal cells adjacent.

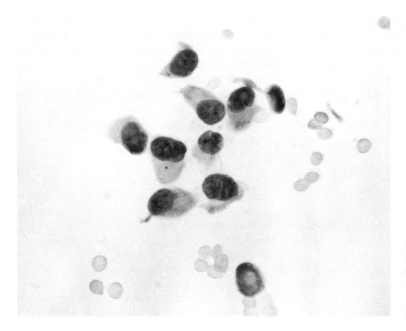

Fig. 6-24 Metastatic melanoma in breast showing single tumor cells with occasional intranuclear cytoplasmic inclusions. Rare cells contained pigment (Papanicolaou ×160).

dase or esterases on air-dried smears can also be useful. The cytologic characteristics of lymphoma cells depend on the histologic subtype of the lymphoma. Cell size ranges from that of a normal lymphocyte to the size of a histiocyte or larger. Nuclei may be round or clefted. Lymphoglandular bodies may be seen in the background. Comparison with the patient's original lymphoma slides is recommended. Immunocytochemistry for leukocyte common antigen and lymphoid antigens may be useful to confirm the diagnosis. Lymphomas must be differentiated from benign intramammary lymph nodes; the latter have a mixed population of lymphocytes as well as tingible-body histiocytes.

Malignant melanoma may have a variety of cytologic appearances (Fig. 6-24). The most common is single large cells with eccentric nuclei, frequent multinucleation, prominent eosinophilic nucleoli, and occasional intranuclear cytoplasmic inclusions. Cytoplasm is usually moderate to abundant and may show pigment. Cells may have an epithelioid or spindled appearance. Immunocytochemistry is often useful if the diagnosis cannot be made on the basis of cytologic features and comparison with the previous primary tumor.

Metastatic carcinomas may present a characteristic picture for the primary site. For example, renal carcinoma often shows cells with granular or clear cytoplasm and round nuclei with central nucleoli. Small cell undifferentiated carcinoma from the lung shows oval or angulated cells with scant cytoplasm, molding, and coarse chromatin. Metastatic gynecologic tumors may be difficult to differentiate from primary breast carcinomas, how-ever (Fig. 6-25). We have seen examples of metastatic ovarian cancer initially interpreted as papillary breast carcinomas.

Breast secretions

Nipple secretions related to physiologic disturbances, fibrocystic disease, and duct ectasia show overlapping features.[32] A proteinaceous background is seen with scattered foam cells and a variable number of clustered ductal cells (Fig. 6-26). Foam cells are especially common with duct ectasia.[73] Secretions related to intraductal papillomas usually show clusters of ductal cells and occasionally apocrine cells. The epithelial cells may show slightly atypical or degenerative features.[73] Red cells may be seen in the background. Numerous inflammatory cells are seen with mastitis. Secretions from patients with carcinoma show poor cell cohesion with loose clusters or individual cells.[73] Malignant nuclear criteria are present, as described in sections on FNA findings (see Fig. 6-20). Blood may be seen in the background.

RESULTS OF FINE-NEEDLE ASPIRATION
Terminology for reporting fine-needle aspiration results

The terminology used in reporting FNA results should convey the degree of certainty in the diagnosis. The terminology used must provide the clinician with recommendations on patient follow-up and the need for surgical biopsy.

A "positive for malignancy" diagnosis in our institution means that the clinician can proceed

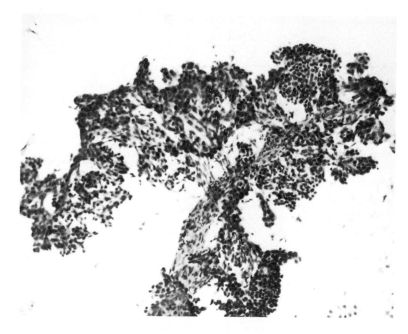

Fig. 6-25 Metastatic papillary ovarian carcinoma in breast FNA (Papanicolaou ×33); features may overlap those of a primary breast cancer.

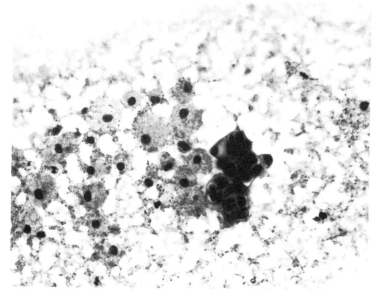

Fig. 6-26 Spontaneous breast discharge with foam cells and cluster of degenerated ductal cells in a proteinaceous background (Papanicolaou ×100).

with definitive cancer therapy such as mastectomy, lumpectomy, or chemotherapy. No frozen-section diagnosis of cancer is required in such situations. For this reason, no false-positive diagnoses are desirable. To help prevent false-positive results, such aspirates are reviewed by two or three cytopathologists.

A "suspicious for carcinoma" diagnosis means that most but not all diagnostic criteria for malignancy are present. These specimens are usually less cellular, show more cell cohesion, or have fewer malignant nuclear criteria than positive specimens. A frozen section or other biopsy procedure is recommended before definitive cancer therapy. All suspicious diagnoses require some additional evaluation in a timely fashion.

An atypical diagnosis means the overall cytologic impression is benign, but some of the cells show atypical features. An excisional biopsy or close clinical follow-up is recommended.

A benign diagnosis is given when adequate cells are obtained and the cytologic features are that of a benign process, which correlates with the physical findings.

A "nondiagnostic" result is given when there is concern that the cytologic findings do not explain the physical findings. Such terminology is also used when the cytologic features are not recognized as any specific pathologic process or when the specimen is scantly cellular.

An "unsatisfactory" diagnosis is given when insufficient cellular material is obtained (see section on criteria for adequate specimens).

Atypical, benign, and nondiagnostic cytologic reports should include some description of the cellular elements identified. For example, a benign or negative report may read "apocrine cells, foam cells, and ductal cells, most consistent with fibrocystic disease." In some cases, a differential diagnosis may be listed, such as "fibrocystic disease versus fibroadenoma."

Since there is always a possibility that the lesion was not properly sampled, a benign, nondiagnostic, or unsatisfactory result does not exclude the possibility of carcinoma. If there is any clinical or mammographic suspicion of carcinoma, another form of biopsy is recommended after a negative FNA result.

False-negative and false-positive results

Reasons for false-negative results are listed in Box 6-5. Inexperience of the aspirator is one of the most important reasons for both false-negative results and unsatisfactory specimens, as discussed previously. The size of the lesion is also important. Small lesions (less than 1 cm) and large lesions

---

BOX 6-5 REASONS FOR FALSE-NEGATIVE ASPIRATES

Inexperience of aspirator
Size and location of mass: small, large, or deep seated
Necrosis, hemorrhage, and cystic change
Extensive desmoplasia
Specific types of cancer associated with higher rates of false-negative diagnoses:
    Lobular carcinoma
    Tubular or well-differentiated carcinomas
    Intraductal carcinomas
    Papillary carcinomas
    Colloid carcinoma

(greater than 4 cm) may both be associated with false-negative results.[106,109] Large lesions may be more difficult to delineate and are often associated with necrosis and/or hemorrhage. Cystic lesions and desmoplastic lesions often yield a sparsely cellular specimen.[106] Interpretive errors account for the minority of false-negative results and may be due to observer inexperience.[95,111] However, well-differentiated or tubular carcinomas, colloid carcinomas, papillary carcinomas, and lobular carcinomas account for a significant number of false-negative diagnoses in many series.[105,106] As discussed earlier, these carcinomas may show minimal nuclear criteria of malignancy. Lobular carcinomas may also be associated with sparse cellularity.

False-positive or suspicious diagnoses may be due to improper preparation of the specimen, including air drying and distortion of cells. Inexperience and lack of clinical history are also important factors. Some of the lesions cited in the literature as recurring causes of false-positive results are listed in Box 6-6.[51,104,106] Proliferative fibrocystic disease and fibroadenomas with atypia are frequent causes, since they are relatively common lesions. Fat necrosis may clinically mimic a carcinoma and be associated with atypical histiocytes and reactive epithelial cells. Most of the other lesions have been discussed earlier in this chapter.

Results of large series of breast fine-needle aspirations

Many large series of breast FNAs have been published, including more than 30,000 cases total. Giard and Hermans recently analyzed 29 series in the English literature.[100] A few of the larger or more detailed series are summarized in Table 6-1.

BOX 6-6 LESIONS ASSOCIATED WITH FALSE-POSITIVE OR SUSPICIOUS DIAGNOSES

Fibrocystic disease: proliferative or atypical
Fibroadenomas
Fat necrosis
Lactational changes
Papillomas
Radiation changes
Organizing hematoma
Gynecomastia

Series from U.S. hospitals are listed at the top, and foreign series are at the bottom. Many of the largest series are from European centers, where clinical practices may differ slightly from standards of care in the United States.

Methods for calculating sensitivity and specificity vary somewhat in different series, so this is important to note when evaluating results. Most series calculate sensitivity by considering both malignant and suspicious results to be true-positives. If the calculation is based only on malignant results, the sensitivity is usually considerably lower. Atypical or nondiagnostic results are considered negative in some series, whereas other investigators consider atypia abnormal or exclude both from statistical analysis. If sensitivity is calculated only on satisfactory specimens, FNA appears to be a better technique than if calculated on both sat-

Table 6-1 **Sensitivity of breast FNA in detection of cancer**

Author	Series total	Proven cancers	Cytology positive (%)	Suspicious (%)	Cytology negative (%)	Sensitivity (%)	Insufficient*
Eisenberg (1986)[97]	1906	1390	76	9†	5	85	11%
Feldmen (1985)[98]	300	100	84	16	0	100	5%
Frable (1984)[3]	853	331	83	9	8	92	2%
Kline (1985)[72]	2623	327	80	11	9	91‡	1%
Oertel (1987)[51]	3605	857	80	9§	6	89	17%
Deschennes (1978)[96]	2050	114	81	11	8	92	3%
Fessia (1987)[99]	7495	650	66	12	12	78	10%
Halevy (1987)[103]	1953	355	90	4	6	94	NG
Lamb (1989)[105]	1318	1318	78	14	8	92	11%
Palombini (1988)[108]	1956	492	92	5	3	97	1%
Schondorf (1978)	2519	307	92	6	2	98	NG
Zajdela (1975)[109]	2772	1745	93	3	4	96	5%
Zajicek (1970)[110]	2111	1068	80	13	7	93	3%

*Insufficient rate is based on cancers, if given, or on entire FNA series.
†Additional 10% called atypical.
‡Increases to 94% if cancers <1 cm are excluded.
§Additional 5% called atypical.
NG = not given.

isfactory and unsatisfactory specimens. For example, the sensitivity decreases from 92% to 82% if unsatisfactory aspirates were included in one series.[105] In Table 6-1 the sensitivities are based only on satisfactory specimens and include both malignant and suspicious results as true-positives. The range in this table for sensitivity is 78% to 100%. Some papers report sensitivities of less than 70% but have included unsatisfactory specimens in their calculations.

The percentage of negative FNA results in patients with proven breast cancer is 0% to 8% in this table. Not included are some of the atypical or inconclusive results in a few of the series. The rate of insufficient specimens shows considerable variation and depends on both FNA technique and criteria to define specimen adequacy. In general, greater expertise of the aspirator leads to a lower rate of inadequate specimens. Lee and colleagues[107] found that a single experienced aspirator had a 9.8% technically inadequate rate, whereas several inexperienced aspirators had an overall inadequate rate of 45.9%. In Oertel's series, the pathologist aspirator had an inadequate rate of 0.7% out of 1230 FNAs, compared with the internist rate of 50% out of 246 aspirates.[51] The percentage of unsatisfactory specimens is usually lower for malignant lesions than for benign lesions.

False-positive results are based on the number of malignant FNA results with benign follow-up. False suspicious results are enumerated in many series but are usually not included when specificity is calculated. The false-positive rate in the literature is about 1% to 3% but is usually well under 1%. About 1% to 5% of benign specimens have false suspicious FNA diagnoses in most series.

The statistical results of FNA vary somewhat according to the medical practices. If definitive therapy is based on a malignant FNA result, the number of false-positive results must approach zero. This is reflected in many of the larger series reported from the United States. In such circumstances, the number of suspicious FNA results is usually higher. Over 75% of suspicious FNA results will prove malignant in our experience and that of others.

Statistical results also vary somewhat depending on the population studied. The predictive value of an abnormal or suspicious result may be lower in a young population with less breast cancer.[102] Conversely, as the prevalence of cancer increases in the population aspirated, the percentage of false suspicious aspirates decreases.

REFERENCES

1. Bell DA, Hajdu SI, Urban JA, et al: Role of aspiration cytology in the diagnosis and management of mammary lesions in office practice, *Cancer* 51:1182, 1983.
2. Berg JW, Robbins GF: A late look at the safety of aspiration biopsy, *Cancer* 15:826, 1962.
3. Frable WJ: Needle aspiration of the breast, *Cancer* 53:671, 1984.
4. Franzen S, Zajicek J: Aspiration biopsy in diagnosis of palpable lesions of the breast: critical review of 3479 consecutive biopsies, *Acta Radiol* 7:241, 1968.
5. Frisell J, Eklund G, Nilsson R, et al: Additional value of fine-needle aspiration biopsy in a mammographic screening trial, *Br J Surg* 76:840, 1989.
6. Koss LG, Woyke S, Olszewski W: *Aspiration biopsy: cytologic interpretation and histologic bases*, ed 2, New York, 1992, Igaku-Shoin.
7. Lopes Cardozo P: Atlas of clinical cytology. Targa BVs—Hertogenbosch, published by author, distributed by JB Lippincott, Philadelphia, 1976.
8. Martin HE, Ellis EB: Biopsy by needle puncture and aspiration, *Ann Surg* 92:169, 1930.
9. Preece PE, Hunter SM, Duguid HL, et al: Cytodiagnosis and other methods of biopsy in the modern management of breast cancer, *Semin Surg Oncol* 5:69, 1989.
10. Silverman JF, Lannin DR, O'Brien K, et al: The triage role of fine needle aspiration biopsy of palpable breast masses: diagnostic accuracy and cost-effectiveness, *Acta Cytol* 31:731, 1987.
11. Soderstrom N: *Fine needle aspiration biopsy*, New York, 1966, Grune & Stratton.
12. Stewart FN: The diagnosis of tumors by aspiration, *Am J Pathol* 9:801, 1933.

Fine-needle aspiration techniques

13. Abele JS, Miller TR, King EB, et al: Smearing techniques for the concentration of particles from fine needle aspiration biopsy, *Diagn Cytopathol* 1:59, 1985.
14. Auer GU, Caspersson TO, Wallgren AS: DNA content and survival in mammary carcinoma, *Anal Quant Cytol Histol* 2:161, 1980.
15. Azavedo E, Svane G, Auer G: Stereotactic fine-needle biopsy in 2594 mammographically detected nonpalpable lesions, *Cancer* 68:2007, 1991.
16. Bolmgren J, Jacobson B, Nordenstrom B: Stereotaxic instrument for needle biopsy of the mamma, *AJR* 129:121, 1977.
17. Charpin C, Andrac L, Habib MC, et al: Immunodetection in fine-needle aspirates and multiparametric (SAMBA) image analysis, *Cancer* 63:863, 1989.
18. Ciatto S, Cariaggi P, Bulgaresi P: The value of routine cytologic examination of breast cyst fluids, *Acta Cytol* 31:301, 1987.
19. Ciatto S, Del Turco MR, Bravetti P: Nonpalpable breast lesions: stereotaxic fine-needle aspiration cytology, *Radiology* 173:57, 1989.
20. Ciatto S, Catanio S, Bravetti P, et al: Fine-needle cytology of the breast: a controlled study of aspiration versus nonaspiration, *Diagn Cytopathol* 7:125, 1991.
21. Daum GS, Kline TS, Artymyshyn RL, et al: Aspiration biopsy cytology of occult breast lesions using the "scouting needle": a prospective study of 261 cases. *Cancer* 67:2150, 1991.
22. Davey DD, Banks ER, Jennings CD, et al: Comparison of nuclear grade and DNA cytometry in breast carcinoma aspirates to histologic grade in excised cancers, *Am J Clin Pathol* (in press).

23. Dowlatshahi K, Gent HJ, Schmidt R, et al: Nonpalpable breast tumors: diagnosis with stereotaxic localization and fine-needle aspiration, *Radiology* 170:427, 1989.

24. Dundas SA, Sanderson PR, Matta H, et al: Fine needle aspiration of palpable breast lesions: results obtained with cytocentrifuge preparation of aspirates, *Acta Cytol* 32:202, 1988.

25. Edelman AS, Waisman J: Stability of estrogen receptors in air-dried smears of mammary tumors, *Acta Cytol* 35:605, 1991.

26. Evans WP, Cade SH: Needle localization and fine-needle aspiration biopsy of nonpalpable breast lesions with use of standard and stereotactic equipment, *Radiology* 173:53, 1989.

27. Flowers JL, Burton GV, Cox EB, et al: Use of monoclonal antiestrogen receptor antibody to evaluate estrogen receptor content in fine needle aspiration breast biopsies, *Ann Surg* 203:250, 1986.

28. Fornage BD, Faroux MJ, Simatos A: Breast masses: US-guided fine-needle aspiration biopsy, *Radiology* 162:409, 1987.

29. Gent HJ, Sprenger E, Dowlatshahi K: Stereotaxic needle localization and cytological diagnosis of occult breast lesions, *Ann Surg* 204:580, 1986.

30. Hann L, Ducatman BS, Wang HH, et al: Nonpalpable breast lesions: evaluation by means of fine-needle aspiration cytology, *Radiology* 171:373, 1989.

31. Jackson VP, Bassett LW: Stereotactic fine-needle aspiration biopsy for nonpalpable breast lesions, *Am J Radiol* 154:1196, 1990.

32. Johnson TL, Kini SR: Cytologic and clinicopathologic features of abnormal nipple secretions: 225 cases, *Diagn Cytopathol* 7:17, 1991.

33. Katz RL, Patel S, Sneige N, et al: Comparison of immunocytochemical and biochemical assays for estrogen receptor in fine needle aspirates and histologic sections from breast carcinomas, *Breast Cancer Res Treat* 15:191, 1990.

34. Keebler C: *Cytopreparatory techniques*. In Bibbo M, editor: *Comprehensive cytopathology*, Philadelphia, 1991, WB Saunders.

35. Keshgegian AA, Inverso K, Kline TS: Determination of estrogen receptor by monoclonal antireceptor antibody in aspiration biopsy cytology from breast carcinoma, *Am J Clin Pathol* 89:24, 1988.

36. Klemi PJ, Joensuu H: Comparison of DNA ploidy in routine fine needle aspiration samples and paraffin-embedded tissue samples, *Anal Quant Cytol Histol* 10:195, 1988.

37. Kline TS, Kline IK: *Guides to clinical aspiration biopsy: breast*, New York, 1989, Igaku-Shoin.

38. Kopans DB: Fine-needle aspiration of clinically occult breast lesions, *Radiology* 170:313, 1989.

39. Layfield LJ, Parkinson B, Wong J, et al: Mammographically guided fine-needle aspiration biopsy of nonpalpable breast lesions. Can it replace open biopsy? *Cancer* 68:2007, 1991.

40. Lofgren M, Andersson I, Lindholm K: Stereotactic fine-needle aspiration for cytologic diagnosis of nonpalpable breast lesions, *AJR* 154:1191, 1990.

41. Lofgren M, Anderson I, Bondeson L, et al: X-ray guided fine-needle aspiration for the cytologic diagnosis of nonpalpable breast lesions, *Cancer* 61:1032, 1988.

42. Lozowski M, Greene GL, Sadri D, et al: The use of fine needle aspirates in the evaluation of progesterone receptor content in breast cancer, *Acta Cytol* 34:27, 1990.

43. Ljung B: *Fine needle aspiration cytology of the breast*. In Astarita RW, editor: *Practical cytopathology*, New York, 1990, Churchill Livingstone.

44. Lundy J, Lozowski M, Sadri D, et al: The use of fine needle aspirates of breast cancers to evaluate hormone receptor status, *Arch Surg* 125:174, 1990.

45. Marshall CJ, Schuman GB, Ward JH, et al: Cytologic identification of clinically occult proliferative breast disease in women with a family history of breast cancer, *Am J Clin Pathol* 95:157, 1991.

46. Martin AW, Davey DD: C-erbB-2 oncogene expression in breast adenocarcinomas: a comparison of fine needle aspirates and tissue sections, *Acta Cytol* 34:730, 1990.

47. Masood S: Use of monoclonal antibody for assessment of estrogen receptor content in fine-needle aspiration biopsy specimen from patients with breast cancer, *Arch Pathol Lab Med* 113:26, 1989.

48. Masood S: Estrogen and progesterone receptors in cytology: A comprehensive review, *Diagn Cytopathol* 8:475, 1992.

49. Masood S: *Sex steroid hormone receptors in cytologic material*. In Schmidt WA and others, editors: *Cytopathology annual 1992*, Baltimore, 1992, Williams & Wilkins.

50. Masood S, Frykberg ER, McLellan GL, et al: Prospective evaluation of radiologically directed fine-needle aspiration biopsy of nonpalpable breast lesions, *Cancer* 66:1480, 1990.

51. Oertel YC: *Fine needle aspiration of the breast*, Boston, 1987, Butterworths.

52. Pennes DR, Naylor B, Rebner M: Fine needle aspiration biopsy of the breast: influence of the number of passes and the sample size on the diagnostic yield, *Acta Cytol* 34:673, 1990.

53. Ramzy I: *Clinical cytopathology and aspiration biopsy*, Norwalk, Conn, 1990, Appleton & Lange.

54. Reiner A, Reiner G, Spona J, et al: Estrogen receptor immunocytochemistry for preoperative determination of estrogen receptor status on fine-needle aspirates of breast cancer, *Am J Clin Pathol* 88:399, 1987.

55. Remvikos Y, Magdelenat H, Zajdela A: DNA flow cytometry applied to fine needle sampling of human breast cancer, *Cancer* 61:1629, 1988.

56. Takeda T, Matsui A, Sato Y, et al: Nipple discharge cytology in mass screening for breast cancer, *Acta Cytol* 34:161, 1990.

57. Zajdela A, Zillhardt P, Voillemot N: Cytological diagnosis by fine needle sampling without aspiration, *Cancer* 59:1201, 1987.

Interpretation of fine-needle aspirate specimens

58. Abendroth CS, Wang HH, Ducatman BS: Comparative features of carcinoma in situ and typical ductal hyperplasia of the breast on fine-needle aspiration biopsy specimens, *Am J Clin Pathol* 96:654, 1991.

59. Bibbo M, Scheiber M, Cajulis R, et al: Stereotaxic fine needle aspiration cytology of clinically occult malignant and premalignant breast lesions, *Acta Cytol* 32:193, 1988.

60. Bondeson L: Aspiration cytology of radiation-induced changes of normal breast epithelium, *Acta Cytol* 31:309, 1987.

61. Bondeson L, Lindholm K: Aspiration cytology of tubular breast carcinoma, *Acta Cytol* 34:15, 1990.

62. Bottles K, Chan JS, Holly EA, et al: Cytologic criteria for fibroadenoma: a step-wise logistic regression analysis, *Am J Clin Pathol* 89:707, 1988.

63. Dawson AE, Mulford DK, Dvoretsky PM, et al: Aspiration cytology of tubular carcinomas: diagnostic features with mammographic correlation, *Acta Cytol* 34:713, 1990.

64. Duane GB, Kanter MH, Branigan T, et al: A morphologic and morphometric study of cells from colloid carcinoma of the breast obtained by fine needle aspiration: distinction from other breast lesions, *Acta Cytol* 31:742, 1987.

65. Dusenbery D, Frable WJ: Fine needle aspiration cytology of phyllodes tumor: Potential diagnostic pitfalls. *Acta Cytol* 36:215, 1992.

66. Filomena CA, Jordan AG, and Ehya H: Needle aspiration cytology of the irradiated breast, *Diagn Cytopathol* 8:327, 1992.

67. Galblum LI, Oertel YC: Subareolar abscess of the breast: diagnosis by fine-needle aspiration, *Am J Clin Pathol* 80:496, 1983.

68. Grenko RT, Lee KP, Lee KR: Fine needle aspiration cytology of lactating adenoma of the breast: a comparative light microscopic and morphometric study, *Acta Cytol* 34:21, 1990.

69. Howell LP, Kline TS: Medullary carcinoma of the breast: an unusual cytologic finding in cyst fluid aspirates, *Cancer* 65:277, 1990.

70. Johnson TL, Kini SR: The significance of atypical apocrine cells in fine needle aspirates of the breast, *Acta Cytol* 32:785, 1988.

71. Kline TS, Kannan V: Papillary carcinoma of the breast: a cytomorphologic analysis, *Arch Pathol Lab Med* 110:189, 1986.

72. Kline TS, Kannan V, Kline IK: Appraisal and cytomorphologic analysis of common carcinomas of the breast, *Diagn Cytopathol* 1:188, 1985.

73. Koss LG: *Diagnostic cytology and its histopathologic bases*, ed 4, Philadelphia, 1992, JB Lippincott.

74. Ku NNK, Mela NJ, Cox CE, et al: Diagnostic pitfalls in aspiration biopsy cytology of papillary breast lesions, *Acta Cytol* 35:612, 1991.

75. Leach C, Howell LP: Cytodiagnosis of classic lobular carcinoma and its variants, *Acta Cytol* 36:199, 1992.

76. Lilleng R, Hagmar BM, Farrants G: Low-grade cribriform ductal carcinoma in situ of the breast: fine needle aspiration cytology in three cases. *Acta Cytol* 36:48, 1992.

77. Lilleng R, Hagmar B: The comedo subtype of intraductal carcinoma: Cytologic characteristics, *Acta Cytol* 36:345, 1992.

78. Lowhagen T, Rubio CA: The cytology of the granular cell myoblastoma of the breast: report of a case, *Acta Cytol* 21:314, 1977.

79. Mazzara PF, Flint A, Naylor B: Adenoma of the nipple: cytopathologic features, *Acta Cytol* 33:188, 1989.

80. Novotny NB, Maygarden SJ, Shermer RW, et al: Fine needle aspiration of benign and malignant breast masses associated with pregnancy, *Acta Cytol* 35:676, 1991.

81. Peterse JL, Thunnissen FBJM, van Heerde P: Fine needle aspiration cytology of radiation-induced changes in nonneoplastic breast lesions: possible pitfalls in cytodiagnosis, *Acta Cytol* 33:176, 1989.

82. Peterse JL, Koolman-Schellekens MA, van de Peppel-van de Ham T, et al: Atypia in fine-needle aspiration cytology of the breast: a histologic follow-up study of 301 cases, *Semin Diagn Pathol* 6:126, 1989.

83. Pinedo F, Vargas J, de Agustín P, et al: Epithelial atypia in gynecomastia induced by chemotherapeutic drugs, *Acta Cytol* 35:229, 1991.

84. Rao CR, Narasimhamurthy NK, Jaganathan K, et al: Cystosarcoma phyllodes: Diagnosis by fine needle aspiration cytology, *Acta Cytol* 36:203, 1992.

85. Rogers LA, Lee KR: Breast carcinoma simulating fibroadenoma or fibrocystic change by fine-needle aspiration: A study of 16 cases, *Am J Clin Pathol* 98:155, 1992.

86. Salhany KE, Page DL: Fine-needle aspiration of mammary lobular carcinoma in situ and atypical lobular hyperplasia, *Am J Clin Pathol* 92:22, 1989.

87. Silverman JF: *Breast.* In Bibbo M, editor: *Comprehensive cytopathology*, Philadelphia, 1991, WB Saunders.

88. Silverman JF, Geisinger KR, Frable WF: Fine-needle aspiration cytology of mesenchymal tumors of the breast, *Diagn Cytopathol* 4:50, 1988.

89. Silverman JF, Feldman PS, Covell JL, et al: Fine needle aspiration cytology of neoplasms metastatic to the breast, *Acta Cytol* 31:291, 1987.

90. Simi U, Moretti D, Iacconi P, et al: Fine needle aspiration cytopathology of phyllodes tumor: differential diagnosis with fibroadenoma, *Acta Cytol* 32:63, 1988.

91. Sneige N: *Current issues in fine needle aspiration of the breast: cytologic features of in situ lobular and ductal carcinomas and clinical implications of nuclear grading.* In Schmidt WA and others, editors: *Cytopathology annual 1992*, Baltimore, 1992, Williams & Wilkins.

92. Tabbara SO, Mesonero C, Sidawy MK: Ductal adenoma: a potential pitfall in fine needle aspiration of the breast, *Acta Cytol* 35:610, 1991.

93. Wang HH, Ducatman BS, Eick D: Comparative features of ductal carcinoma in situ and infiltrating ductal carcinoma of the breast on fine-needle aspiration biopsy, *Am J Clin Pathol* 92:736, 1989.

94. Wilson SL, Ehrmann RL: The cytologic diagnosis of breast aspirations, *Acta Cytol* 22:470, 1978.

Results of fine-needle aspiration

95. Cohen MB, Rodgers RP, Hales MS, et al: Influence of training and experience in fine-needle aspiration biopsy of breast, *Arch Pathol Lab Med* 111:518, 1987.

96. Deschênes L, Fabia J, Meisels A, et al: Fine needle aspiration biopsy in the management of palpable breast lesions, *Can J Surg* 21:417, 1978.

97. Eisenberg AJ, Hajdu SI, Wilhelmus J, et al: Preoperative aspiration cytology of breast tumors, *Acta Cytol* 30:135, 1986.

98. Feldman PS, Covell JL: *Fine needle aspiration cytology and its clinical applications: breast and lung*, Chicago, 1985, American Society of Clinical Pathologist Press.

99. Fessia L, Botta G, Arisio R, et al: Fine-needle aspiration of breast lesions: role and accuracy in a review of 7495 cases, *Diagn Cytopathol* 3:121, 1987.

100. Giard RWM, Hermans J: The value of aspiration cytologic examination of the breast: A statistical review of the medical literature, *Cancer* 69:2104, 1992.

102. Gupta RK, Dowle CS, Simpson JS: The value of needle aspiration cytology of the breast, with an emphasis on the diagnosis of breast disease in young women below the age of 30, *Acta Cytol* 34:165, 1990.

103. Halevy A, Reif R, Bogokovsky H, et al: Diagnosis of carcinoma of the breast by fine needle aspiration cytology, *Surg Gynecol Obstet* 164:506, 1987.

104. Kline TS, Joshi LP, Neal HS: Fine-needle aspiration of the breast: diagnoses and pitfalls: a review of 3545 cases, *Cancer* 44:1458, 1979.

105. Lamb J, Anderson TJ: Influence of cancer histology on the success of fine needle aspiration of the breast, *J Clin Pathol* 42:733, 1989.

106. Layfield LJ, Glasgow BJ, Cramer H: Fine-needle aspiration in the management of breast masses, *Pathol Annu* 24:23, 1989.

107. Lee KR, Foster RS, Papillo JL: Fine needle aspiration of the breast: importance of the aspirator, *Acta Cytol* 31:281, 1987.

108. Palombini L, Fulciniti F, Vetrani A, et al: Fine-needle aspiration biopsies of breast masses: a critical analysis of 1956 cases in 8 years (1976–1984), *Cancer* 61:2273, 1988.

109. Zajdela A, Ghossein NA, Pilleron JP, et al: The value of aspiration cytology in the diagnosis of breast cancer: experience at the Foundation Curie, *Cancer* 35:499, 1975.

110. Zajicek J, Caspersson T, Jakobsson P, et al: Cytologic diagnosis of mammary tumors from aspiration biopsy smears: comparison of cytologic and histologic findings in 2111 lesions and diagnostic use of cytophotometry, *Acta Cytol* 14:370, 1970.

111. Zarbo RJ, Howanitz PJ, Bachner P: Interinstitutional comparison of performance in breast fine-needle aspiration cytology, *Arch Pathol Lab Med* 115:743, 1991.

Additional readings

Frable WJ: Needle aspiration biopsy: past, present, and future, *Hum Pathol* 20:504, 1989.

Frable WJ: *Thin-needle aspiration biopsy.* In Bennington JL, editor: *Major problems in pathology,* vol 14, Philadelphia, 1983, WB Saunders.

Hammond S, Keyhani-Rofagha S, O'Toole RV: Statistical analysis of fine needle aspiration cytology of the breast: a review of 678 cases plus 4265 cases from the literature, *Acta Cytol* 31:276, 1987.

Kahky MP, Rone VR, Duncan DL, et al: Needle aspiration biopsy of palpable breast masses, *Am J Surg* 156:450: 1988.

Knight DC, Lowell DM, Heimann A, et al: Aspiration of the breast and nipple discharge cytology, *Surg Gynecol Obstet* 163:415, 1986.

Linsk JA, Franzen S: *Clinical aspiration cytology,* Philadelphia, 1983, JB Lippincott.

Schondorf H: *Aspiration cytology of the breast,* Philadelphia, 1978, WB Saunders.

Strawbridge HTG, Bassett AA, Foldes I: Role of cytology in management of lesions of the breast, *Surg Gynecol Obstet* 152:1, 1981.

Preoperative Mammographic Localization of Nonpalpable Breast Lesions

Carol B. Stelling

Mammographically directed preoperative localization of nonpalpable breast lesions, a common procedure, will continue to be utilized for accurate diagnosis of nonpalpable mammographic lesions, particularly microcalcifications. The basic concept of placing an internal marker to direct a surgical biopsy has not changed over the past 15 years, but technical advances now permit more accurate localization. This chapter discusses the indications for performing and for cancelling the procedure. A brief historical survey of the mammographic techniques that have developed is followed by a detailed protocol to achieve successful localization and excision of nonpalpable mammographic abnormalities. The multidisciplinary team approach is emphasized. A review of the literature documents trends in cancer yield (positive predictive value). The last section presents pitfalls that may be encountered in the procedure.

Specimen radiography and handling of the tissue in the surgical pathology laboratory are discussed in Chapter 8. The reader is strongly encouraged to read this additional section in detail because many pitfalls in accurate tissue diagnosis (i.e., lack of orientation, question of free margins, calcium loss, or failure to include diagnostic areas on permanent section) may occur after the tissue is excised. Localization also may be

accomplished by guidance with ultrasonography or computed tomographic (CT) scan. These approaches are discussed in Chapter 3.

INDICATIONS FOR PERFORMING A LOCALIZATION PROCEDURE

There are well-established radiographic criteria for recommending a preoperative localization procedure and biopsy for a mammographic abnormality (Box 7-1).[6] The yield for cancer from such a biopsy is a function of the degree of radiographic suspicion and the age of the patient.[2] In addition to these well-recognized radiographic criteria for recommending a preoperative localization, there are several special circumstances that may justify this procedure (Box 7-2).

In a busy mammographic practice, there are occasional patients who, because of extreme anxiety, often due to cancerphobia, insist on excision of a nonpalpable mammographic abnormality that is not considered suspicious. The radiologist may be able to assuage the patient's anxiety after a one-to-one consultation and explanation of her mammographic findings. This is preferable to performing a biopsy that is not indicated. Despite such personal reassurance, the woman or her physician may insist on a biopsy, particularly if the level of anxiety generated by follow-up mammography is

BOX 7-1 INDICATIONS FOR PREOPERATIVE LOCALIZATION OF NONPALPABLE BREAST LESIONS

Calcifications without a mass
    Suspicious microcalcifications
    Indeterminate cluster[3-5]

Masses
    Spiculated with or without calcifications
    Knobby or lobulated
    Ill defined or fuzzy margins
    Masses solid by ultrasonography ≥ 1 cm^2
    Solid mass increasing in size
    Parenchymal distortion
    New density[1,5]

Focal asymmetric density (not asymmetric parenchyma)

Single dilated duct[5,8]—if associated with spontaneous discharge a galactogram may also be done

BOX 7-2 SPECIAL CIRCUMSTANCES FOR PREOPERATIVE LOCALIZATION

Nonpalpable radiographic abnormality of low probability for cancer in an anxious patient

Palpable lesion not easily felt in supine position

Direction of diagnostic biopsy of nonpalpable lesion adjacent to palpable lesion (i.e., intramammary lymph node, calcification, or multicentric mass)

considered intolerable, given her personal health profile (personal history of breast cancer, strong family history of breast cancer, or mental condition). Every center has a few localizations that are "overkill," but it is best to keep these to a minimum. Open and frank communication with the referring physician and surgeon is essential. A clearly worded mammographic report with specific recommendations will deter ambiguous recommendations for biopsy and resultant patient anxiety.

An unusual but necessary situation that requires a preoperative localization procedure is the woman with a mass or thickening palpable in the sitting position but not palpable in the supine position. For surgical excision, a mass must also be palpable in the supine position. Infiltration of the tissues with local anesthetic can obscure palpation of vague masses or areas of thickening. If the surgeon judges that the mass will be difficult to locate in the supine position, he or she may request a preoperative localization. These circumstances are infrequent but almost invariably involve the upper half of the breast tissue (i.e., cephalad to the mid-nipple level). These lesions may be easy to palpate in a pendulous breast with the patient sitting and with the examiner using both hands to sandwich the lesion between the opposing fingers, but quite difficult to feel in a supine position (Fig. 7-1).

Another indication for a preoperative localization procedure is to direct adequate excision of nonpalpable suspicious lesions adjacent to an obviously palpable lesion. An example would be to include an enlarged intramammary lymph node or a focus of microcalcification that lies within a few centimeters of an obvious cancer, for example, to direct a complete and adequate excision (Fig. 7-2). The use of two needles to bracket a lesion for lumpectomy is particularly helpful if the area encompassed is several centimeters in length, as is the case with some comedocarcinomas involving a branching duct segment (Fig. 7-3).[7]

INDICATIONS FOR CANCELLING A LOCALIZATION PROCEDURE

Not only must a mammographic consultation clearly determine which patients merit a recommendation for preoperative localization and biopsy, but also the radiologist must be as clear in excluding those patients who do not require localization procedures. The best way to prevent an unnecessary preoperative localization is to require that the mammograms be previewed by the mammographer before scheduling the procedure to determine if sufficient criteria are present to justify the biopsy.[13] If additional problem-solving maneuvers are required such as true lateral views (to triangulate the lesion), skin calcium localization (to differentiate benign skin calcifications from parenchymal clusters), or breast ultrasonography (to detect cystic versus solid mass), these techniques can be performed before scheduling the localization. These maneuvers are somewhat time-consuming, but if the results indicate a low level of suspicion for cancer, the patient has been spared unnecessary biopsy and anxiety.

In our experience of nearly 15 years of performing preoperative localizations there are sev-

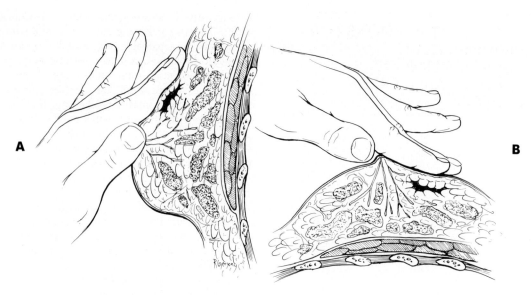

Fig. 7-1 Mass in the upper breast may be palpable with the patient sitting **(A)** but difficult to feel in the supine position **(B).** A preoperative localization procedure may be needed.

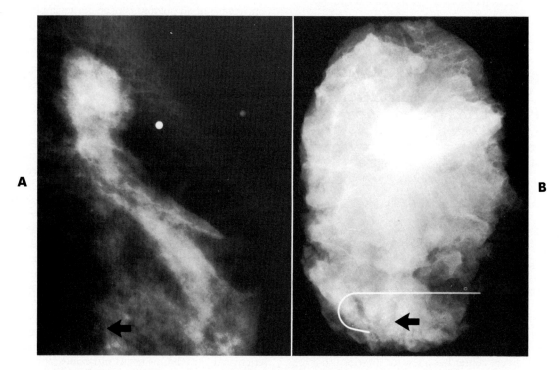

Fig. 7-2 A, A small focus of microcalcifications *(arrow)* was detected within 5 cm of a palpable carcinoma. **B,** The calcifications were included in the lumpectomy specimen with preoperative wire guidance *(arrow).* The pathologic diagnosis was invasive ductal carcinoma (palpable mass) and incidental focus of sclerosing adenosis (calcifications).

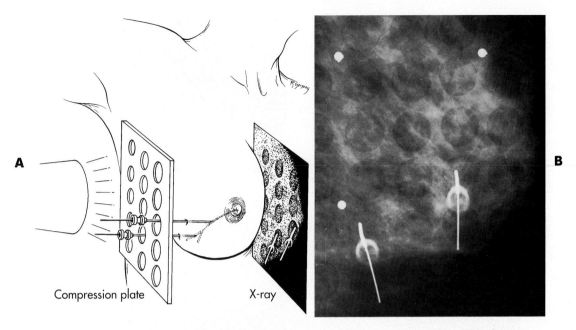

Fig. 7-3 A, To monitor complete excision of suspicious calcifications in a segmental distribution, two needles with wires may be placed to bracket the lesion. **B,** Lateral radiograph showing two needles with wires on end.

BOX 7-3 INDICATIONS FOR CANCELLING PREOPERATIVE LOCALIZATION

Lesion not confirmed	Pseudomass Artifacts (deodorant, adhesive tape)
Lesion not suspicious	Superficial skin lesion Normal structure Benign lesions
Lesion resolved	Ruptured cyst Resolved abscess or hematoma
Lesion palpable in retrospect	Targeted physical examination
Patient factors	Failure to keep appointment Preoperative medications given Anxiety reaction Nonfasting state Unstable medical condition

eral circumstances that are indications for cancelling the procedure (Box 7-3). The pseudomass is a "lesion" apparent in one projection but not confirmed in a projection orthogonal to the first (Fig. 7-4). These densities are caused by a band of normal tissue "telescoped" or projected upon itself in one view only. Additional views fail to confirm the abnormality. Most cases of pseudomass are easily recognized, and it is infrequent that such a case will be scheduled for preoperative localization. The requirement that all mammograms be previewed before scheduling of localization procedure will prevent inappropriate scheduling of a "pseudomass" for excisional biopsy.

Similarly, a critical preview of "abnormal" mammograms may suggest that problem-solving maneuvers such as focal coned compression with magnification or specially tailored views can resolve the "suspicious" area to a normal structure or benign condition that does not merit biopsy (Box 7-4). In our practice we have had women present with "abnormal" mammograms who had a nevus, milk of calcium, and benign skin calcifications.[9,11] Most radiologists are now familiar with the notched appearance of the fatty hilum seen with normal intramammary lymph nodes.

Another normal structure that must not be misinterpreted is the medial insertion of the pectoral muscle that may on occasion simulate a mass in

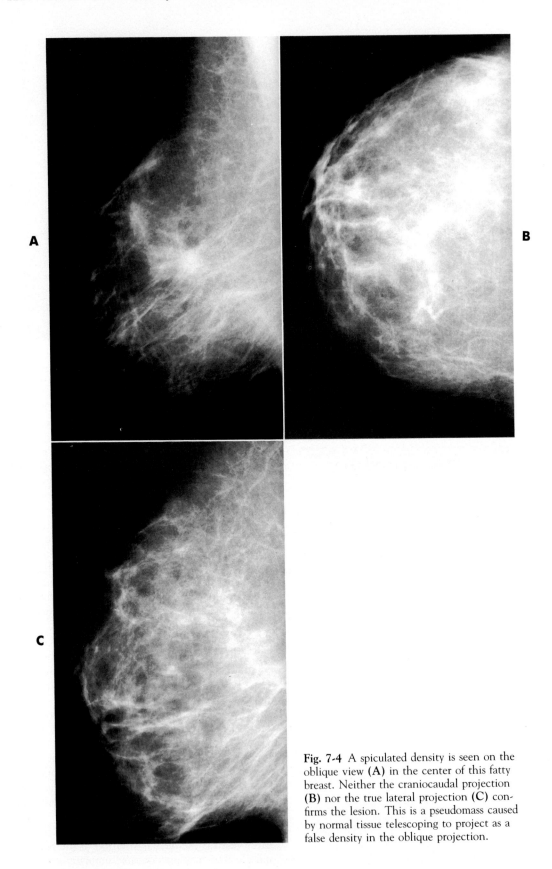

Fig. 7-4 A spiculated density is seen on the oblique view **(A)** in the center of this fatty breast. Neither the craniocaudal projection **(B)** nor the true lateral projection **(C)** confirms the lesion. This is a pseudomass caused by normal tissue telescoping to project as a false density in the oblique projection.

BOX 7-4 MAMMOGRAPHIC "LESIONS" THAT DO NOT MERIT BIOPSY

Superficial skin lesion	Mole, keloid, skin calcifications, sebaceous cyst
Normal structures	Intramammary node Looping vein Medial pectoral muscle insertion
Lesions with low suspicion	Peripheral calcifications of fibroadenoma Stable "benign" mass Vascular calcifications Milk of calcium Asymmetric parenchyma without distortion or palpable abnormalities Mass proven cystic by ultrasonography

the medial breast on the craniocaudal view (Fig. 7-5).[10] Demonstration of continuity of muscle fibers on a craniocaudal view will confirm the pectoral muscle as the cause of this "mass." Craniocaudal positioning, exaggerated for the medial breast, may be required. With dedicated equipment the experienced technologist may include the pectoral muscle on the craniocaudal views more often than in the past.

Not only may old mammograms confirm the benign nature of an intramammary lymph node or a medial pectoral muscle insertion, but old films may also confirm that a mammographic lesion has been stable in appearance for 2 or more years. This type of additional information most often leads to a decision to observe a lesion. Caution necessitates continued surveillance of benign masses because cases of carcinoma that are slow to change radiographically have been reported.[12] Data concerning outcome of the decision to perform a biopsy or to observe a lesion should be part of a professional quality assurance program of a mammography practice.[14]

It is also possible that a lesion may resolve over

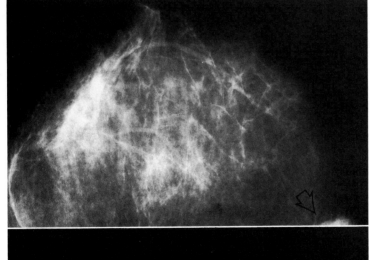
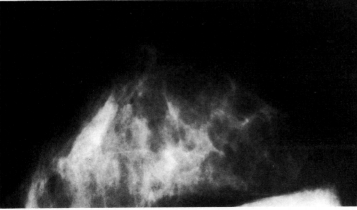

Fig. 7-5 On the craniocaudal projection (**A**), the medial pectoral muscle may project as a rounded soft-tissue density *(arrow)*. This should not be misinterpreted as an abnormality. Additional views may show confluence with the more central muscle fibers (**B**).

the several weeks between detection and preoperative localization procedure. Such a scenario might suggest a rupture or aspiration of a cyst, a resolved hematoma or treated abscess, or an artifact.[15]

Another strong indication for cancelling the preoperative localization is the discovery that the mammographic lesion is palpable. It is usually the domain of the surgeon to decide which abnormalities require preoperative localization and which are palpable. However, in a busy clinical practice, miscommunication may result in the occasional scheduling of a palpable mass for preoperative localization. If the radiologist feels that the localization procedure is not required, then the surgical team should be consulted. For masses that manifest only as slight asymmetric thickening, the localization procedure is usually performed since infiltration of the area with local anesthetic may make a barely palpable lesion become nonpalpable.

Lastly, a cooperative patient in good condition is an obvious requirement for completing a successful localization procedure and surgical excision of a suspicious lesion. Procedures for patients who have received excessive preoperative medications, are nonfasting, have an unstable medical condition, or have an acute anxiety reaction should be cancelled and rescheduled with correction of the problem or condition.

REVIEW OF DEVELOPMENT OF MAMMOGRAPHIC LOCALIZATION TECHNIQUES

Since the 1960s the preoperative localization techniques in the breast have progressed from quadrantectomy to sophisticated needle and wire placement using freehand, template, or stereotaxic guidance.[16–19]

Spot localization

The use of a colored dye to mark nonpalpable breast lesions was first described by Simon in 1972.[22] This was a modification of a technique originally used in the 1940s to localize lung abscesses. The technique requires transfer of coordinate measurements from the mammogram to the compressed breast and placement of a straight needle to the correct depth. Postplacement craniocaudal and mediolateral films are used to verify the relationship of the lesion to the needle tip and permit repositioning as needed. A solution of equal parts of colored dye and radiopaque contrast material is injected in a small quantity (0.1 ml) through a small (tuberculin) syringe. Repeat mammograms are reviewed with the surgeon to direct excision of the lesion. It is recommended that the biopsy follow within 4 hours of the injection since

there is diffusion of dye within the tissues. This technique is easy to perform and gives good results.[16,21] Blue dyes that have been used for spot localization include Evans blue, sky blue,[21] toluidine blue, and methylene blue.[20] When a prolonged interval between radiographic localization and surgical excision is anticipated, toluidine blue or a sterile aqueous suspension of carbon powder is recommended.[20,23]

Freehand localization

During the 1970s and early 1980s it became commonplace for the preoperative localization device, whether needle, wire, or a combination, to be placed using a freehand approach.[29] This approach is still used in some centers and is particularly useful for some lesions in the inferior breast.[17] Location of the lesion from craniocaudal and true lateral mammographic images is transferred to skin coordinates by measuring distances from the center of the nipple. The coordinates are transferred to the breast skin surface, which may be compressed manually to simulate the compression achieved during roentgenographic exposure, thereby improving accuracy. Either a linear or an arc method can be used to transfer the coordinates to the breast.[24,27] The needle may be placed perpendicular to the chest wall so that compression during postlocalization films in the craniocaudal and lateral projections does not interfere with the protruding hub.[28] Some lesions are approached using the arc method with the needle perpendicular to the skin, particularly if this is the shortest distance (Fig. 7-6).

If the patient is supine during placement of the needle, caution must be used to avoid placing the needle into the pectoral muscle[26] or the pleural cavity.[25] It is recommended that the breast be lifted away from the chest wall. Alternatively, it is possible to place the needle perpendicular to the chest wall with the patient seated. This helps keep the lesion away from the chest wall, allowing a safer placement of the needle. In the sitting position a pendulous contour of the breast may distort the skin coordinates. Adjustment can be accomplished by taking coordinate measurements from the mid-nipple axis on the lateral projection.[27]

The freehand method is still performed wherever template localization devices are not available and is the approach preferred by some surgeons. It may also be adapted to localize a lesion in a retroareolar area where angling of the localization device is needed to avoid placing a needle through the sensitive areolar skin. Moreover, some mammography units do not allow template guidance of needle placement from a caudal approach. The radiologist may then elect to do a

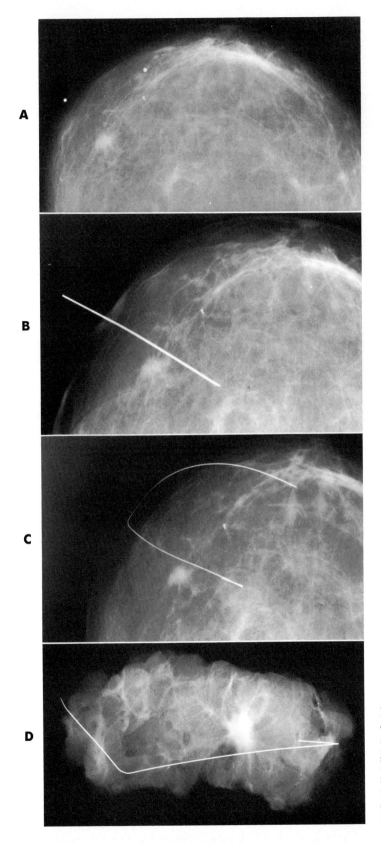

Fig. 7-6 A freehand localization procedure may be used for selected cases. **A,** Two skin markers were used to judge the preferred entry point. **B,** Needle placed perpendicular to the skin (arc method). **C,** Wire placement confirmed. **D,** Specimen x-ray confirms successful excision of spiculated carcinoma.

freehand placement from the inferior breast[17] or approach the lesion from the lateral or medial side using a template for guidance.

Template guidance

In 1974 a device for more precise needle placement for biopsy or preoperative localization was reported from Sweden.[32] This compression device was affixed to a standard mammographic unit and contained 70 holes, 7 mm in diameter, marked by a coordinate system of engraved letters. Additional reports from Sweden and modifications reported in the United States[31,33] spurred interest in the use of templates with perforations or a rectangular coordinate system. Such localization devices are now commercially available with most mammography units.

Such a guidance system improves the accuracy of wire and needle placement as compared with a freehand method.[34] With the freehand method it was not uncommon for the needle to be 1.0 to 1.5 cm from the lesion. This was considered adequate, particularly in a large breast. A template-guided procedure requires less repositioning than the freehand method, and in expert hands the wire and needle has been reported to transfix the lesion or lie within 2 mm in as many as 96% of cases.[30] The use of a template guide permits the needle to be inserted parallel to the chest wall and is therefore safer than freehand placement of a needle perpendicular to the chest wall.

Stereotaxic needle guidance

With the development of stereotaxic devices, reports of needle localization by stereotaxis have begun to appear. Major advocates of stereotaxis are exploring the accuracy of fine-needle aspiration cytology and needle core biopsy for histologic diagnosis via stereotaxic-guided needle placement. Additional references concerning stereotaxic-guided core biopsy and fine-needle aspiration cytology are listed at the end of this chapter under Suggested Readings.

The original prototype was developed in Sweden at the Karolinska Institute.[35] With this very sophisticated instrument, a sampling precision of ± 1 mm is possible in 90 percent of patients.[39] Failures occurred in patients when the lesion was too close to the chest wall, the breast was too small to be held firmly by the compression unit, the lesion had resolved, or the needle tip was deviated because of firm encapsulated tumor such as fibroadenoma.

A more recent study by Dowlatshahi and others reports localization within 2 mm in 90% of patients using this stereotaxic mammography unit.[37] The authors have performed 528 such localizations and emphasize that a single target point

must be selected in the lesion toward which the needle can be aimed. Even with this precise equipment the success of fine-needle aspirates was very operator dependent. Others have not been able to reproduce this accuracy of preoperative localization.[40] The hook may not be as close to the lesion as anticipated once the compression is released.

Less expensive devices have been devised to attach to existing standard mammography units.[36,38] The need for a redesign of the standard mammography unit to permit the tube to pivot relative to the film holders has been suggested to permit stereotaxic procedures without purchase of a supplementary device.[41]

In any case, the interest in stereotaxis arises not so much to improve localization accuracy for excisional biopsy but to permit nonoperative tissue diagnosis. The technique, advantages, and disadvantages of fine-needle aspiration cytology are discussed in Chapter 6. The clinical role of stereotaxic-guided fine needle aspiration cytology and needle core biopsy of mammographic abnormalities is rapidly developing. Refining the criteria for the procedures and cost benefit analysis is expected. Meanwhile it is expected that wire and needle localization procedures will continue to be performed in North America, particularly in facilities of moderate size.

PREOPERATIVE MAMMOGRAPHIC LOCALIZATION PROCEDURE: A PROTOCOL

No where is the concept of the multidisciplinary breast team approach more important than in wire directed biopsy of clinically occult mammographic lesions. Responsibility for different phases of this multistep procedure rests separately with the radiologist, surgeon and surgical pathologist. Overall coordination, however, usually depends upon the radiologist to ensure successful diagnosis.

This section provides a step-by-step description of the preoperative wire and needle localization procedure, including modifications recommended for special situations. At our institution we recognize three phases including eight separate steps in the process (Box 7-5). The first four steps and the sixth and eighth steps are discussed in this chapter. Step 5, which covers the biopsy procedure itself, is discussed in Chapter 5 and includes placement of the biopsy incision and orientation of the specimen for the pathologist. Step 7, processing the tissue, includes handling the specimen—for example, inking the margins—correlation of gross appearance, and indications for doing a frozen section or recuts. This step is presented in Chapter 8. Close cooperation of the breast team is essential for accurate diagnosis.

Step 1. Review the case

A review of the mammograms is the initial step in preparation for a localization procedure. In fact, this review is best performed when the recommendation for the localization procedure is generated. One should be confident that the lesion is suspicious enough to warrant biopsy, that it is not palpable, and that its location has been confirmed in two orthogonal views. It may be desirable to obtain a true lateral view at this time (orthogonal to a craniocaudal projection) to estimate lesion depth. It is useful to have the true lateral view before the localization procedure in order to select the needle and wire length and to plan direction of approach.[44] We usually tape a skin marker over the lesion as determined by the craniocaudal projection. From the true lateral projection we are able to measure depth of the lesion from the skin surface (denoted by skin marker) (Fig. 7-7). This maneuver is particularly helpful for lesions in the upper inner quadrant because the oblique projection may overestimate the depth of the lesion (Fig. 7-8). The technologist should take the appropriate true lateral projection with the lesion closest to the receptor (e.g., for a medial lesion, the projection is lateral to medial and for a lateral lesion the film is placed on the lateral side).

A review of prior mammograms is essential when the patient has had mammograms at another location. It is not uncommon for the biopsy to be cancelled if the review or additional problem-solving views confirm a benign condition such as an intramammary lymph node, a cluster of skin calcifications, or milk of calcium. It is advisable to review the case before scheduling the biopsy because once the patient and her surgeon are mentally prepared to proceed, it may be difficult to cancel the procedure.[13]

BOX 7-5 PREOPERATIVE LOCALIZATION PROCEDURE

Phase 1: Mammographic localization

1. Review the case
2. Prepare the patient
3. Place the localization wire and needle
4. Communicate with the team

Phase 2: Surgical excision

5. Remove the specimen
6. Confirm lesion removal (specimen radiography)

Phase 3: Pathologic evaluation

7. Process the tissue
8. Review the pathology

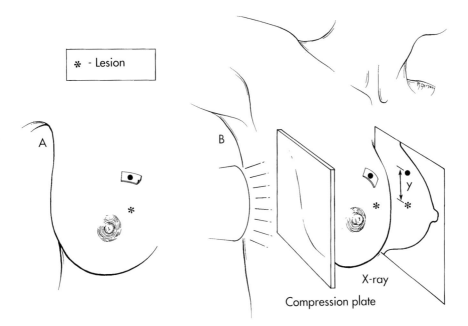

* - Lesion

Fig. 7-7 Use of a skin marker to measure true depth of the lesion. **A,** Skin marker taped to breast over approximate entry point as determined from craniocaudal view. **B,** Lateral projection obtained (film closest to lesion). The distance between the skin marker and the lesion on this projection (y) is the minimal length of needle required for the localization procedure.

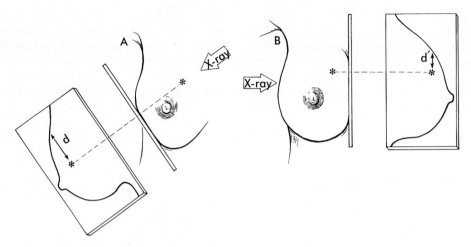

Fig. 7-8 The depth of a lesion in the upper inner quadrant may be overestimated (*d* in **A**) on the oblique projection. A true lateral projection **(B)** is required to judge the true depth (*d'*) of the lesion.

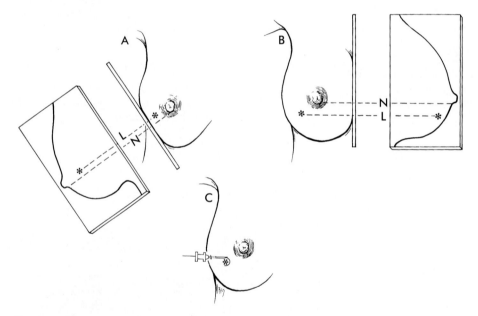

Fig. 7-9 A lesion in the lower outer quadrant of the breast may project superior to the nipple on the oblique view **(A)**, when in fact it lies caudad to the nipple in the true lateral view **(B)**. In the inferior breast, a lateral needle approach is often used **(C)**. L = lesion; N = nipple.

The procedures of preoperative localization and breast biopsy are scheduled by the surgical team and are dependent on availability of operating room time. At our institution an hour is allowed for a localization procedure in the radiology department. If the patient requires a bilateral procedure, we allow 90 minutes.

The mammograms must be available the morning of the procedure. On the day before any needle and wire localizations, we like to confirm that we have the mammograms in hand. Usually, we retain any outside studies in anticipation of this need. At this time, we often draw the lesion on a diagram illustrating the three-dimensional relationship. We plan our approach and select the needle length (Figs. 7-9 to 7-11). This preparation is particularly valuable when the case is difficult or if the radiologist performing the procedure is not familiar with the case. The transposing of the lesion location to a diagram helps prevent in-

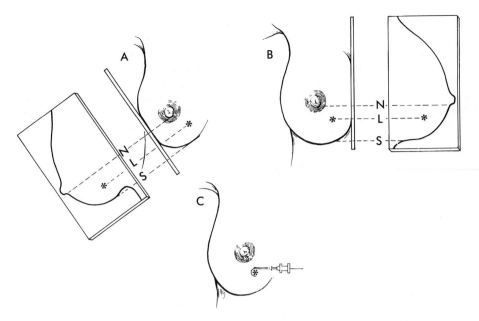

Fig. 7-10 A lesion in the lower inner quadrant of the breast may not change much in position between the oblique **(A)** and lateral **(B)** projections. A medial approach with the localization needle is most often planned **(C)**. L = lesion; N = nipple; S = skin.

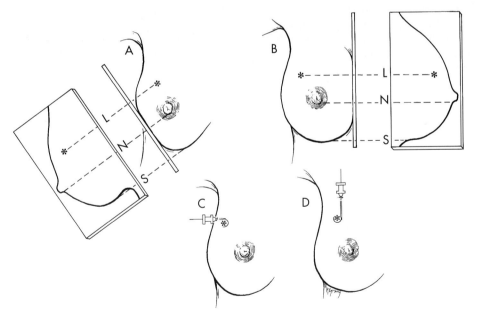

Fig. 7-11 A lesion in the upper outer quadrant will project above the nipple on both the oblique projection **(A)** and the true lateral projection **(B).** One must choose between the lateral approach **(C)** and the craniocaudal approach **(D)** for needle placement. L = lesion; N = nipple; S = skin.

advertent localization in the wrong breast or quadrant.

Step 2. Prepare the patient
It is important to explain the procedure to the patient before placement of the wire and needle.

Ideally, this is accomplished before the day of the biopsy so that she and her family have had an opportunity to ask questions and have all their concerns addressed.

There are several ways in which this preparation can be accomplished. We briefly explain the concept of placing an internal marker to assist the surgeon in locating the lesion when the need for the biopsy is first discussed with the patient. We also provide a form letter explaining the value of preoperative localization so that she and her family can understand the plan *before* talking with the surgical team. By the time the referring physician and surgeon have seen the patient and scheduled the biopsy, the patient and her family understand that the area is nonpalpable and a tissue diagnosis is being considered.

The timing of the biopsy and selection of anesthesia are determined by the surgical team. Preoperative instructions are given. It is important to note here that any medication should not be given to the patient until after the localization procedure has been completed. It is imperative that the patient remain alert and fully cooperative for the localization procedure.

It is not customary to require a separate consent form for the preoperative localization procedure. Any potential complications are largely those of the surgical biopsy and anesthesia and are covered in the surgical consent form.

On the morning of the localization, the patient is reassured that the procedure is simple, relatively painless, and necessary for diagnosis. We begin by explaining that the placement of the needle and wire is about as uncomfortable as a venipuncture. We indicate that in most cases the area of concern may be too small for a frozen-section diagnosis and the final diagnosis will be rendered on the basis of the permanent sections. We tell the family that they will be notified of the diagnosis in 3 or 4 days. This permits sufficient time for histologic recuts and appropriate pathologic consultation for most cases. In fact, most women receive the results in 2 days.

We frequently inform the patient that there is a small failure rate (2% to 3%). The chance of failure is particularly pertinent if the lesion is very deep in a large breast with fatty replacement. For further discussion of the frequency and causes of localization failures, see pages 138–139.

Some might wonder whether we are overeducating the patient about this procedure. It is our philosophy that the patient has a right to know what will happen and what the potential limitations are. Using this approach, we find that our patients for the most part are cooperative and less fearful than if they have been referred for preoperative localization without sufficient explanation. It is always worthwhile to take the extra time to answer the patient's concerns and questions before beginning the localization procedure. In a busy practice it is helpful if the surgical nurse can as-

sist in patient preparation and education. Pamphlets and videotapes are now commercially available that explain the localization procedure in nontechnical terms.

Step 3. Place the localization wire

Planning the approach. The location and depth of the lesion will determine the direction in which the needle and wire are to be placed into the breast tissue. The general rule of thumb is to select an entry point that is closest to the lesion; for example, use the shortest needle and wire possible (Fig. 7-12). Usually, the localizing template is positioned over the cranial, medial, or lateral breast surface. An inferior approach is possible on some mammography units. However, an inferior approach is often awkward for both the patient, who must straddle the tube head, and for the radiologist, who may need to kneel on the floor to insert the needle. For lesions in the inferior breast, an approach from the lateral or medial side is usually performed. A freehand placement of the needle is an alternative for lesions in the inferior breast.[17]

The length of needle and wire required can be estimated from the mammogram. The role of a true lateral mammogram with a skin marker to help judge depth has already been discussed. It is preferable to overestimate the length required. Passage of the needle and wire beyond the lesion is recommended in the fatty breast, where anchoring of the hook is less firm than in the dense breast.[56] A needle and wire that are too short may lead to difficulty in removing the appropriate area. A second longer needle should be placed if the distance between the lesion and the wire is considered unacceptable (more than 1.5 cm).

Selecting the localization device. Once the depth of the lesion is determined, the type of needle and wire device is selected. There are many commercially available hooked or barbed wires, both retractable and nonretractable.[45,46,48,53,55] Straight needles or modifications of straight needles are also widely used[47,49,50,51,54] The selection depends on the radiologist's and surgeon's preferences, availability, and cost.[18,43] The length of the needle desired may also influence selection, because some brands have a better selection of short lengths while others have longer lengths. Long spinal needles will suffice if needed. Many devices now come with markings etched every centimeter on the needle shaft to help improve accuracy of depth placement.

A combination of different localizing devices may be required if two sites are localized in the same breast. It is best if there are some distinguishing characteristics in the wire type, hub design, or other feature to permit differentiation on the

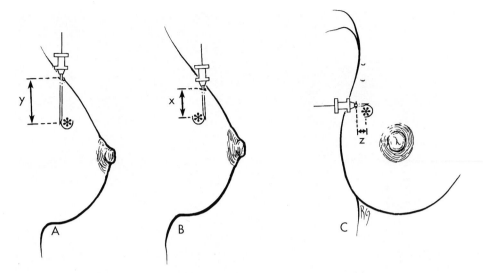

Fig. 7-12 A lateral projection can be used to plan placement of the needle from a craniocaudal approach (**A** or **B**). If the needle is placed posterior to the mass, a surprisingly long needle (y>×>z) may be required to accommodate the slope of the skin near the chest wall (**A**). A horizontal approach (**C**) is often preferred to minimize the distance and to help keep the biopsy scar within any potential mastectomy flap area.

radiograph. Another option would be to leave the needle on one wire and remove it from the second wire if like devices and lengths are used.

With experience it has become evident that some of the needle and wire devices are preferable, depending on the type of breast parenchyma. It is difficult to firmly anchor any device in fatty tissue, because fat is nearly liquid at body temperature. We prefer the retractable J-hook with the needle left in place for very fatty breasts. We also recommend that the dissection be done by dissecting back toward the J-hook rather than in a core down around the needle or wire. Inadvertent retraction of the localization device during a core biopsy may occur in a fatty breast and result in a failure of excision.

In very dense parenchymal tissue, some needles may be difficult to advance. We select those devices that have the most angled bevel when the tissue appears very fibrous. A wire that can be set by withdrawing the needle rather than by advancing the wire may be easier to place in firm, fibrous tissue. A barbed wire can be placed more accurately and with less discomfort.

Positioning the template localizer. Most dedicated mammography units are available with a template localizer made of nonattenuating material. Both perforated and grid coordinate plates are available. If a perforated plate is used, the holes should be large enough in diameter to allow the hub of the localizing needle to pass, thereby permitting the template to be easily removed while the needle remains in position.

The template should be placed over the skin surface closest to the lesion and moderate compression applied. The compression should be tight enough to remind the patient not to move but not as tight as that used for a standard mammographic exposure since she must remain in this position for 5 to 10 minutes. We often mark the skin with ink at the margins of the field to detect any motion that may inadvertently occur between the first exposure and needle placement. If the patient moves, we repeat the exposure.

While this localizing film is being processed, we prepare the skin surface with a povidone-iodine (Betadine) and alcohol wash. Some experts recommend Hibiclens, which is said to be less deleterious to the compression plate over the long term. During this wait we also try to distract the patient by pleasant conversation. We do not leave her unattended in the mammography room but have someone with her at all times. The assistant may keep light pressure on her back or shoulder to remind her not to move and provide needed emotional support.

The localizing film is then reviewed (Fig. 7-13A). The area of concern is identified and the film is oriented. Care is needed at this step to be sure that the correct quadrant is selected. The site of entry is selected. This site is usually directly over the lesion so that the needle transfixes the lesion or passes immediately adjacent to it.

If local anesthesia is used, it should be infiltrated into the dermis at this point in the procedure. We have omitted this step during the last 5

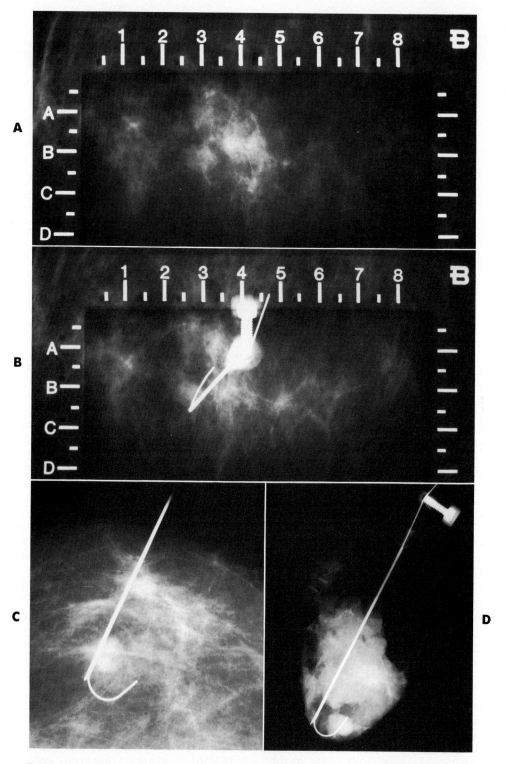

Fig. 7-13 Localization procedure. **A,** Template film is reviewed to select needle entry point at 3B in this case. **B,** After placement of the needle and wire, the localization view is repeated, confirming that the tip of the needle and wire is adjacent to the lesion. **C,** After the template is removed, an orthogonal view confirms appropriate depth of the wire and needle. **D,** Specimen radiograph confirms removal of the lesion. The pathologic diagnosis is fibroadenoma.

years. The expense, time, and discomfort to the patient do not seem to justify taking this additional step. Most women are compliant when told that the local anesthetic is more painful than the direct needle stick. Rarely will a patient insist on the use of local anesthesia for needle and wire placement.

The needle is placed with a swift, deliberate puncture of the skin. Some authors have recommended that the needle be rotated during insertion to minimize any deflection of the needle caused by tissue resistance. We try to pass the needle to depth with one motion because this tends to minimize patient discomfort. An occasional woman will flinch or pull back at the moment of needle insertion. Having her turn her head so that she cannot see the needle and a gentle, yet firm pressure on her back may minimize this tendency to move.

The position of the needle, angle, and depth should be reevaluated after placement (Fig. 7-13B). An obvious deflection or angulation may be corrected at this point. If the position looks acceptable, a second radiographic exposure is obtained to confirm appropriate position relative to the lesion. Frequently, a small mass or an area of microcalcifications is obscured by the hub or device on this confirmation film. This indicates that the needle is "on target."

An orthogonal film is then obtained to confirm appropriate depth of the needle (Fig. 7-13C). During this exposure the hub of the needle should be protected by sterile gauze to maintain antiseptic procedure. Use of a spot compression device to replace the fenestrated template is recommended to permit access to the hub of the needle.[52] The wire is then advanced and inserted into the tissue, and a repeat film is obtained to confirm final position.

If a retractable wire and needle device is used, the wire may be advanced immediately after the initial placement of the needle. Repositioning is then possible if subsequent orthogonal views show an unsatisfactory placement.

Uncommonly a patient may develop a vasovagal reaction during the procedure. It is best to have the patient seated at all times and to minimize unnecessary roughness or compression. A pleasant distracting conversation can do much to avert this tendency. These patients respond readily to a rest in the supine position.[42]

Step 4. Communicate with the team

Several steps follow, all of which consolidate and coordinate the success of the entire procedure. At the completion of the localization, we alert the operating room that the patient is ready and the surgical pathology laboratory that a breast biopsy requiring a specimen radiograph is in the offing. We do this to ensure that adequate film is on hand for the specimen radiograph and appropriate personnel are in attendance. We offer to show the patient and her family the localization radiographs.

As an important step, we prepare our films and radiograph jacket with both a diagram and a word picture of the location of the area to be removed relative to the internal marker. We prefer to communicate in person with the head of the surgical team, because miscommunication or misunderstanding by students or physicians in training may lead to a delay in the operating room or a failure of excision.

We hang the films on the view box in an orientation the surgeon would see when standing at the side of the patient. The nipple is clearly marked and appropriate labels are added (e.g., cranial, caudal, medial, lateral). We outline the lesion to be removed by a wax marker on the film and describe its exact location relative to the wire tip on the radiograph jacket, which accompanies the patient to the operating room.

Step 6. Confirm lesion removal

A specimen radiograph is obtained on *all* wire-directed biopsies (Fig. 7-13D).[16] The procedure is not dictated until the specimen radiograph has been reviewed. In this way the success or possible failure of the entire procedure can be documented in the final dictated report. Calcifications are often more dramatic on the specimen radiograph than on the mammogram (Fig. 7-14A to C).

The radiologist remains accessible to see the specimen radiograph as soon as it is processed. The tissue should not be sectioned until after the specimen radiograph and inking of margins have been completed.[58] If there is difficulty in seeing the lesion, the specimen radiograph should be repeated with more penetration, more compression of the tissue, or a rotation of the tissue by 90 degrees (Fig. 7-15).[57,59,60] All or a combination of any two of these three suggestions may be used (Box 7-6). It is particularly valuable to compress the specimen or perform an x-ray examination of it surrounded by water if the lesion is a noncalcified mass. These maneuvers decrease the surface lobularity and make noncalcified lesions more evident. If uncertainty remains concerning adequacy of excision, it may be necessary to section the tissue to inspect for a lesion corresponding in density and size to the abnormality detected on the mammogram. The tissue must not be cut until the margins have been inked. A frozen section is not usually performed.[28]

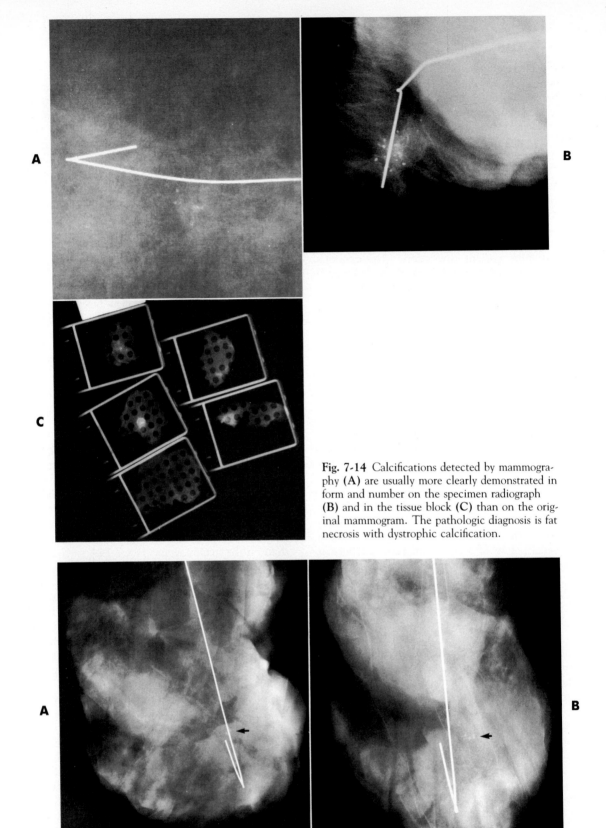

Fig. 7-14 Calcifications detected by mammography **(A)** are usually more clearly demonstrated in form and number on the specimen radiograph **(B)** and in the tissue block **(C)** than on the original mammogram. The pathologic diagnosis is fat necrosis with dystrophic calcification.

Fig. 7-15 The focus of calcifications (*arrow*) was obscured on the initial specimen radiograph **(A)**. The calcifications (*arrow*) are confirmed on a repeat radiograph **(B)** obtained after rotating the tissue 90 degrees.

BOX 7-6 PROBLEMS ENCOUNTERED WITH SPECIMEN RADIOGRAPHS

Lesion removal uncertain	Rotate specimen 90 degrees and retake radiograph
Mass difficult to see	Flatten tissue and retake radiograph Correlate with gross appearance at "cut-in" Repeat mammogram in 6 to 8 weeks
Wire transected	Alert surgeon Use portable x-ray equipment as needed

It is the duty of the radiologist to inform the surgeon about the status of the specimen radiograph.[58] A request for additional tissue may be indicated if:

1. The lesion is not seen in the specimen radiograph.
2. The lesion is demonstrated to be close to a free margin (Fig. 7-16).
3. The lesion has been transected and only a portion is included in the specimen.
4. The wire has been cut and pieces are not all accounted for (Fig. 7-17).

In any of these circumstances it is helpful for the surgeon to have some indication of which areas should be excised as the second piece. Preservation of the specimen's orientation during transport and during the specimen radiograph helps to ensure that all the lesion is excised with adequate margins. In our institution the orientation is written on the towel next to the specimen and radiodense markers are laid in the corresponding locations before specimen radiography. Further recommendations relative to tissue processing are discussed in Chapter 8.

Step 8. Review the pathology

The preoperative localization procedure is not completed until the radiologist and surgeon review the histopathologic results. This is necessary to ensure that the area of mammographic abnormality has been appropriately examined histologically. Recuts or review may be needed if the radiographic lesion seen does not correspond to the histopathologic appearance.

The pathologic results should be collated and summarized. This type of data may serve as part of a professional quality assurance program. Certainly the feedback thus gained produces more experienced mammographers.

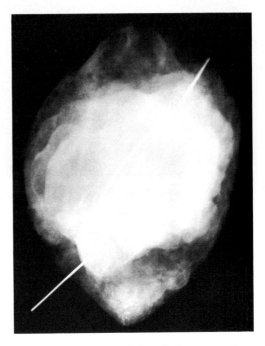

Fig. 7-16 The location of the calcifications at the edge of the specimen prompted the radiologist to request that the surgeon take a second specimen along this margin. The pathologic diagnosis was comedocarcinoma in the first specimen. No cancer was found in the second specimen.

RESULTS OF PREOPERATIVE LOCALIZATION PROCEDURE
Yield for cancer

A review of preoperative localization and biopsy results should include detailed information about the type of pathology found. If cancer is discovered, the data should reflect whether it is ductal or lobular in origin and in situ or invasive in extent. The size of the cancer and status of the axillary lymph nodes are also pertinent.

If the pathology report does not diagnose cancer, it is of interest to note whether the lesion was a fibroadenoma, sclerosing adenosis, or fat necrosis. Radial scars are of special interest in that they mimic spiculated carcinomas mammographically. If fibrocystic disease is present, the degree of hyperplasia should be noted (Fig. 7-18). Subtypes of fibrocystic disease, including atypical lobular and ductal hyperplasia, and their significance are discussed in further detail in Chapter 11.

The results of 291 preoperative needle localizations are presented in Box 7-7. These data are a compilation of all wire-directed biopsies performed over a 9-year interval at our institution. During the early years it was customary to perform biopsies of all solid breast masses greater than 1 cm in diameter and all isolated clusters of suspicious or indeterminate microcalcifications. With these liberal criteria our positive biopsy rate for cancer averaged 19%. Beginning in the late 1980s there has been a national trend toward observing some mammographic lesions of low-level suspicion.

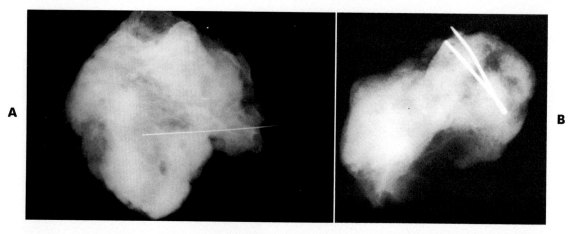

Fig. 7-17 The first specimen radiograph **(A)** showed that the wire had been transected. The surgeon was alerted and could palpate the retained wire. The second specimen radiograph **(B)** confirms removal of the entire wire.

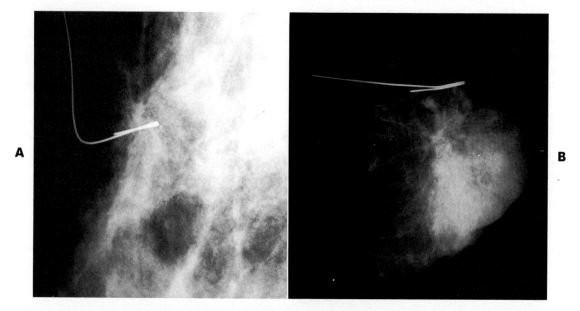

Fig. 7-18 Parenchymal distortion **(A)** required a preoperative wire localization. The specimen radiograph **(B)** confirmed successful excision. The pathologic diagnosis was florid proliferative fibrocystic disease with ductal hyperplasia.

With these more strict criteria, our biopsy yield for cancer has risen to 30%. The availability of magnification mammography has assisted in resolving the fine detail needed to characterize calcifications and some masses. Refinements in criteria for recommending biopsies continue to be developed.

As the criteria for biopsy of mammographic abnormalities are refined, the positive yield for cancer is rising (Table 7-1). The positive predictive value (PPV) of mammography is a reflection not only of the mammographic criteria used to rec- ommend biopsy but also of the patient population being studied.[69] In most American series the PPV ranges between 20% and 30% compared with a reported PPV of 50% to 70% for a "positive" mammogram in Europe, where repetitive screening trials are the norm.[68] In the United States, an ever expanding screening population, the desire to diagnose cancer as early as possible, and concern over the litigation implications of a delay in diagnosis have produced a lower biopsy yield. It is also difficult to compare data from an organized European screening trial with data grouped in a mixed

BOX 7-7 WIRE LOCALIZATION RESULTS
UNIVERSITY OF KENTUCKY MEDICAL CENTER

Histopathology	Percentage for 1981–1989 (291 total)	Percentage for 1990* (51 total)
Cancer	19	31
Atypia	5	10
Proliferative FCD	38	17
Bland FCD	20	16
Fibroadenoma	12	20
Other	4	6
Failure	2	0
Total	100%	100%

*Mammographic follow-up of lobular masses with smooth margins and clusters of punctate calcifications.
FCD, Fibrocystic disease

Table 7-1 **Summary of preoperative localization series**

Source	Year of procedures	Cumulative experience (years)	Number of procedures	Cancer yield (%)	Failures (%)
Libshitz[58]	1976	—	83	22	0
Homer[44]	1972–1982	5	80	18	10
Schwartz[77]	1977	1	189	27	—
Rasmussen[75]	1980–1982	2	42	13.5	—
Hall[64]	1980–1984	4	70	13	<2
Meyer[72]	1978–1983	5½	500	23.4	—
Gisvold[42]	1980–1982	2	343	27	3
Pitzen[74]	1974–1984	10	63	27	—
Ciatto[61]	1970–1985	15	512	30	—
Tinnemans[79]	1975–1983	8	335	30	—
Hermann[66]	1982–1985	3	220	35	—
Rosenberg[76]	1974–1985	12	927	29	—
Marrujo[70]	1986	—	237	27	—
Hall[65]	1984–1987	2	400	30	5–10
Meyer[73]	1987	1	601	18	<2
Silverstein[7]	1983–1987	5	1014	20	—
Gallagher[30]	1987–1988	1	100	24	1

population of symptomatic and asymptomatic women.[40] The implications of defining the patient population are further underscored by the observations that in a select group of women who have had definitive radiation therapy for early-stage carcinoma of the breast, the PPV of an abnormal mammogram in the presence of a normal physical examination was 66%.[78]

Magnification mammography is strongly recommended to fully characterize mammographic lesions to improve separation of suspicious from probably benign lesions. Importantly, the positive predictive value (PPV) of recommended biopsies should be accompanied by a description of the size and stage of cancers being diagnosed. Lobular carcinoma in situ should not be included in the cancer statistics. Ductal carcinoma in situ should be tracked separately from invasive cancers. The percentage of cancers less than 1 cm in diameter, the interval cancer rate, the false-negative rate and the frequency of cancers diagnosed per 1000 women at first screen and then subsequent screen are all useful to assess the significance of a PPV[69].

There is increasing interest in decreasing the proportion of negative biopsies without missing small cancers. It has been recommended that equivocal lesions be reviewed with a colleague. Two names on a mammographic report or on a surgical note may provide better psychological and legal support for a recommendation to observe a lesion by mammography rather than biopsy.[63] If a decision to observe a lesion by serial mammography is instituted, appropriate caution must be exercised. In a recent report by Franceschi and others concerning result of biopsy for microcalcifications (nonmagnification technique) 36% of the cancers were found in biopsies of microcalcifications classified as having minimal or low suspicion of malignancy.[62] A long-term program of follow-up (3 or more years) is recommended because some cancers that fail to change radiographically in 2 years have been described.[67,71]

Moreover, it is wise to be relatively lenient in assigning a nonpalpable, probably benign lesion to close mammographic surveillance, otherwise subtle malignancies may be assigned to the normal group and result in a delay in diagnosis. The reader is referred to suggested readings concerning follow-up strategies for low suspicion mammographic abnormalities at the end of this chapter. The editorial by D'Orsi listed in the suggested readings is particularly recommended. The desirability of operating at a low rate of false negative findings on the typical receiver operator characteristic (ROC) curve is emphasized when screening for early stage breast cancer. The corollary is that the false-positive rate may necessarily be higher as a trade-off for a given lower false-negative rate due to the reciprocal relationship of these values on the ROC curve.

Failures and complications

Published series in the literature document a failure rate for preoperative localization of 1% to 10% (see Table 7-1). If the lesion is not confirmed to be removed by specimen radiography or close inspection of all the excised tissue, failure is suspected. A postbiopsy mammogram is recommended in 6 to 8 weeks to determine if the lesion remains in the breast.[85] The subsequent course of action, whether rebiopsy or long-term mammographic follow-up, is determined by consultation between the radiologist and the surgeon.

Some reasons for failure are listed in Box 7-8 with suggested solutions. Nearly every radiologist has been fooled once by clustered dermal calcifications. A high degree of suspicion that any lesion within 1 cm of the skin surface could be dermal should prompt the appropriate skin localization maneuvers.[9]

Poor communication between members of the patient care team is not usually a problem except in the beginning of setting up a service. This is likely to be more of a concern in large institutions where many individuals may be rotating onto the team. We have found that an accurate three-dimensional drawing is valuable for the surgeon to see in the operating room during dissection. The films are also labeled and oriented for reference in the operating room but are often more confusing than a three-dimensional sketch. Direct communication between the radiologist and surgeon is recommended.

The difficulty of anchoring the wire and needle in fatty tissue remains the main cause of the occasional failure in our practice. These failures mostly occur for small lesions deep in fatty breasts. Despite all efforts to avoid dislodging the wire, the surgeon may lose orientation if the first or second specimen does not contain the lesion. The surgeon then decides when a prudent amount of tissue has been excised and the procedure is terminated. The suggestion to support the large fatty breast during transport makes a great deal of sense. We also strongly recommend inserting the wire and needle at least 1 cm beyond the lesion when fatty tissue is predominant. The surgeon must make every effort not to pull or retract on the wire during dissection of the specimen.

It is essential that the wire be removed in situ so that it continues to serve as an internal marker on the specimen radiograph of the oriented specimen. This procedure facilitates directing removal of a second piece of tissue if the first specimen fails

BOX 7-8 SOME CAUSES OF LOCALIZATION FAILURE

Problem	Solution
Poor understanding of location[80]	Three-dimensional drawing
Dislodgement in fatty breast	Anchor wire beyond lesion Support breast during transport Avoid retracting wire
Loss of orientation of specimen[44]	Remove wire in situ with specimen Orient specimen and label
Superficial lesion[44]	Be suspicious Check for dermal calcifications before scheduling biopsy
Wire pulled out prematurely by assistant[45]	Train new operating room personnel about proper procedure
Ruptured cyst	Look for cyst wall on histopathology Increase use of preoperative ultrasound examination

to contain the entire lesion. Retaining orientation of the tissue and wire together with accurate wire placement will do much to reduce the number of failures. A success rate of 96% to 98% should be achievable.[30]

The incidence of significant complications after wire-directed biopsy of nonpalpable mammographic abnormalities is low. There have been occasional reports of wire transection, wire migration, pneumothorax, hematoma, and infection (Box 7-9). A question of breast tumor seeding along the guide-wire track parallel to the chest wall has been raised but not observed.[82–84] Vasovagal reactions are usually minor and respond to rest.[42,83]

Wire migration has been reported in six cases: one in the breast, one in the pleural cavity, three in distant subcutaneous tissues, and one that ended up in the muscles of the neck.[25,81,86] This last case occurred when the hook was lodged in the pectoral muscle and the end of the wire was lost in the subcutaneous tissues. It is believed that muscular action caused migration of the wire into the soft tissues of the upper neck as demonstrated by a CT scan. Using a long wire and securing it to the skin by kinking the wire first and taping or clamping the external end have been recommended to avoid this complication.[26,86,87]

Wire transection may occur, particularly if scissors are used for tissue dissection. A retained fragment may be suspected if the specimen radiograph shows a slight curve at the end of the wire in the excised tissue.[81] The surgeon should be informed of suspected transection. If the retained fragment cannot be palpated, a portable chest x-ray ma-

BOX 7-9 COMPLICATIONS OF WIRE-DIRECTED BIOPSY

Vasovagal reactions
Wire migration
Wire transection
Pneumothorax
Hematoma
Infection

chine or C-arm fluoroscopy in the operating room may assist in locating the fragment. Some localizing wires are more resistant to transection than others.

The incidence of hematoma and infection should be about the same as for any breast biopsy procedure.[30] These surgical complications are seldom addressed in the radiographic literature. An occasional hematoma is caused by placing the needle for localization.[42] Most postbiopsy radiographic changes represent uncomplicated seromas, which resolve over 3 to 12 months.

PROBLEMS AND PITFALLS IN PREOPERATIVE LOCALIZATION PROCEDURE

This section discusses special circumstances (Box 7-10) that sometimes arise and require a more innovative approach than the standard method. Where available, literature references are provided for a more detailed discussion. Individual radiologists will undoubtedly develop their own favorite solutions.

BOX 7-10 PROBLEMS IN LOCALIZATION PROCEDURE

Trouble in triangulating a lesion
Difficult approach
Inaccurate needle length
More than one area to be localized
Difficulty in advancing the wire

Trouble in triangulating a lesion

The issue of problems in triangulating a lesion seen in one view only has received considerable attention in the literature. Fortunately, this circumstance is not frequent because most "lesions" seen in one view only are in fact a "pseudomass." A normal band of parenchyma may be telescoped upon itself in a single projection, producing a pseudomass or density in one view only. With experience, this appearance is easily recognized. A *slight* change in angulation of the x-ray beam will cause the "lesion" to dissipate and reveal the diffuse nature of the normal breast parenchyma.[91] Addition of focal spot compression with magnification to this additional view with slightly modified beam orientation can also be elected. If a mass or density is real, a slight angulation of the beam will *not* cause it to disappear; it will persist. With increasing intervals of angulation it may be possible to follow such a lesion through the breast structures in order to find it on an orthogonal position. An alternative is to rotate the breast slightly around the nipple axis to shift the lesion.[92]

Because the mediolateral oblique view is less than 90 degrees from the craniocaudal view, it is desirable to triangulate the lesion using a true lateral view. If this projection does not pinpoint the lesion, the ability to "think oblique" must be used.[91]

Another approach is to devise creative orthogonal views to permit a nontraditional localization approach. The standard methodology is to use a craniocaudal and a true lateral projection. Equally effective is to pair a 45-degree oblique view with a 45-degree lateromedial oblique view or a −45-degree mediolateral oblique view.[88,93] A Cleopatra view or an exaggerated craniocaudal view can be used to locate a deep lesion in the tail seen only on the oblique view.[88] If the lesion is not lateral, a craniocaudal view exaggerated for the deep medial tissues or a cleavage view is the next step.

At times calcifications are easily detected in one projection and not the other. This may be a situation where the calcifications are in the skin or subcutaneous parenchyma. A careful search with a bright light at the appropriate distance behind the nipple will usually locate the cluster near the skin surface. If the cluster of calcification is still not seen, one should apply the principle of geometric unsharpness. The unsharpness of the calcifications is a measure of their distance from the film. For instance, very small distinct microcalcifications easily seen on a craniocaudal view are most often in the inferior breast. If these are not seen easily on the mediolateral oblique projection, they may not be lateral but may be medial in location. A view with the medial breast closest to the film (a lateral to medial true lateral) may confirm the calcifications' location.

Rarely, a suspicious lesion can be seen only on a single projection in spite of repeated attempts to disclose its location by creative angled and orthogonal views. Parallax techniques have been described for nondedicated[94] and dedicated mammography units to meet this dilemma[89,92] For women with mobile skin and subcutaneous tissues the skin-pinch technique may successfully localize lesions seen in one view only, or lesions in the inferior breast.[90] Alternatively, placement of a guide wire using ultrasonography or CT for guidance is feasible, provided the lesion can be pinpointed three-dimensionally by these imaging techniques.

Difficult approach

Some mammographic abnormalities are a particular challenge for preoperative wire placement. Three special circumstances are discussed: the deep lesion close to the chest wall, the lesion in the inferior breast, and lesions immediately retroareolar in location.

Very deep mammographic lesions are a particular problem because it may be difficult to image the area by orthogonal views, and once the lesion is imaged, the wire is usually placed in fatty tissue, where a dislodgement leading to failure may occur. Exaggerated craniocaudal views for the lateral breast are recommended for directing placement of a wire from the craniocaudal approach for a lesion close to the chest wall in the tail of the breast. If the lesion is medial, an exaggerated craniocaudal view for deep medial tissues is used, or a cleavage view. The placement of the wire parallel to the chest wall is believed to be safe and less likely to result in inadvertent placement of a hooked wire into the pectoral muscle.[48] Dislodgement is often a concern if the deep tissue is primarily fatty. It is recommended to advance the wire beyond the lesion so that, should the wire be withdrawn during dissection by inadvertent traction, the area will still lie along the path of the slightly retracted wire.[44] Support of the heavy, pendulous breast during transport from the radiology department to the surgery suite is also suggested to minimize movement of the wire in the large fatty breast. In addition, some centers may wish to inject blue dye around the wire through the needle into the tissue for a "belt and suspenders approach" to more difficult lesions. Many centers advocate the use of general anesthesia for removing deep lesions.[48]

Mammographic abnormalities in the inferior breast may be approached in one of several ways: a medial or a lateral approach, freehand placement from below, a template-guided caudocranial approach or the skin-pinch technique. Most radiographers use the lateral or medial approach, choosing to insert the needle so that the shortest distance of breast tissue is traversed. A freehand approach perpendicular to the chest wall can also be used with the needle inserted to the hub so that a postlocalization craniocaudal view can be safely obtained.[17] In some centers caudocranial projections are feasible, and this approach may be the most direct. A word of caution, however, is suggested. If the patient must stand to straddle the tube head assembly in a caudocranial projection, she may be more prone to a vasovagal reaction. In our center we prefer a lateral to medial or a medial to lateral approach so that the patient may remain seated during needle placement.

Lastly, it is conceivable that a nonpalpable lesion may lie so close to the nipple–areolar complex that a template-guided needle placement would require placing the needle through the pigmented areolar skin. The areola has a high number of nerve endings and should be avoided. We recommend entering the skin at a periareolar location and angling the tip of the needle as needed to provide an optimal localization in the retroareolar area.

Inaccurate needle length

Selection of the localization device depends not only on the radiologist's and surgeon's preferences for the type of hook or wire but also on the availability of appropriate needle lengths. It is best to err on the side of having a needle that is too long rather than one too short. Because the breast is spheroid in shape, a skin marker placed over the lesion will permit the most accurate estimate of the lesion depth on an orthogonal view. The value of obtaining a true lateral view with a skin marker on the superior surface of the breast at the needle entry site has already been stressed.[44] This view also helps detect any abnormality that may be originating in the skin because the lesion will project quite close to the superficial marker, alerting the radiologist to a possible dermal location.

More than one area to be localized

Circumstances may necessitate that more than one area be localized in a single patient. If the areas are in separate breasts, we prefer to perform the easiest localization first to optimize the patient's first experience. It is wise to plan the approach so that the wires do not interfere with one another. We usually choose the most direct approach.

If there are two separate areas in the same breast, it is required that the needle and wire devices be distinguishable from each other on the postlocalization films. Different types of needles can be selected, or some external marker can be placed to identify which wire goes to which lesion. If both are placed from the same direction, there is no difficulty in obtaining an orthogonal film to evaluate depth. If differing orientations are needed, careful preplanning is necessary so that the first wire or hub does not interfere with the projection needed to guide placement of the second wire. Situations in which two wires are required might include nonpalpable synchronous multicentric carcinoma in different quadrants, a long lesion such as segmental involvement by comedocarcinoma to direct a complete lumpectomy, or two lesions lying in the same quadrant but more than 1.5 cm from each other.

Difficulty in advancing the wire

In our experience, occasionally it is difficult to advance some wire localization devices through very dense tissue. This is infrequent, occurring in less than 5% of all cases.[48] Suggestions to avoid this difficulty include changing the approach of the needle so that it traverses fat rather than dense parenchyma, rotating the needle and readvancing the wire, and changing to a different needle with a sharper bevel or to a hook that can be engaged by withdrawing the needle rather than by advancing the wire. Rarely, the principal difficulty is in penetrating the external skin. A small nick by a scalpel blade after infiltration by local anesthesia is recommended if needed.

REFERENCES
Indications for performing a localization procedure

1. Martin JE, Gallager HS: Mammographic diagnosis of minimal breast cancer, *Cancer* 28:1519, 1971.
2. Moskowitz M: The predictive value of certain mammographic signs in screening for breast cancer, *Cancer* 51:1007, 1983.
3. Murphy WA, DeSchryver-Kecskemeti K: Isolated clustered microcalcifications in the breast: radiologic-pathologic correlation, *Radiology* 127:335, 1978.
4. Rogers JV, Powell RW: Mammographic indications for biopsy of clinically normal breasts: correlation with pathologic findings in 72 cases, *AJR Am J Roentgenol* 115:794, 1972.

5. Sickles EA: Mammographic features of "early" breast cancer, AJR Am J Roentgenol 143:461, 1984.

6. Sickles EA: Mammographic features of 300 consecutive nonpalpable breast cancers, AJR Am J Roentgenol 146:661, 1986.

7. Silverstein MJ, Gamagani P, Colburn WJ, et al: Nonpalpable breast lesions: diagnosis with slightly overpenetrated screen-film mammography and hook wire-directed biopsy in 1,014 cases, Radiology 171:633, 1989.

8. Wolfe JN: Mammography: ducts as a sole indicator of breast carcinoma, AJR Am J Roentgenol 89:206, 1967.

Indications for cancelling a localization procedure

9. Berkowitz JE, Gatewood OMB, Donovan GB, et al: Dermal breast calcifications: localization with template-guided placement of skin marker, Radiology 163:282, 1987.

10. Britton CA, Baratz AB, Harris KM: Carcinoma mimicked by the sternal insertion of the pectoral muscle, AJR Am J Roentgenol 153:955, 1989.

11. Kopans DB, Meyer JE, Homer MJ, et al: Dermal deposits mistaken for breast calcifications, Radiology 149:592, 1983.

12. Meyer JE, Kopans DB: Stability of a mammographic mass: a false sense of security, AJR Am J Roentgenol 137:595, 1981.

13. Meyer JE, Sonnenfeld MR, Greenes RA, et al: Cancellation of preoperative breast localization procedures: analysis of 53 cases, Radiology 169:629, 1988.

14. Murphy WA Jr, Destouet JM, Monsees BS: Professional quality assurance for mammography screening programs, Radiology 175:319, 1990.

15. Pennes DR, Homer MJ: Disappearing breast masses caused by compression during mammography, Radiology 165:327, 1987.

Review of development of mammographic localization techniques

16. Hall FM, Frank HA: Progress in radiology: preoperative localization of nonpalpable breast lesions, AJR Am J Roentgenol 132:101, 1979.

17. Homer MJ: Preoperative needle localization of lesions in the lower half of the breast: needle entry from below, AJR Am J Roentgenol 149:43, 1987.

18. Kopans DB, Swann CA: Progress in radiology: preoperative imaging-guided needle placement and localization of clinically occult breast lesions, AJR Am J Roentgenol 152:1, 1989.

19. Stevens GM, Jamplis RW: Mammographically directed biopsy of nonpalpable breast lesions, Arch Surg 102:292, 1971.

Spot Localization

20. Czarnecki DJ, Feider HK, Splittgerber GF: Toluidine blue dye as a breast localization marker, AJR Am J Roentgenol 153:261, 1989.

21. Horns JW, Arndt RD: Percutaneous spot localization of nonpalpable breast lesions, AJR Am J Roentgenol 127:253, 1976.

22. Simon J, Lesnick GJ, Lerer WN, et al: Roentgenographic localization of small lesions of the breast by the spot method, Surg Gynecol Obstet 134:572, 1972.

23. Svane G: A sterotaxic technique for preoperative marking of non-palpable breast lesions, Acta Radiol 24:145, 1983.

Freehand Localization

24. Becker W: Stereotactic localization of breast lesions, Radiology 133:238, 1979.

25. Bristol JB, Jones PA: Case reports: transgression of localizing wire into pleural cavity prior to mammography, Br J Radiol 54:139, 1981.

26. Davis PS, Wechsler RJ, Feig SA, et al: Migration of breast biopsy localization wire, AJR Am J Roentgenol 150:787, 1988.

27. Feig SA: Localization of clinically occult breast lesions, Radiol Clin North Am 21:155, 1983.

28. Frank HA, Hall FM, Steer ML: Preoperative localization of nonpalpable breast lesions demonstrated by mammography, N Engl J Med 295:259, 1976.

29. Threatt B, Appelman H, Dow R, et al: Percutaneous needle localization of clustered mammary microcalcifications prior to biopsy, AJR Am J Roentgenol 121:839, 1974.

Template Guidance

30. Gallagher WJ, Cardenosa G, Rubens JR, et al: Minimal-volume excision of nonpalpable breast lesions, AJR Am J Roentgenol 153:957, 1989.

31. Goldberg RP, Hall FM, Simon M: Preoperative localization of nonpalpable breast lesions using a wire marker and perforated mammographic grid, Radiology 146:833, 1983.

32. Muhlow A: A device for precision needle biopsy of the breast at mammography, AJR Am J Roentgenol 121:843, 1974.

33. Tabar L, Dean PB: Interventional radiologic procedures in the investigation of lesions of the breast, Radiol Clin North Am XVII:607, 1979.

34. Tinnemans JGM, Wobbes T, Hendriks JHCL, et al: Localization and excision of nonpalpable breast lesions: a surgical evaluation of three methods, Arch Surg 122:802, 1987.

Stereotaxic Needle Localizations

35. Bolmgren J, Jacobson B, Nordenstrom B: Stereotaxic instrument for needle biopsy of the mamma, AJR Am J Roentgenol 129:121, 1977.

36. Chen HH, Bernstein JR, Paige ML, et al: Needle localization of nonpalpable breast lesions with a portable dual-grid compression system, Radiology 170:687, 1989.

37. Dowlatshahi K, Gent HJ, Schmidt R, et al: Nonpalpable breast tumors: diagnosis with stereotaxic localization and fine-needle aspiration, Radiology 170:427, 1989.

38. Evans WP, Cade SH: Needle localization and fine-needle aspiration biopsy of nonpalpable breast lesions with use of standard and stereotactic equipment, Radiology 173:53, 1989.

39. Gent HJ, Sprenger E, Dowlatshahi K: Stereotaxic needle localization and cytological diagnosis of occult breast lesions, Ann Surg 204:580, 1986.

40. Kopans DB: Preoperative localization of nonpalpable breast lesions, Curr Opin Radiol 1:200, 1989.

41. Yagan R, Weisen E, Skubic S, et al: Needle localization of nonpalpable breast lesions with current dedicated mammographic systems, Radiology 172:580, 1989.

Preoperative mammographic localization: a protocol

42. Gisvold JJ, Martin JH Jr: Prebiopsy localization of nonpalpable breast lesions, AJR Am J Roentgenol 143:477, 1984.

43. Hall FM, Tobey DM: Cost of localization devices, AJR Am J Roentgenol 152:1340, 1989.

44. Homer MJ: Localization of nonpalpable breast lesions: technical aspects and analysis of 80 cases, AJR Am J Roentgenol 140:807, 1983.

45. Homer MJ: Nonpalpable breast lesion localization using a curved-end retractable wire, Radiology 157:259, 1985.

46. Homer MJ: Localization of nonpalpable breast lesions with the curved-end retractable wire: leaving the needle in vivo, AJR Am J Roentgenol 151:919, 1988.

47. Homer MJ, Fisher DJ, Sugarman JH: Post-localization needle for breast biopsy of nonpalpable lesions, *Radiology* 140:241, 1981.
48. Homer MJ, Pile-Spellman ER: Needle localization of occult breast lesions with a curved-end retractable wire: technique and pitfalls, *Radiology* 161:547, 1986.
49. Jensen SR, Luttenegger TJ: Wire localization of nonpalpable breast lesions, *Radiology* 132:484, 1979.
50. Kalisher L: An improved needle for localization of nonpalpable breast lesions, *Radiology* 128:815, 1978.
51. Kopans DB, DeLuca S: A modified needle-hookwire technique to simplify preoperative localization of occult breast lesions, *Radiology* 134:781, 1980.
52. Kopans DB, Lindforsk, McCarthy KA, et al: Spring hookwire breast lesion localizer: use with rigid-compression mammographic systems, *Radiology* 157:537, 1985.
53. Kopans DB, Meyer JE: Versatile spring hookwire breast lesions localizer, *AJR Am J Roentgenol* 138:586, 1982.
54. Loh CK, Perlman H, Harris JH Jr, et al: An improved method for localization of nonpalpable breast lesions, *Radiology* 130:244, 1979.
55. Urrutia EJ, Hawkins MC, Steinbach BG, et al: Retractable-barb needle for breast lesion localization: use in 60 cases, *Radiology* 169:845, 1988.
56. Welch JS: Editorial comment, *Arch Surg* 117:68, 1982.
57. Chilcote WA, Davis GA, Suchy P, et al: Breast specimen radiography: evaluation of a compression device, *Radiology* 168:425, 1988.
58. Libshitz HI, Feig SA, Fetouh S: Needle localization of nonpalpable breast lesions, *Radiology* 121:557, 1976.
59. Rebner M, Pennes DR, Baker DE, et al: Two-view specimen radiography in surgical biopsy of nonpalpable breast masses, *AJR Am J Roentgenol* 149:283, 1987.
60. Stomper PC, Davis SP, Sonnenfeld MR, et al: Efficacy of specimen radiography of clinically occult noncalcified breast lesions, *AJR Am J Roentgenol* 151:43, 198

Results of preoperative localization procedure

Yield for Cancer

61. Ciatto S, Cataliotti L, Distante V: Nonpalpable lesions detected with mammography: review of 512 consecutive cases, *Radiology* 165:99, 1987.
62. Franceschi D, Crowe J, Zollinger R, et al: Breast biopsy for calcifications in nonpalpable breast lesions, *Arch Surg* 125:170, 1990.
63. Hall FM: Mammographic second opinions prior to biopsy of nonpalpable breast lesions, *Arch Surg* 125:298, 1990.
64. Hall WC, Aust JB, Gaskill HV, et al: Evaluation of nonpalpable breast lesions, experience in a training institution, *Am J Surg* 151:467, 1986.
65. Hall FM, Storella JM, Silverstone DZ, et al: Nonpalpable breast lesions: recommendations for biopsy based on suspicion of carcinoma at mammography, *Radiology* 167:353, 1988.
66. Hermann G, Janus C, Schwartz IS, et al: Nonpalpable breast lesions: accuracy of rebiopsy mammographic diagnosis, *Radiology* 165:323, 1987.
67. Homer MJ: Nonpalpable mammographic abnormalities: timing the follow-up studies, *AJR Am J Roentgenol* 136:923, 1981.
68. Homer MJ: Nonpalpable breast abnormalities: a realistic view of the accuracy of mammography in detecting malignancies, *Radiology* 153:831, 1984.
69. Kopans DB: Perspective: the positive predictive value of mammography. *AJR Am J Roentgenol* 158:521, 1992.
70. Marrujo G, Jolly PC, Hall MH, et al: Nonpalpable breast cancer: needle-localized biopsy for diagnosis and considerations for treatment, *Am J Surg* 151:599, 1986.
71. Meyer JE, Kopans DB: Stability of a mammographic mass: a false sense of security, *AJR Am J Roentgenol* 137:595, 1981.
72. Meyer JE, Kopans DB, Stomper PC, et al: Occult breast abnormalities: percutaneous preoperative needle, *Radiology* 150:335, 1984.
73. Meyer JE, Sonnenfeld MR, Greenes RA, et al: Preoperative localization of clinically occult breast lesions: experience at a referral hospital, *Radiology* 169:627, 1988.
74. Pitzen RH, Urdaneta LF, Al-Jurf AS, et al: Specimen xeroradiography after needle localization and biopsy of noncalcified, nonpalpable breast lesions, *Am Surg* 51:50, 1985.
75. Rasmussen OS, Seerup A: Preoperative radiographically guided wire marking of nonpalpable breast lesions, *Acta Radiol* 25:13, 1984.
76. Rosenberg AL, Schwartz GF, Feig SA, et al: Clinically occult breast lesions: localization and significance, *Radiology* 162:167, 1987.
77. Schwartz GF, Feig SA, Patchefsky AS: Clinicopathologic correlations and significance of clinically occult mammary lesions, *Cancer* 41:1147, 1978.
78. Solin LJ, Fowble BL, Schultz DJ, et al: The detection of local recurrence after definitive irradiation for early stage carcinoma of the breast, *Cancer* 65:2497, 1990.
79. Tinnemans JGM, Wobbes T, vander Sluis RF, et al: Multicentricity in nonpalpable breast carcinoma and its implication for treatment, *Am J Surg* 151:334, 1986.

Failures and Complications

80. Bigongiari LR, Fidler W, Skerker LB, et al: Percutaneous localization of breast lesions prior to biopsy: analysis of failures, *Clin Radiol* 28:419, 1977.
81. Bronstein AD, Kilcoyne RF, Moe RE, et al: Complications of needle localization of foreign bodies and nonpalpable breast lesions, *Arch Surg* 123:775, 1988.
82. Fajardo LL: Breast tumor seeding along localization guide wire tracks, *Radiology* 169:580, 1988.
83. Helvie MA, Ikeda DM, Adler DD: Localization and needle aspiration of breast lesions: complications in 370 cases. *AJR Am J Roentgenol* 157:711, 1991.
84. Kopans DB, Gallagher WJ, Swann CA, et al: Does preoperative needle localization lead to an increase in local breast cancer recurrence? *Radiology* 167:667, 1988.
85. Meyer JE, Kopans DB: Preoperative roentgenographic guided percutaneous localization of occult breast lesions, *Arch Surg* 117:65, 1982.
86. Owen AWMC and Kumar EN: Migration of localizing wires used in guided biopsy of the breast, *Clinical Radiology* 43:251, 1991.
87. Wales LR: Prevention of migration of breast biopsy localization wire, *AJR Am J Roentgenol* 151:413, 1988.

Problems and pitfalls in preoperative localization procedure

88. Goodrich WA: The Cleopatra view in xeromammography: a semireclining position for the tail of the breast, *Radiology* 128:811, 1978.
89. Kopans DB, Waitzkin ED, Linetsky L, et al: Localization of breast lesions identified on only one mammographic view, *AJR Am J Roentgenol* 149:39, 1987.
90. Pollack AH: Localization of breast lesions identified on one mammographic view: the skin-pinch technique, *Radiology* 185:278, 1992.
91. Sickles EA: Practical solutions to common mammographic problems: tailoring the examination, *AJR Am J Roentgenol* 151:31, 1988.
92. Swann CA, Kopans DB, McCarthy KA, et al: Localization of occult breast lesions: practical solutions to problems of triangulation, *Radiology* 163:577, 1987.

93. Vyborny CJ, Merrill TN, Geurkink RE: Difficult mammographic needle localizations: use of alternative orthogonal projections, *Radiology* 161:839, 1986.
94. Yagan R, Wiesen E, Bellon EM: Mammographic needle localization of lesions seen in only one view, *AJR Am J Roentgenol* 144:911, 1985.

SUGGESTED READINGS
Stereotaxic needle guidance

Burbank F, Belville J: Core breast biopsy, research, and what not to do. *Radiology* 185:639, 1992.

Dowlatshahi K, Yaremko ML, Kluskens LF, Jokich PM: Nonpalpable breast lesions: findings of stereotaxic needle-core biopsy and fine-needle aspiration cytology. *Radiology* 181:745, 1991.

Dronkers DJ: Stereotaxic core biopsy of breast lesions. *Radiology* 183:631, 1992.

Fajardo LL, Davis JR, Wiens JL, Trego DC: Mammography-guided stereotactic fine-needle aspiration cytology of nonpalpable breast lesions: prospective comparison with surgical biopsy results. *AJR Am J Roentgenol* 155:977, 1990.

Franquet T, Cozcolluela R, DeMiguel C: Stereotaxic fine-needle aspiration of low-suspicion, nonpalpable breast nodules: valid alternative to follow-up mammography. *Radiology* 183:635, 1992.

Harter LP, Curtis JS, Ponto G, Craig PH: Malignant seeding of the needle track during stereotaxic core needle breast biopsy. *Radiology* 185:713, 1992.

Helvie MA, Baker DE, Adler DD et al: Radiographically guided fine-needle aspiration of nonpalpable breast lesions. *Radiology* 174:657, 1990.

Jackson VP, Reynolds HE: Stereotaxic needle-core biopsy and fine-needle aspiration cytologic evaluation of nonpalpable breast lesions. *Radiology* 181:633, 1991.

Meyer JE: Value of large-core biopsy of occult breast lesions. *AJR Am J Roentgenol* 158:991, 1992.

Parker SH: When is core biopsy really core? *Radiology* 185:641, 1992.

Parker SH, Lovin JD, Jobe WE, Burke BJ et al: Nonpalpable breast lesions: Stereotactic automated large-core biopsies. *Radiology* 180:403, 1991.

Yield for cancer

Adler DD, Helvie MA, Ikeda DM: Nonpalpable, probably benign breast lesions: follow-up strategies after initial detection on mammography. *AJR Am J Roentgenol* 155:1195, 1990.

Datoc PD, Hayes CW, Conway WF et al: Mammographic follow-up of nonpalpable low-suspicion breast abnormalities: one versus two views. *Radiology* 180:387, 1991.

D'Orsi CJ: To follow or not to follow, that is the question. *Radiology* 184:306, 1992.

Erickson EJ, McGreevy JM, Muskett A: Selective nonoperative management of patients referred with abnormal mammograms. *Am J Surg* 160:659, 1990.

Hamby LS, McGrath PC, Stelling CB, et al: The management of mammographic indeterminate lesions. *Am Surg* 59:4, 1993.

Helvie MA, Pennes DR, Rebner M, Adler DD: Mammographic follow-up of low-suspicion lesions: compliance rate and diagnostic yield. *Radiology* 178:155, 1991.

Reid SE, Jr., Scanlon EF, Bernstein JR et al: An alternative approach to nonpalpable breast biopsies. *J Surg Oncol* 44:93, 1990.

Sickles EA: Periodic mammographic follow-up of probably benign lesions: results in 3,184 consecutive cases. *Radiology* 179:463, 1991.

Ancillary Techniques for Breast Biopsy Specimens

Michael L. Cibull
C. Darrell Jennings

Mamographically directed wire localization
Estrogen and progesterone receptors
Cell cycle and DNA content
Cathepsin D, oncogenes, and other biologic markers

In this chapter, we address techniques for examining breast tissue beyond those employed in routine histopathology. One technique, mammographically directed wire localization, is useful for ensuring that nonpalpable, often grossly invisible lesions identified by mammography are adequately excised and examined. The other techniques discussed are used not primarily for diagnosis but in an attempt to provide information useful for prognosis and therapeutic decision making once a carcinoma has been identified in the specimen. In this regard, mammary carcinoma is one of the most intensively studied human tumors, both because of its high frequency and because routine histopathology has proved imperfect in providing complete prognostic and therapeutic information. It should be emphasized, however, that these techniques are ancillary and do not replace adequate gross and histologic examination. Information regarding tumor size, tumor type and grade, and lymph node status remains the cornerstone of breast cancer care and are discussed in Chapter 12.

MAMMOGRAPHICALLY DIRECTED WIRE LOCALIZATION

Improvements in mammographic technique and interpretation have made it possible to identify areas of abnormal density or microcalcification that are likely to represent in situ or small invasive mammary carcinomas—that is, carcinomas at a potentially highly curable stage.[6] These lesions are usually nonpalpable and often virtually unrecognizable at the level of gross specimen examination. This makes it difficult for both the surgeon and pathologist to identify the lesion at the time of biopsy and necessitates close cooperation between the radiologist, surgeon, and pathologist to ensure that the lesion has been excised and that, once it is excised, it is adequately evaluated. The numerous, seemingly complex steps described subsequently are best understood when viewed in the light of these two simple principles.

Mammographically directed biopsy evaluation can be divided into three phases as outlined in Box 7-5. In the first phase, mammographic localization, the radiologist places a marker in proximity to the lesion. In our institution, a hooked wire is used, but injection of a visible dye may also be employed. In the second phase, surgical excision, the marker (presumably with the lesion) is excised by the surgeon and an x-ray examination is done to ensure that the lesion has been completely removed. We employ a small specimen x-ray device, but if such a device is unavailable, x-ray equipment in the radiology department may be employed. Once it is confirmed radiographically that the suspicious area has been excised, the surgeon can close the biopsy site. If the lesion has been incompletely excised, the surgeon extends the biopsy until the lesion is completely removed.

The third phase involves the positive identification of the lesion in the pathologic specimen and confirmation of histologically adequate sampling. This can be accomplished in several ways. After the surface of the specimen is inked so that the adequacy of margins can be assessed if a carcinoma is found, the tissue is sliced and gross lesions are noted. An x-ray examination of the tissue slices is then done, and those slices that con-

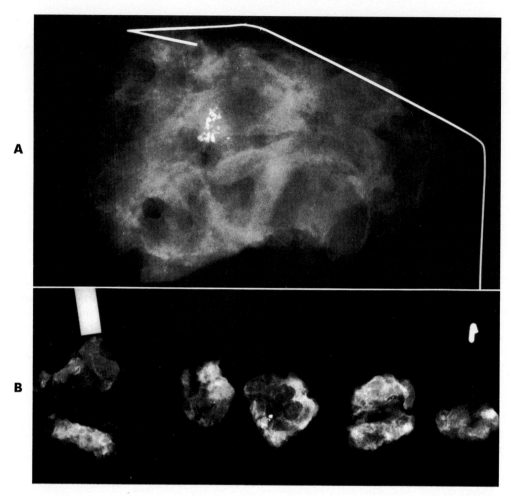

Fig. 8-1 A, X-ray of resected breast tissue. Note wire marker and cluster of suspicious microcalcifications. **B,** The breast tissue has been sliced for placement into cassettes. The cluster of suspicious microcalcifications is present in the middle slice; this block will be identified specifically in the gross dictation.

tain the mammographically suspicious densities or microcalcifications are identified specifically (Fig. 8-1). The biopsy specimen is then submitted for histologic processing, and those blocks that contain the suspicious areas are identified in the dictation. It is our practice to submit virtually all grossly identifiable breast tissue (rather than surrounding fat) for microscopic examination because significant lesions may be present some distance from the radiologically identified suspicious areas. This approach is supported by the work of Owings and colleagues,[2] who found that up to 2% of noninvasive carcinomas and 26% of atypical hyperplasias would be missed if only mammographically suspicious areas are submitted.

If suspicious microcalcifications are the reason for biopsy, evidence of these calcifications must be found microscopically to ensure adequate sam-

pling. If microcalcifications are not found on initial examination, the appropriate blocks are resectioned until the area containing the microcalcification is identified on the slides. It may be necessary to perform an x-ray examination of the paraffin blocks themselves to note at what level the calcifications are located in order to guide further sectioning (Fig. 8-2).[3] The necessity for this time-consuming and labor-intensive approach is illustrated by the study of Snyder and Rosen,[4] who found that 6% of carcinomas were missed if the suspicious microcalcifications were not observed in the histologic sections. In up to 17% of cases clinically significant calcifications noted on radiographs are composed of calcium oxalate, which may be largely dissolved in processing and identified only by the use of polarized light microscopy.[1,7]

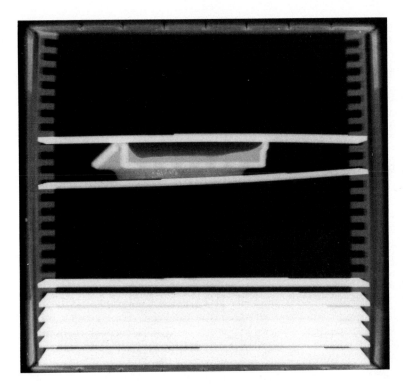

Fig. 8-2 Microcalcifications were not seen in several sections of the appropriate block. The block was x-rayed and the majority of microcalcifications are still a considerable distance from the face of the block.

BOX 8-1 WIRE-LOCALIZATION BIOPSY: PITFALLS IN TISSUE HANDLING

Problem	Solution
Question of clear margins	Ink margins *always* before sectioning Orient specimen at all steps
Lesion too small for ER/PR	Do not do a frozen section Do ER/PR by immunochemistry on permanent sections
Question if calcium is lost	Do not shave block before sectioning Re-radiograph blocks before and after recuts

Two caveats are worth noting in regard to mammographically directed biopsy processing. First, unless a grossly suspicious lesion is identified, examination by frozen section is strongly discouraged. It is unlikely that a definite diagnosis will be rendered on frozen section, and the artifactual distortion caused by freezing may make it difficult or impossible to establish a diagnosis upon subsequent paraffin processing. We have found touch preparations to be useful in some cases, and this procedure does not adversely affect tissue for further processing. The second caveat concerns the misinterpretation of minimal microcalcifications as those identified by mammography. Extremely small calcifications are not identified by mammography (the limit of detection is 0.3 mm); if any question of adequacy of sampling exists, further sectioning of the appropriate blocks is suggested (Box 8-1).

This approach to breast biopsy processing appears well justified in view of the high degree of curability for early lesions identified by mammography. For processing to be optimally effective, however, close cooperation between the radiologist, surgeon, and pathologist as well as between the pathologist and histotechnologist is mandatory. Specimen radiographs may also be useful in cases where x-ray localization has not been done if the specimen is large or if atypical hyperplasia or noninvasive carcinoma is found in routine sections.[5]

In the remainder of the chapter, we turn our attention to various tests that may provide information useful in therapeutic decision making and in establishing prognosis.

ESTROGEN AND PROGESTERONE RECEPTORS

The utility of identifying the presence of and quantifying the number of estrogen (ER) and progesterone (PR) receptors in breast cancer tissue has been thoroughly evaluated as an ancillary technique for supplying useful information not available by routine gross and microscopic examination. ER levels with or without PR levels have been used with variable success as independent predictors of disease-free and overall survival in patients with breast cancers at various stages.* Moreover, their utility in predicting response to hormonal therapy has been established; those patients whose tumors show a low level of expression of ER have little chance of responding to hormonal manipulation, whereas those with very high ER levels frequently show such a response. Additionally, those patients who express both ER and PR are much more likely to respond to hormonal manipulation than those who express ER receptors only.

Steroid hormonal receptor analysis may be done either as a biochemical assay or by immunohistochemistry. The former technique is long established and represents the gold standard against which immunohistochemical methods have been validated. The biochemical cytosol steroid receptor assay has both advantages and disadvantages. Advantages include the fact that it produces quantitative data that correlate well with the probability of response to endocrine therapy. Patients with tumors containing ER values of less than 10 fmol/mg of cytosol protein have a less than 10% chance of responding to hormonal manipulation, while those whose tumors have values greater than 100 fmol/mg of protein have a greater than 75% chance of such response. Patients with intermediate levels have an intermediate likelihood of response.[26]

Disadvantages of the bioassay include the relatively large amount of tissue needed for routine techniques (0.5 g) and the lability of ER protein.[28,30,41] Delays in freezing tissue, improper handling, or low tumor cellularity[35] may cause false-negative results. Moreover, since the assay is done on cytosol, it may be difficult to be sure that tumor is being assayed; contamination with nonmalignant breast tissue may cause false-negative or false-positive results.[8,25,32,41] For this reason we recommend histologic examination of tissue adjacent to that taken for ER and PR studies to confirm that tumor is being assayed. ER expression may be heterogeneous within a tumor, so that some portions of the tumor may express high ER levels and other portions may have no ER.[12,35] This tissue variability may help to explain hormonal response in those cases with apparently low ER values or lack of hormonal response in those cases with higher values.

More recently, immunohistochemical techniques have become available for determining ER and PR status using both frozen-section and paraffin-embedded material.* Advantages include the small amount of tissue required for analysis and the fact that one can positively identify the cells showing immunoreactivity as tumor cells. Moreover, one can assess such tissue in a semiquantitative fashion using image analysis techniques in addition to assessing tumor tissue heterogeneity with regard to ER and PR expression.[9,19,20,21] Immunohistochemistry agreement with cytosol assay is in the range of 80% to 90% using frozen-section technique.[34] Several recent studies have shown that methods are available to achieve comparable results with paraffin-embedded material. That very little tumor tissue is necessary for performing ER and PR determination by immunohistochemical methods is highlighted by the fact that these studies can be accomplished using material obtained by fine-needle aspiration (FNA).[29,43] This is particularly useful if one anticipates neoadjuvant chemotherapy on tumors diagnosed by FNA when confirmatory biopsy is not anticipated. Although biochemical ligand-binding assays are still the preferred methodology for tumors of sufficient size, immunohistochemical techniques are now not only quantitatively comparable but also are being used in clinical studies.[8a] Because many breast cancers now diagnosed and treated are too small to permit biochemical analysis, immunohistochemistry may in a relatively short time become the method of choice for ER and PR determination in breast tumors.[8b]

CELL CYCLE AND DNA CONTENT

Tumor cells frequently undergo alterations in their DNA content that are not part of normal alter-

---

*References 10, 11, 14, 15, 18, 22, 23, 24, 33, 35, 42.

*References 13, 16, 17, 27, 31, 36-40.

ations in the cell cycle. Examples of such change are chromosome deletion, duplication, and translocation. Many of these changes result in a cell whose G0/G1 DNA content is different from the DNA content of a normal human diploid cell; that is, they are aneuploid. Such a genetic alteration may give rise to a survival or proliferative advantage and result in a subpopulation of the tumor with clonal aneuploid DNA content.

DNA analysis of tumors identifies aneuploid cell populations and gauges the proliferative capacity of the tumor by measuring the proportion of cells in different parts of the cell cycle, particularly the active DNA-synthesizing portion, the S phase. The fundamental assumption underlying the use of this technique is that tumors containing expanded clones with aneuploid DNA content and tumors with elevated proliferative fractions will display more aggressive biologic behavior than tumors lacking these features. For many common human tumors this assumption appears to be largely correct.[65] The data on breast cancer are both extensive and controversial, and after a brief discussion of several important technical points, the remainder of this section will review the relevant data correlating ploidy and cell cycle analysis with patient outcome.

Flow cytometry is the most frequently used method for ploidy and S-phase analysis. In this technique, a single cell suspension is made to flow in laminar fashion, one cell at a time, through an optical chamber. The cells are labeled with a fluorescent dye that binds stoichiometrically to DNA. The emitted fluorescence is proportional to cellular DNA content, and its magnitude is quantified on a per cell basis. Most current instruments use a laser for fluorescent excitation and also measure basic light scattering properties of the cells, allowing an estimation of cell size and cytoplasmic complexity. This method allows the measurement of total DNA content of many cells in a relatively short period, and thus gives a profile of the DNA content of a tumor population. Because cells in the G0/G1, S, and G2M phases of

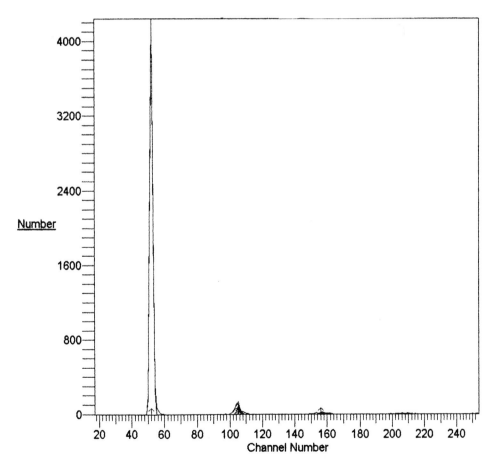

Fig. 8-3 This histogram illustrates a normal diploid population (channel 52) with small G_2M population (channel 104), a very low S-phase fraction.

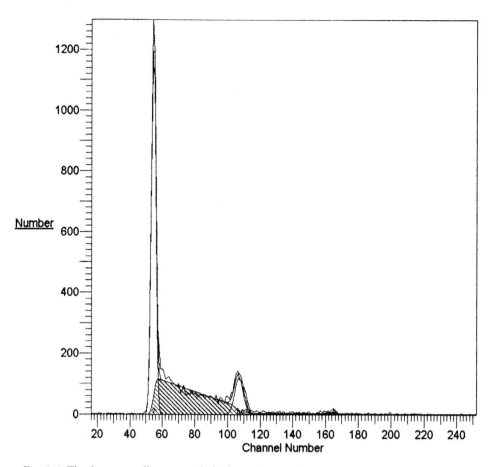

Fig. 8-4 This histogram illustrates a diploid population (channel 54) with modest G_2M (channel 107) and large S-phase fraction (area shaded with diagonal lines).

the cell cycle as well as aneuploid populations have different DNA contents, the relative proportion of tumor cells in each of these groups can be determined, as illustrated in Figs. 8-3 to 8-5.

Flow cytometric DNA analysis may be done on fresh or frozen tumor tissue or on fixed paraffin-embedded blocks. In general, fresh tissue gives technically superior results but has the disadvantage of needing to be performed before the standard pathologic examination is completed, so that some assays may be performed for patients who will not benefit from DNA analysis. Good communication between primary physician, surgical pathologist, and the flow cytometry laboratory can minimize these unnecessary assays. Frozen tissue gives almost identical results as fresh tissue and allows time to consider the histopathologic findings before doing DNA analysis but requires storage at $-70°$ C. Paraffin-embedded tissue offers the greatest flexibility in selecting both the timing of the assay and the most relevant portion of the specimen to study but has the disadvantage of in-

ferior technical quality. Nevertheless, more than 80% of paraffin-embedded tissues yield satisfactory results, and these tissues are a viable alternative to using fresh or frozen tissue. The utility of paraffin-embedded tissue for selecting specific areas of a tumor for study may be particularly relevant if two recent studies implying significant intratumor heterogeneity are shown to be clinically significant.[47,57] However, this finding has been questioned by other investigators.[62]

The S-phase fraction is usually determined by a mathematic calculation from the histogram displaying the DNA content of the tumor cell population. These calculations are affected by the presence of nuclear debris, storage, and the method of processing.

S-phase measurements do not reproduce well between laboratories or tissues, so it is best if individual laboratories determine their own limits for what is considered a high or low S-phase value. Aneuploid populations with DNA content very near the normal diploid population may merge

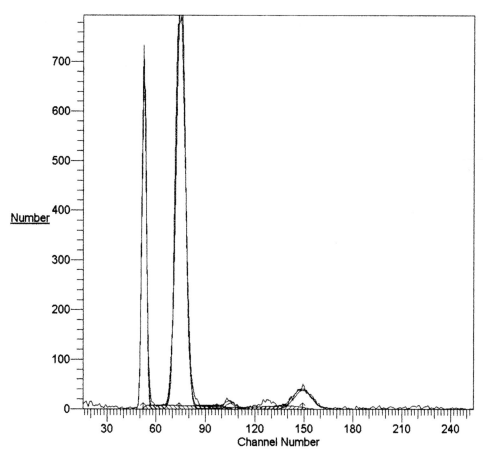

Fig. 8-5 This histogram illustrates diploid population (channel 52) and a large aneuploid population (channel 75) with small diploid G_2M (channel 105) and aneuploid G_2M (channel 149).

with the diploid peak on the DNA histogram, giving what appears to be a widened diploid population. Alternatively, population distributions may appear wide because of technical factors such as partial fixation or excessive flow rates. Each laboratory should have a uniform policy on the interpretation of these types of assays. It is sometimes helpful to analyze normal tissue from the same specimen that is submitted with the tumor. Fresh or frozen lymphocytes or paraffin-embedded lymph nodes or tonsils provide other sources of control material. Until interlaboratory standardization is realized, intralaboratory standardization and attention to principles of good laboratory practice must suffice.

For breast carcinomas, the current understanding of the use of DNA content and cell cycle analysis can be summarized as follows:

1. Tumors with aneuploid populations probably are more aggressive than strictly diploid tumors, but the magnitude of the resulting survival difference may not be sufficient to dictate differential treatment regimens and may not be independent of traditional prognostic factors.

2. Tumor S-phase fraction probably is an independent prognostic factor in early disease and may have a role in delineating patient groups with significantly different prognoses.

3. Both ploidy status and S phase may play some role in conjunction with other prognostic factors in defining patient groups with exceptionally good or unusually poor survival who may then be candidates for conservative or aggressive therapy, respectively.

Several early studies highlighted the relationship between abnormal S phase, aneuploidy, and poor overall and disease-free survival.* However, more recent large series have not confirmed the

*References 48-50, 52-54, 58, 60, 61, 64, 66, 70.

role of ploidy as an independent prognostic indicator in multivariate analysis.[46,56,61a,71] In contrast, S phase has been found to be a powerful predictor of prognosis.* For example, when S-phase data were combined with PR status and tumor size, Sigurdsson and colleagues[69] found that patients with favorable indicators had a 5-year overall survival rate of 92%, which did not differ from the expected age-adjusted rate for Swedish women. Although S-phase data appear useful in early-stage disease, recent studies suggest that the information may not be useful in patients with advanced disease.[63,72]

Tumor proliferative activity may also be assessed by immunohistochemical methods that employ the monoclonal antibody Ki-67 or a monoclonal antibody that identifies proliferating cell nuclear antigen (PCNA), also known as cyclin. Ki-67 identifies a nuclear antigen that is expressed during the G1, S, G2, and M phases of the cell cycle, and PCNA is maximally expressed during the S phase. In spite of this apparent difference in expression, Dervan and associates[51] have shown that the percentage of cells that express PCNA is equivalent to the percentage that expressed Ki-67 for a wide variety of tumors, including carcinoma of the breast. Both antigens show strong correlation with other measures of proliferative activity such as S phase by flow cytometry, mitotic count, and thymidine labeling index. However, insufficient data are available to determine if Ki-67 or PCNA immunohistochemistry will offer independent prognostic information in multivariate analysis. If shown to be useful, immunohistochemistry offers significant advantages over flow cytometry or thymidine labeling, in terms of both cost and simplicity.[59,67]

CATHEPSIN D, ONCOGENES, AND OTHER BIOLOGIC MARKERS

Cathepsin D (CD) is a ubiquitous, estrogen-inducible 52-K lysosomal protease that appears to be overexpressed in malignant but not benign breast tissue.[94,97] It has been hypothesized that CD acts by dissolving tissue basement membrane and stroma to facilitate tumor invasion and/or that it functions as a mitogen.[97] Many,[93,97,98] but not all,[80a,80,95] reported studies have shown that a high level of CD in tumor tissue is an independent predictor of poor disease-free and overall survival.

CD levels are generally measured by radioimmunoassay on tumor cytosol; therefore, one may use material in excess of that needed for ER and PR receptor analysis. CD determination requires approximately 0.05 g of fresh or fresh-frozen tissue. CD may also be identified by immunohistochemical means using frozen- or paraffin-section technique. Unfortunately, immunohistochemistry as opposed to cytosol analysis has not shown a high level of correlation between the presence of CD and prognosis.[73,80,95] It is interesting, however, that some immunohistochemical studies have shown that CD is present in tumor stroma as well as the neoplastic epithelium (Fig. 8-6), and at least one study suggests that stromal expression may, in fact, be more important than tumor cell expression in determining tumor aggressiveness.[99] This would support the hypothesis that CD is important in connective tissue lysis and facilitates invasive behavior.

Recent advances in tumor biology have shed considerable light on the molecular events of oncogenesis. Cellular oncogenes and their protein products have played a pivotal role in these studies, and this has led to an attempt to correlate oncogene amplification or overexpression with disease progression in breast cancer. The most closely scrutinized oncogene in breast cancer is c-erbB-2 (HER-2/neu). c-erbB-2 is a cellular oncogene present on chromosome 17 that encodes for a 185-Kd transmembrane glycoprotein thought to be the receptor for an as yet not fully defined tissue growth factor.[86] As such, it is hypothesized that amplification and/or overexpression of this gene is related to increased tumor aggressiveness. Approximately 20% to 30% of breast cancers or breast cancer cell lines studied show overexpression of c-erbB-2. Slamon and coworkers[96] as well as others* have shown shortened disease-free and overall survival in breast cancer patients who show gene amplification, particularly in patients with node-positive disease. This relationship has not been universally confirmed.[74,100] The relative importance of variability of c-erbB-2 expression versus variability in methodology in these disparate results is unclear.[92] It is clear, however, that methodologic concerns must be addressed before this controversy can be resolved.[89]

c-erbB-2 may be studied by Southern blot analysis to detect gene amplification as well as by immunohistochemistry to detect the presence of its protein product. The former is generally performed on fresh or frozen tissue, and the latter may be performed by frozen-section or paraffin-embedded techniques.

Other oncogenes, including c-myc,[77,83] H-ras,[101] int,[104] and c-myb,[75] have been studied, and there is some evidence that overexpression of

---

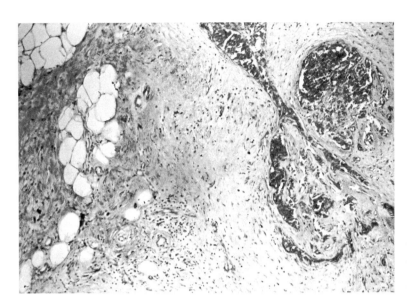

Fig. 8-6 Both the neoplastic epithelium and the stroma of this infiltrating ductal carcinoma stain for cathepsin D.

these oncogenes may be seen in aggressive breast cancers. Their role in prognosis is undefined, however.[75] Also undefined is the role of abnormalities in tumor suppressor genes such as p53, which is present on chromosome 17. Abnormalities in p53 may play a significant role in the pathogenesis of familial breast cancer,[82] although its role in tumor progression is unclear. The presence of other tumor markers, such as carcinoembryonic antigen, kappa casein, alpha lactalbumin, pregnancy-specific beta-1-glycoprotein, human chorionic gonadotropin, and placental lactogen, has not proved to be prognostically significant when examined in tissue.[76,81] Epidermal growth factor receptor, heat shock proteins, plasminogen activators, and the metastasis suppressor gene NM23 are factors currently under study and shown to have some role in identifying prognostic subgroups of patients with node-negative breast cancer.[85] Recent publications suggest that tumor angiogenesis as measured by microvessel immunochemical identification and counting is a highly significant indicator of prognosis in early stage breast cancer.[102] Other putative prognostic indicators such as the nucleolar antigen P120 appear to offer useful information,[78] but more extensive clinical studies are required before their roles are defined.

From the preceding discussion it should be clear that, apart from ER and PR analysis, the study of biologic markers in breast cancer tissue is an evolving area of investigation. The ultimate role of the markers described and other as yet undefined markers in therapeutic decision making is unclear. McGuire[87] highlighted the need for careful clinical studies to evaluate the merits of proposed prognostic indicators and, with cowork-

ers,[88] has suggested an algorithm, which includes both pathologic and biologic parameters that might be useful in decision making for individual patients. Although they are of questionable practicality at this time, it is possible to foresee the use of such information as tumor grade, nodal status, ER/PR, S-phase data, amplification of oncogenes, and presence of CD to specifically define the risk of relapse in subgroups of breast cancer patients. For example, a patient with a small, node-negative breast cancer of low histologic grade but absent ER and PR, high S-phase, increased levels of CD, and amplification of c-erb B-2 may be at significantly greater risk for relapse than patients with a similar tumor showing more favorable biologic markers. The former may be a more reasonable candidate for aggressive adjuvant chemotherapy than the latter.

The exact role of these markers and those yet to be identified will require extensive clinical study before their utility is optimized. In this regard, it is an interesting footnote to our health care system that the tests described are currently available commercially, either singly or as panels.

REFERENCES
Mammographically directed wire localization

1. D'Orsi CJ, Reale FR, Davis MA, et al: Breast specimen microcalcifications: radiographic validation and pathologic-radiologic correlation, *Radiology* 180:397, 1991.
2. Owings DV, Hann L, Schnitt SJ: How thoroughly should needle localization breast biopsies be sampled for microscopic examination: a prospective mammographic/pathologic correlative study, *Am J Surg Pathol* 14:578, 1990.
3. Rebner M, Helvie MA, Pennes DR, et al: Paraffin tissue block radiography: adjunct to breast specimen radiography, *Radiology* 173:695, 1989.

4. Snyder RE, Rosen P: Radiography of breast specimens, *Cancer* 28:1608, 1971.
5. Stein MA, Karlan MS: Calcifications in breast biopsy specimens: discrepancies in radiologic-pathologic identification, *Radiology* 179:111, 1991.
6. Tabar L: Control of breast cancer through screening mammography, *Radiology* 174:655, 1990.
7. Truong LD, Cartwright J, Alpert, L: Calcium oxalate in breast lesions biopsied for calcification detected in screening mammography: incidence and clinical significance, *Mod Pathology* 4:146-152, 1992.

Estrogen and progesterone receptors

8. Allegra JC, Lippman ME, Green L, et al: Estrogen receptor value in patients with benign breast disease, *Cancer* 44:228, 1979.
8a. Allred DC, Bustamante MA, Daniel CO, et al: Immunocytochemical analysis of estrogen receptors in human breast carcinomas. Evaluation of 130 cases and a review of the literature regarding concordance with the biochemical assay and clinical revelance. *Arch Surg* 125:107, 1990.
8b. Allred DC: Should immunohistochemical examination replace biochemical hormone receptor assays in breast cancer? *Am J Clin Pathol* 99:1, 1993.
9. Baddoura FK, Cohen C, Unger ER, et al: Image analysis for quantitation of estrogen receptor in formalin-fixed paraffin-embedded sections of breast carcinoma, *Mod Pathol* 4:91, 1991.
10. Bloom ND, Tobin EH, Schreibman B, et al: The role of progesterone receptors in the management of advanced breast cancer, *Cancer* 45:2992, 1980.
11. Butler JA, Bretsky S, Menendez-Botet C, et al: Estrogen receptor protein of breast cancer as a predictor of recurrence, *Cancer* 55:1178, 1985.
12. Charpin C, Martin PM, DeVictor B, et al: Multiparametric study (Samba 200) of estrogen receptor in microhistochemical assay in 400 human breast carcinomas: analysis of estrogen receptors' distribution heterogeneity in tissues and correlations with dextran coated charcoal assays and morphological data, *Cancer Res* 48:1578, 1988.
13. Cheng L, Binder SW, Yao SF, et al: Methods in laboratory investigation: demonstration of estrogen receptors by monoclonal antibody in formalin-fixed breast tumors, *Lab Invest* 58:346, 1988.
14. Chevallier B, Heintzmann F, Mosseri V, et al: Prognostic value of estrogen and progesterone receptors in operable breast cancer: results of a univariate and multivariate analysis, *Cancer* 62:2517, 1988.
15. Clark GM, McGuire WL, Hubay CA, et al: Progesterone receptors as a prognostic factor in stage II breast cancer, *N Engl J Med* 309:1343, 1983.
16. Cudahy TJ, Boeryd BR, Franlund BK, et al: A comparison of three different methods for the determination of estrogen receptors in human breast cancer, *Am J Clin Pathol* 90:583, 1988.
17. DeRosa CM, Ozzello L, Greene GL, et al: Immunostaining of estrogen receptor in paraffin sections of breast carcinomas using monoclonal antibody D775P3y: effects of fixation, *Am J Surg Pathol* 11:943, 1987.
18. Early Breast Cancer Trialists' Collaborative Group: Effects of adjuvant tamoxifen and of cytotoxic therapy on mortality in early breast cancer: an overview of 61 randomized trials among 28,896 women. *N Engl J Med* 319:1681, 1988.
19. El-Badawy N, Cohen C, DeRose PB, et al: Immunohistochemical estrogen receptor assay: quantitation by image analysis, *Mod Pathol* 4:305, 1991.
20. Esteban JM, Kandalaft PL, Menta P, et al: Improvement of the quantification of estrogen and progesterone receptors in paraffin-embedded tumors by image analysis. *Am J Clin Pathol* 99:32, 1993.
21. Esteban JM, Battifora H, Warsi Z, et al: Quantification of estrogen receptors on paraffin-embedded tumors by image analysis, *Mod Pathol* 4:53, 1991.
22. Feldman JG, Pertshuk LP, Carter AC, et al: Histochemical estrogen binding: an independent predictor of recurrence and survival in stage II breast cancer, *Cancer* 57:911, 1986.
23. Fisher B, Fisher ER, Redmond C, et al: Tumor nuclear grade, estrogen receptor, and progesterone receptor: their value alone or in combination as indicators of outcome following adjuvant therapy for breast cancer, *Breast Cancer Res Treat* 7:147, 1986.
24. Fisher ER, Redmond C, Fisher B, et al: Pathologic findings from the national surgical adjuvant breast and bowel projects (NSABP): prognostic discriminants for 8-year survival for node-negative invasive breast cancer patients, *Cancer* 65:2121, 1990.
25. Giani C, D'Amore E, Delarve JC, et al: Estrogen and progesterone receptors in benign breast tumors and lesions: relationship with histological and cytological features, *Int J Cancer* 37:7, 1986.
26. Heuson JC, Longeval E, Mattheim WH, et al. Significance of quantitation assessment of estrogen receptors for endocrine therapy in advanced breast cancer. *Cancer* 39:1971-1977.
27. Hiort O, Kwan PW, DeLellis RA: Immunohistochemistry of estrogen receptor protein in paraffin sections: effects of enzymatic pretreatment and cobalt chloride intensification, *Am J Clin Pathol* 90:559, 1988.
28. Leung B, Manaugh LC, Wood DC: Estradiol receptors in benign and malignant disease of the breast, *Clin Chem Acta* 46:69, 1973.
29. Masood S: Use of monoclonal antibody for assessment of estrogen receptor content in fine-needle aspiration biopsy specimen from patients with breast cancer, *Arch Pathol Lab Med* 113:26, 1989.
30. McGuire WH, Chamness GC, Costlow ME, et al: Progress in endocrinology and metabolism: hormone dependence in breast cancer. *Metabolism* 23:75, 1974.
31. Nenci I: Estrogen receptor cytochemistry in human breast cancer: status and prospects, *Cancer* 48:2674, 1981.
32. Netto GJ, Cheek JH, Zachariah NY, et al: Steroid receptors in benign mastectomy tissue, *Am J Clin Pathol* 94:14, 1990.
33. Night WE III, Livingston RB, Gregory EJ, et al: Estrogen receptor as an independent prognostic factor for early reccurrence in breast cancer, *Cancer Res* 37:4669, 1977.
34. Parl FP, Posey YF. Discrepancies of the biochemical and immunohistochemical estrogen receptor assays in breast cancer, *Hum Pathol* 19:960, 1988.
35. Parl FF, Schmidt BP, Dupont WD, et al: Prognostic significance of estrogen receptor status in breast cancer in relation to tumor stage, axillary node metastasis, and histopathologic grading, *Cancer* 54:2237, 1984.
36. Perrot-Applanat M, Grayer-Picard MT, Vu Hai MT, et al: Immunocytochemical staining of progesterone receptor in paraffin sections of human breast cancers, *Am J Pathol* 135:457, 1989.
37. Pertschuk LP Eisenberg KB, Carter AC, et al: Immunohistologic localization of estrogen receptors in breast cancer with monoclonal antibodies, *Cancer* 55:1513, 1985.
38. Pertschuk LP, Feldman JC, Eisenberg KB, et al: Immunocytochemical detection of progesterone receptor in breast cancer with monoclonal antibody, *Cancer* 62:342, 1988.

39. Pertschuk LP, Kim DS, Nayer K, et al: Immunocytochemical estrogen and progestin receptor assays in breast cancer with monoclonal antibodies, *Cancer* 66:1663, 1990.

40. Raam S, Nemeth E, Tamura H, et al: Immunohistochemical localization of estrogen receptors in human mammary carcinoma using antibodies to the receptor protein, *Eur J Cancer* 18:1, 1982.

41. Raynaud JP and others: *Progesterone receptors in normal and neoplastic tissues: estrogen and progesterone receptors in human breast cancer.* In McGuire WL, Raynaud JP, Baulier EE, editors: *Progress in cancer research and therapy*, vol 4, New York, 1977, Raven Press.

42. Vollenweider-Zerargui L, Barrelet L, Wong Y, et al: The predictive value of estrogen and progesterone receptors' concentrations on the clinical behavior of breast cancer in women: clinical correlation on 547 patients, *Cancer* 57:1171, 1986.

43. Weintraub J, Weintraub D, Redard M, et al: Evaluation of estrogen receptors by immunocytochemistry on fine-needle aspiration biopsy specimens from breast tumors, *Cancer* 60:1163, 1987.

44. Reference deleted in proof.

45. Reference deleted in proof.

Cell cycle and DNA content

46. Beerman H, Kluin PM, Hermans J, et al: Prognostic significance of DNA-ploidy in a series of 690 primary breast cancer patients, *Int J Cancer* 45:34, 1990.

47. Beerman H, Smit V, Kluin PM, et al: Flow cytometric analysis of DNA stemline heterogeneity in primary and metastatic breast cancer, *Cytometry* 12:147, 1991.

48. Clark GM, Dressler LG, Owens MA, et al: Prediction of relapse or survival in patients with node negative breast cancer by DNA flow cytometry, *N Engl J Med* 320:627, 1989.

49. Cornelisse CJ, van der Velde CJH, Caspers RJC, et al: DNA ploidy and survival in breast cancer patients, *Cytometry* 8:225, 1987.

50. Coulson PB, Thornwaite JT, Woolley TW, et al: Prognostic indicators including DNA histogram type, receptor content, and staging related to human breast cancer patient survival, *Cancer Res* 44:4187, 1984.

51. Dervan PA, Magee HM, Buckley C, et al: Proliferating cell nuclear antigen counts in formalin-fixed paraffin-embedded tissue correlate with Ki-67 in fresh tissue, *Am J Clin Pathol* 97(suppl 1):51, 1992.

52. Dressler LG, Seamer LC, Owens MA, et al: DNA flow cytometry and prognostic factors in 1331 frozen breast cancer specimens, *Cancer* 61:420, 1988.

53. Eskelinen M, Nordling S, Puittinen J, et al: The flow cytometric analysis of DNA content and S-phase fraction of human breast cancer, *Path Res Pract* 185:694, 1989.

54. Ewers S, Längström E, Baldetorp B, et al: Flow-cytometric DNA analysis in primary breast carcinomas and clinicopathological correlations, *Cytometry* 5:408, 1984.

55. Fisher B, Gunduz N, Constantino J, et al: DNA flow cytometric analysis of primary operative breast cancer, *Cancer* 68:1465, 1991.

56. Fisher ER, Redmond C, Fisher B, et al: Pathological findings from the national surgical adjuvant breast and bowel projects, *Cancer* 65:2121, 1990.

57. Fuhr JE, Frye A, Kattine AA, et al: Flow cytometric determination of breast tumor heterogeneity, *Cancer* 67:1401, 1991.

58. Hatschek T, Fagerberg G, Stål D, et al: Cytometric characterization and clinical course of breast cancer diagnosed in a population-based screening program, *Cancer* 64:1074, 1989.

59. Isola JJ, Helin HJ, Helle MJ, et al: Evaluation of cell proliferation in breast carcinoma, *Cancer* 65:1180, 1990.

60. Joensuu H, Toikkanen S, Klemi PJ: DNA index and S-phase fraction and their combination as prognostic factors in operable ductal breast carcinoma, *Cancer* 66:331, 1990.

61. Kallioniemi O, Hietanen T, Mattila J, et al: Aneuploid DNA content and high S-phase fraction of tumor cells are related to poor prognosis in patients with primary breast cancer, *Euro J Cancer* 23:277, 1987.

61a. Keyhani-Rofagha S, O'Toole RV, Farrar WB, et al: Is DNA ploidy an independent prognostic indicator in infiltrative node-negative breast adenocarcinoma, *Cancer* 65:1577, 1990.

62. Kute T: Response to Beerman et al., Letter to the editor, *Cytometry* 12:155, 1991.

63. Kute TE, Muss HB, Cooper MR, et al: The use of flow cytometry for the prognosis of stage II adjuvant treated breast cancer patients, *Cancer* 66:1810, 1990.

64. Lewis WE: Prognostic significance of flow cytometric DNA analysis in node-negative breast cancer patients, *Cancer* 65:2315, 1990.

65. Merkel DE, McGuire WL: Ploidy proliferative activity and prognosis, *Cancer* 65:1194, 1990.

66. Muss HG, Kute TE, Case LD, et al: The relation of flow cytometry to clinical and biologic characteristics in women with node negative primary breast cancer, *Cancer* 64:1894, 1989.

67. Sahin AA, Ro JY, El-Naggar AK, et al: Tumor proliferative fraction in solid malignant neoplasms, *Am J Clin Pathol* 96:512, 1991.

68. Reference deleted in proof.

69. Sigurdsson H, Baldetorp B, Borg Ä, et al: Indicators of prognosis in node-negative breast cancer, *N Engl J Med* 322:1045, 1990.

70. Stal O, Wingren S, Carstensen J, et al: Prognostic value of DNA ploidy and S-phase fraction in relation to estrogen receptor content and clinicopathological variables in primary breast cancer, *Eur J Cancer* 25:301, 1988.

71. Toikkanen S, Joensuu H, Klemi P: Nuclear DNA content as a prognostic factor in $T_{1-2}N_o$ breast cancer, *Am J Clin Pathol* 93:471, 1990.

72. Witzig TE, Gonchoroff NJ, Therneau T, et al: DNA content flow cytometry as a prognostic factor for node-positive breast cancer, *Cancer* 68:1781, 1991.

Cathepsin D, oncogenes, and other biologic markers

73. Reference deleted in proof.

74. Allred DC, Tandon AK, Clark GM, et al: *HER-2/neu oncogene amplification and expression in human mammary carcinoma.* In Preslow TG, editors: *Biochemical and molecular aspects of selected cancers*, 1991, Academic Press.

75. Cline M, Battifora HC, Hokota J: Proto-oncogene abnormalities in human breast cancer: correlations with anatomic features and clinical course of disease, *J Clin Oncol* 5:999, 1987.

76. Cohen C, Sharkey FE, Shulman G, et al: Tumor-associated antigens in breast carcinomas: prognostic significance, *Cancer* 60:1294, 1987.

77. Escot C, Theillet C, Lidereau R, et al: Genetic alteration of the c-myc protooncogene (MYC) in human primary breast carcinomas, *Proc Natl Acad Sci USA* 83:4834, 1986.

78. Freeman JW, McGrath P, Bondado V, et al: Prognostic significance of proliferation associated nucleolar antigen P120 in human breast carcinoma, *Cancer Res* 51:1973, 1991.

79. Gullick WJ, Love SB, Wright C, et al: c-erbB-2 protein overexpression in breast cancer is a risk factor in patients

with involved and uninvolved lymph nodes, *Br J Cancer* 63:434, 1991.

80. Henez JA et al: Prognostic significance of the estrogen-regulated protein, cathepsin D in breast cancer, *Cancer* 65:265, 1990.

80a. Kandalaft K, Chang C, Ahn P: Immunohistochemical analysis of cathepsin D in breast cancer: Is it prognostically significant? *Lab Invest* 66:14a, 1992.

81. Lee AK, Rosen PP, DeLellis RA, et al: Tumor marker expression in breast carcinomas and relationship to prognosis: an immunohistochemical study, *Am J Clin Pathol* 84:687, 1985.

82. Lee E: Tumor suppressor genes: a new era for molecular genetic studies of cancer, *Breast Cancer Res Treat* 19:3, 1991.

83. Locker AP, Dowle CS, Ellis IO, et al: C-myc oncogene product expression and prognosis in operable breast cancer, *Br J Cancer* 60:669, 1989.

84. Lovekin C, Ellis IO, Locker A, et al: c-erbB-2 oncoprotein expression in primary and advanced breast cancer, *Br J Cancer* 63:439, 1991.

85. Maguire WL and Clark GM: Prognostic factors and treatment decisions in auxiliary-node-negative breast cancer, *New Engl J Med* 326:1756, 1992.

86. Maguire HC, Greene MI: Neu(c-erbB-2), a tumor marker in carcinoma of the female breast, *Pathobiology* 58:297, 1990.

87. McGuire WL: Breast cancer prognostic factors: evaluation guidelines, *J Natl Cancer Inst* 83:154, 1991.

88. McGuire WL, Tandon AK, Alfred DC, et al.: How to use prognostic factors in axillary node-negative breast cancer patients, *J Natl Cancer Inst* 82:1006, 1990.

89. Naber SP, Tsutsumi Y, Yin S, et al: Strategies for the analysis of oncogene overexpression: studies of the neu oncogene in breast carcinoma, *Am J Clin Pathol* 94:125, 1990.

90. O'Reilly SM, Barnes DM, CampleJohn RS, et al: The relationship between c-erbB-2 expression, S-phase fraction and prognosis in breast cancer, *Br J Cancer* 63:444, 1991.

91. Paik S, Hazan R, Fisher ER, et al: Pathologic findings

from the national surgical adjuvant breast and bowel project: prognostic significance of erbB-2 protein overexpression in primary breast cancer, *J Clin Oncol* 8:103, 1990.

92. Press MF: Oncogene amplification and expression: importance of methodologic considerations, *Am J Clin Pathol* 94:240, 1990.

93. Rochefort H: Cathepsin D in breast cancer, *Breast Cancer Res Treat* 16:3, 1990.

94. Rochefort H, Augereau P, Briozzo P, et al: Structure, function, regulation and clinical significance of the 52K pro-cathepsin D secreted by breast cancer cells, *Biochimie* 70:943, 1988.

95. Sahin A, Sneige N, Ordonez N, et al: Immunohistochemical determination of cathepsin D in node-negative breast carcinoma, *Lab Invest* 66:17A, 1992.

96. Slamon DJ, Godolphin W, Jones LA, et al: Studies of the HER-2/neu proto-oncogene in human breast and ovarian cancer, *Science* 244:707, 1989.

97. Spyratos F, Maudelonde T, Brouillet JP, et al: Cathepsin D: an independent prognostic factor for metastasis of breast cancer, *Lancet*, 335:1115-1118, 1989.

98. Tandon AK, Clark GM, Chamness GC, et al: Cathepsin D and prognosis in breast cancer, *N Engl J Med* 322:297, 1990.

99. Tetu B, Cote C, Brisson J: Cathepsin D in node-positive breast carcinoma, *Lab Invest* 66:18A, 1990.

100. Thor AD, Schwartz LH, Koerner FC, et al: Analysis of c-erbB-2 expression in breast carcinomas with clinical follow up, *Cancer Res* 49:7147, 1989.

101. Watson DM, Elton RA, Jack WJ, et al: The H-ras oncogene product p21 and prognosis in human breast cancer, *Breast Cancer Res Treat* 17:161, 1990.

102. Weidner N, Folkman J, Pozza F, et al: Tumor angiogenesis: A new significant and independent prognostic indicator in early-stage breast carcinoma. *J Natl Cancer Inst* 84:1875, 1992.

103. Winstanley J, Cooke T, George WD, et al: The long term prognostic significance of c-erbB-2 in primary breast cancer, *Br J Cancer* 63:447, 1991.

104. Wolman SR, Pauley RJ, Mohamed AN, et al: Genetic markers as prognostic indicators in breast cancers, *Cancer* 70:1765, 1992.

PART II Atlas of Breast Diseases

CHAPTER 9

Circumscribed Breast Masses

Carol B. Stelling
Deborah E. Powell

Fibroadenoma
    Fibroadenoma variants: giant fibroadenoma and juvenile fibroadenoma
Phyllodes tumor
Adenoma
    Tubular adenoma
    Lactating adenoma
Lipoma
Hamartoma
Galactocele

The lesions discussed in this chapter include fibroadenoma and variants, phyllodes tumor, tubular and lactating adenomas, lipoma, hamartoma, and galactocele. All of these lesions are characterized by smooth, well-defined borders. Although most of these lesions are benign tumors, a few (e.g., galactocele) are not true neoplasms. Other benign tumors are discussed in Chapters 10 and 13. Some malignant neoplasms may present as well-circumscribed masses as well (Table 9-1), and these are discussed in Chapters 10, 12, and 13.

FIBROADENOMA

Fibroadenoma is a benign tumor of the breast consisting of both fibrous and epithelial components. The term *adenofibroma* may be used when the epithelial components are predominant. Two patterns of growth (intracanalicular and pericanalicular) have been described histologically. Radiographically, these two types are indistinguishable, and the distinction is not currently used by most surgical pathologists.

Fibroadenomas are the most common benign breast condition after fibrocystic breast disease and the most common benign breast tumor. In a survey of all hospitals in Israel for 1 year, fibroadenomas were diagnosed in 16.6% of 3734 biopsies. The incidence rate was 48.2 in 100,000 for women of European origin and 54.4 in 100,000 for women of African origin.[3]

Fibroadenoma most often presents in clinical practice as a palpable, firm, smooth, mobile mass in women less than 40 years of age. It is the most common breast mass in the adolescent age group.[2,7] The age range, however, is wide, and fibroadenomas may be present in the elderly, presumably remaining undetected from earlier years. The increasingly widespread use of screening mammography in asymptomatic women results in detection of clinically occult fibroadenomas in women older than 40 years of age. Fortunately, some of these masses demonstrate the characteristic coarse, peripheral calcification pattern that allows a confident radiographic diagnosis of a benign fibroadenoma. Most fibroadenomas are well circumscribed, are round or oval, and have only one or two gentle lobulations.[29] Occasionally, the radiographic appearance (lobulations or calcifica-

Table 9-1 **Differential diagnosis of circumscribed breast masses**

Category	Lesion	Special features
Normal	Intramammary lymph node	Fatty hilum
Cystic	Cyst	Classic sonographic appearance
	Epithelial inclusion cyst	Dermal location on tangential view
	Galactocele	Fat–fluid level when present
Benign neoplasm	Fibroadenoma	Characteristic calcification when present
	Adenoma	None
	Lipoma	Fat surrounded by thin capsule
	Hamartoma	Mixed density
	Phyllodes tumor*	None
Malignant neoplasm	Circumscribed carcinoma	None
	Intracystic papillary carcinoma	Sonographically complex cyst
	Solitary metastasis	None
	Lymphoma	None

*Phyllodes tumors may rarely be malignant. See text.

tions) are suspicious for an occult carcinoma, and excisional biopsy or fine-needle aspiration (FNA) cytology is required for diagnosis. An understanding of the histopathologic features of this lesion may help to explain the spectrum of radiographic appearances.

The patient usually presents with a rubbery, firm mass easily palpable and distinct from surrounding parenchyma. The mass is most often painless. However, occasional cyclic tenderness has been reported.[19] Infarction of a fibroadenoma produces focal discomfort in 50% of cases,[11] but this is a rare finding and is most often seen in pregnant or lactating women.

Fibroadenomas are usually 1 to 4 cm in diameter. An interval increase in size over several months frequently is observed. It has been reported that, in general, fibroadenomas double in size within 6 to 12 months and slow or cease growing when 2 to 3 cm in diameter.[14] If the mass develops cystic change or infarction, it may become less firm to palpation.[31] Conversely, associated inflammatory reaction to an infarct may result in a fixed mass and clinical adenopathy mimicking the findings of infiltrative carcinoma on physical examination.[11]

The clinical finding of a solid, well-circumscribed, round or oval mass in a woman in the second or third decade of life indicates a probable fibroadenoma. The diagnosis is most often confirmed by either an excisional biopsy or FNA cytology. In some cases, small lesions are monitored by physical examination to assess growth, if any. Because hormonal influences (birth control pills, pregnancy, or lactation) may cause enlargement of fibroadenomas, it may be recommended that excisional biopsy be considered as an elective procedure in the young woman of child-bearing years.

The role of mammography in the diagnostic evaluation of fibroadenoma is limited. In the adolescent breast, the lesion may not be visible[12] because the dense breast stroma and parenchyma may obscure the margins of the palpable mass. Occasionally, a portion of the margin is seen projecting into the subcutaneous fatty layer,[12] and focal tangential spot films may be used to demonstrate this feature. Because of the lack of radiographic correlation, the increased radiosensitivity of the adolescent breast, and the low yield for detecting clinically occult breast cancer in young women, mammography is not recommended for evaluation of a questionable fibroadenoma in women younger than 25 to 30 years old. In this young population, breast ultrasonography may be used to confirm a well-circumscribed solid mass suggestive of a fibroadenoma if the clinical examination is uncertain.

Breast ultrasonography of fibroadenomas has been well described. Although some fibroadenomas demonstrate classic ultrasonographic features of a round or oval solid mass with homogeneous internal echoes and a smooth wall, breast ultrasonography is not reliable to differentiate a benign from a malignant solid mass.[6,15,16] Biopsy or FNA is recommended for all solid palpable lesions 1 cm or larger to exclude malignancy. Close clinical and mammographic follow-up is recommended for nonpalpable solid masses with radiographic benign features.[4] Fibroadenomas not identified by ultrasonography are presumed to have echo characteristics identical to those of the surrounding breast parenchyma or fat.

The calcification patterns in fibroadenomas fall into two groups. The most common pattern is that of large, coarse calcifications, often peripheral in distribution and increasing over time. This is the pattern of dystrophic calcification in a degenerating or hyalinized fibroadenoma. The radiographic appearance is sufficiently characteristic to establish a diagnosis provided that the margins of the mass are well circumscribed. A rare circumscribed cancer with coarse calcifications has been described, but critical review of the images demonstrated a slightly irregular margin, making the mass suspicious for carcinoma.[18]

The second pattern is that of linear or branching calcifications simulating the pattern seen in intraductal carcinoma.[19,32] These calcifications represent calcified secretions in ductal spaces of the fibroadenoma, similar to the intraluminal calcification in intraductal cancer. These lesions usually are diagnosed by wire-directed excisional biopsy of the suspicious focus of fine linear and branching microcalcifications. A mass may or may not be demonstrated radiographically.

Fibroadenomas are multiple in 20% to 25% of patients. A familial tendency has been reported.[23,25] Traditionally, the diagnosis of fibroadenoma has not been thought to confer any increased risk for subsequent development of malignancy. However, in the last 15 years there has been some evidence to suggest that fibroadenomas might reflect a moderate risk (three times normal) for breast cancer.[9,17,24]

Cancer arising as an incidental finding within a fibroadenoma has been reported.[1,5,21] The prevalence is low (0.02% in a screening population).[8] Most cases are in situ lesions, usually lobular but occasionally ductal. The radiographic appearance may be indistinguishable from that of a benign fibroadenoma. Radiographic findings that should be considered atypical include large or increasing size, indistinct margins, or clustered microcalcifications within the mass.[1] The low prevalence and in situ nature of the cancers should be stressed. The work-up and follow-up of benign-appearing solid breast masses should not be altered because of this rare incidental occurrence of carcinoma within a few fibroadenomas.

Fibroadenomas may contain many of the usual histopathologic features of fibrocystic change, including apocrine metaplasia and sclerosing adenosis. They are tumors derived from lobules and have a characteristic gross appearance. On cut section they are rubbery and white with occasional flecks of yellow to tan tissue. If the tissue is distorted or bent, small cleftlike spaces can be seen. Microscopically, the tumors lack a capsule but are sharply demarcated from the normal parenchyma. They are composed of glands and fibrous stroma and, not infrequently, the glands are compressed into slitlike spaces. Adipose tissue is only rarely seen in fibroadenomas, helping to differentiate them radiographically and histologically from hamartomas. The glands may show varying degrees of

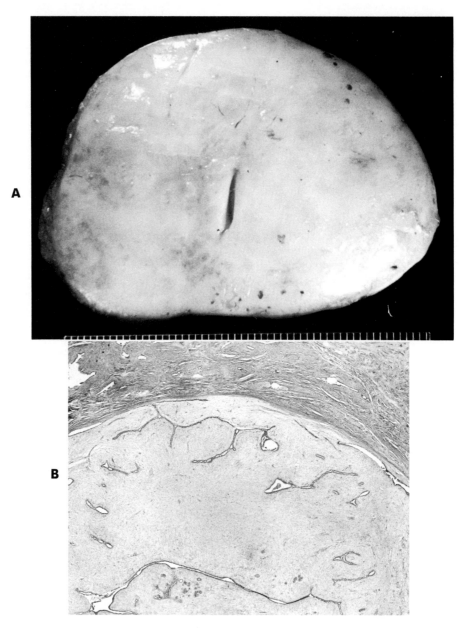

Fig. 9-1 (A) Fibroadenomas grossly are solitary tumors with smooth borders. A somewhat variegated appearance (usually white to yellow) is characteristic of the cut surface. Gland or cyst-like spaces can occasionally be seen grossly. **(B)** Fibroadenomas are characterized by a well-demarcated border that separates them from the surrounding parenchyma. The tumor itself is composed of glands, often compressed by a loose, more cellular stroma as seen in this photomicrograph.

epithelial hyperplasia, similar to that occurring in gynecomastia, and rarely, carcinoma in situ is identified, as mentioned previously. Despite some reports to the contrary, no consistent unusual histologic features are seen in fibroadenomas of long-term users of oral contraceptive pills in large studies of such lesions.[10,20,26] The stroma can vary from resembling closely the normal perilobular stroma to being acellular and hyalinized. This stromal hyalinization is usually found in fibroadenomas of older patients, and the glandular elements may be all or partially obliterated. Likewise, coarse stromal calcification may be present and, occasionally, intraluminal calcification within glands can be seen. In addition, osseous metaplasia[30] and smooth muscle metaplasia[13] have been described within fibroadenomas.

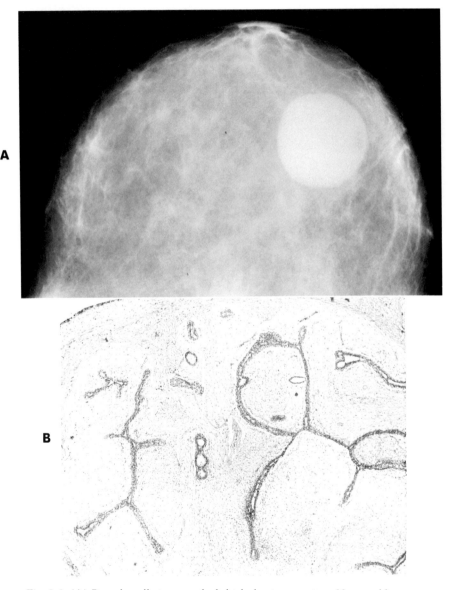

Fig. 9-2 (A) Round, well-circumscribed, high-density mass in a 23-year-old woman. **(B)** The pathologic diagnosis is fibroadenoma. The characteristic cellular stroma of the fibroadenoma is illustrated here. The glandular elements are compressed and show minimal epithelial hyperplasia.

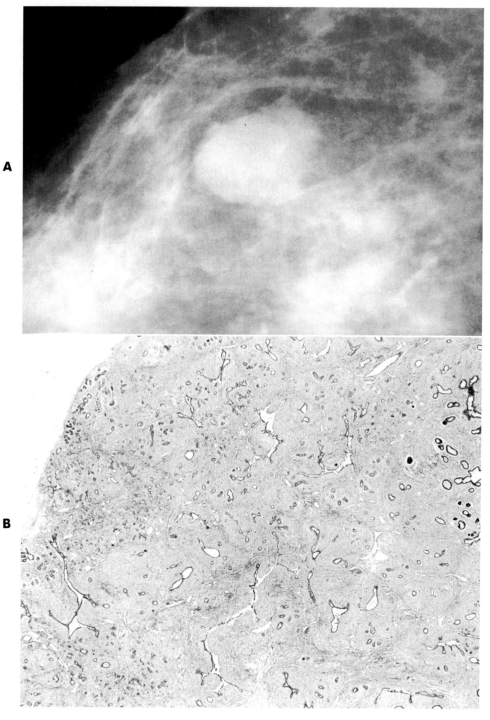

Fig. 9-3 **(A)** Irregular-shaped mass with indistinct margin was solid on ultrasound examination. Wire-directed biopsy in this 45-year-old woman proved the lesion to be a fibroadenoma. **(B)** The glands in this fibroadenoma are less compressed than those previously illustrated, and the stroma is somewhat fibrotic.

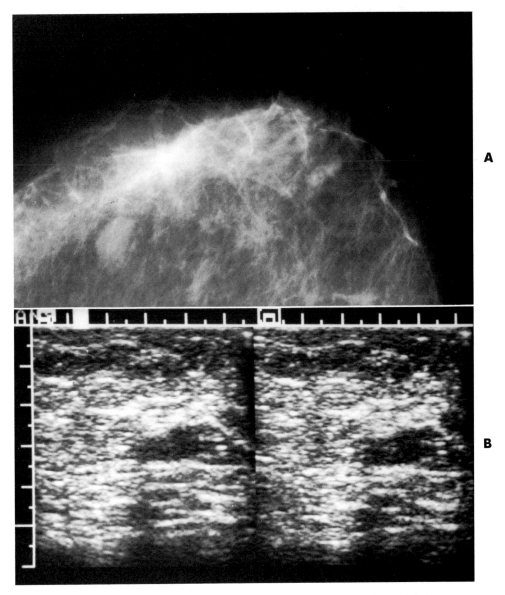

Fig. 9-4 Abnormal screening mammogram in a 50-year-old woman. Low-density lobulate mass with indistinct margins **(A)** was solid on ultrasound examination **(B).** The pathologic diagnosis was fibroadenoma.

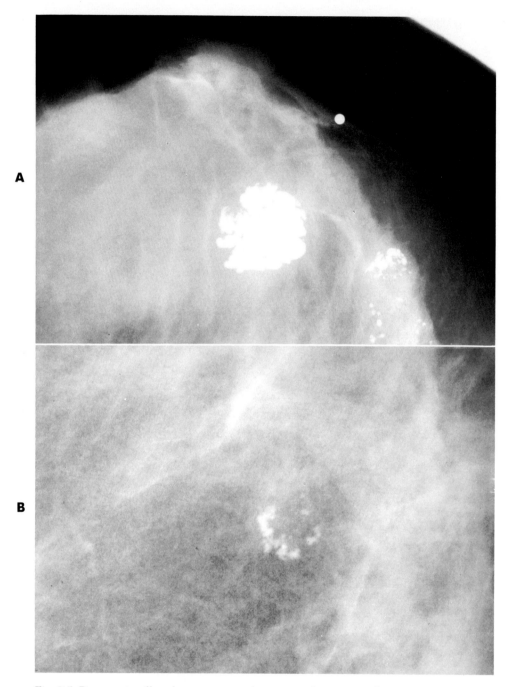

Fig. 9-5 Degenerating fibroadenoma may produce a typical mammographic appearance based on the pattern of calcification. Typical coarse popcorn-type calcifications **(A)** indicate multiple degenerating fibroadenomas, the largest of which was palpable (skin bb). A peripheral location of coarse **(B)** or rounded **(C)** calcifications is typical in some degenerating fibroadenomas. In some patients **(D)**, the pattern of calcification may mimic comedocarcinoma, necessitating a biopsy.

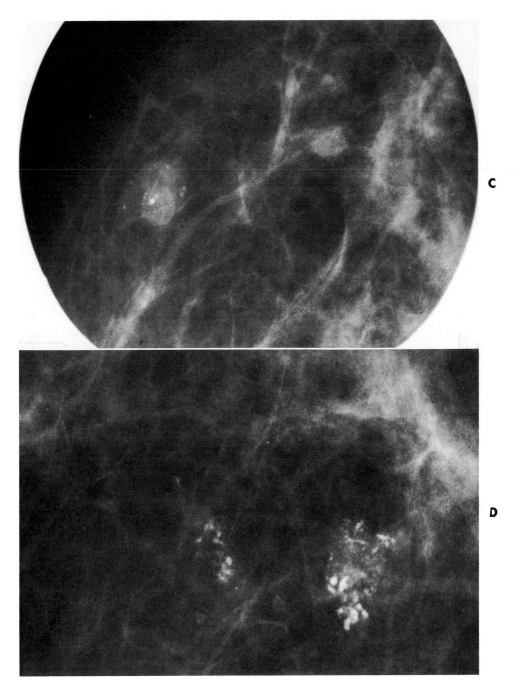

Fig 9-5, cont'd. For legend see opposite page.

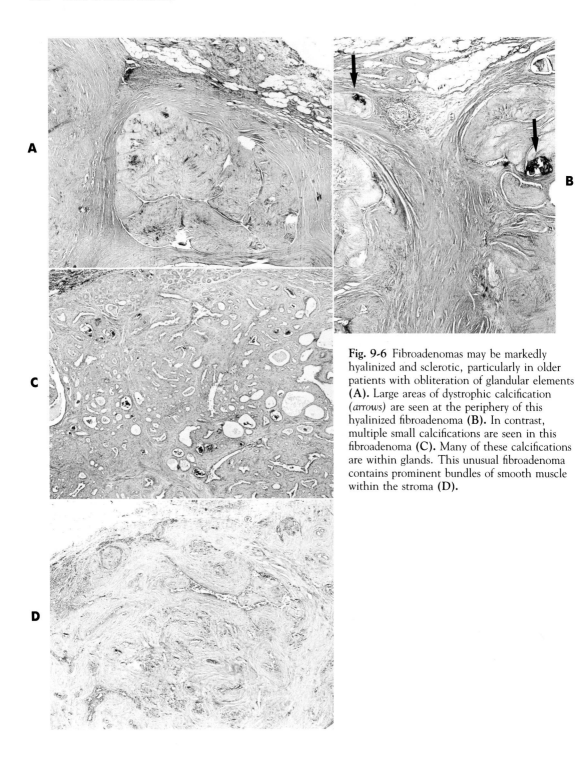

Fig. 9-6 Fibroadenomas may be markedly hyalinized and sclerotic, particularly in older patients with obliteration of glandular elements **(A).** Large areas of dystrophic calcification *(arrows)* are seen at the periphery of this hyalinized fibroadenoma **(B).** In contrast, multiple small calcifications are seen in this fibroadenoma **(C).** Many of these calcifications are within glands. This unusual fibroadenoma contains prominent bundles of smooth muscle within the stroma **(D).**

Fig. 9-7 Low-density, lobulated 2-cm mass with indistinct borders (**A**) was a fibroadenoma with incidental ductal carcinoma in situ. Carcinoma arising in fibroadenomas is most commonly lobular carcinoma in situ, as illustrated in these two low (**B**) and higher magnification (**C**) photomicrographs.

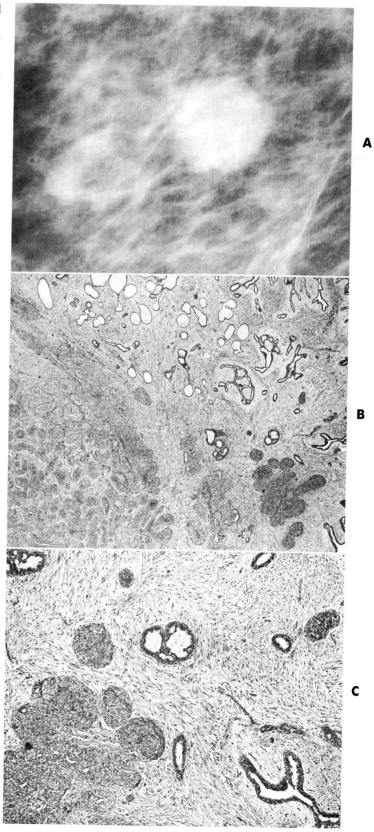

Fibroadenoma variants: giant fibroadenoma and juvenile fibroadenoma

Giant fibroadenoma and juvenile fibroadenoma are fibroadenoma variants (Box 9-1). A giant fibroadenoma is a large benign fibroadenoma, usually 8 to 10 cm in diameter and weighing more than 500 g.[11,28] The histologic features of the stroma are benign by definition.

Juvenile fibroadenoma is a large giant fibroadenoma that also has the following distinctive clinical features. It occurs in an adolescent female; has a rapid growth rate; may enlarge to two to four times the size of the normal breast; and exhibits displacement of the nipple, stretching of the skin, and venous distention. Juvenile fibroadenoma is to be differentiated from adolescent breast hypertrophy, which is bilateral, causes no nipple displacement, and is a diffuse enlargement of the entire breast and not an encapsulated breast mass.[11] Juvenile fibroadenomas often exhibit epithelial hyperplasia of the glands and increased cellularity of the stroma.[22,27]

BOX 9-1 FIBROADENOMA AND VARIANTS

Fibroadenoma
Giant fibroadenoma
Juvenile fibroadenoma
Fibroadenoma with incidental carcinoma in situ

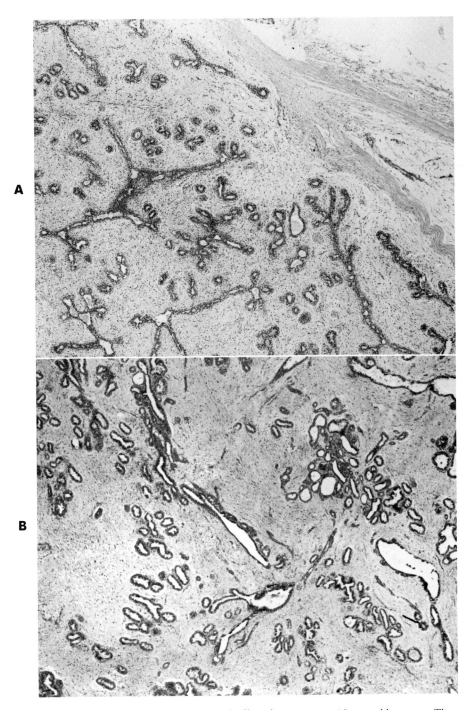

Fig. 9-8 Photomicrographs of a juvenile fibroadenoma in an 18-year-old woman. The tumor measured 10 cm. The glands show moderate epithelial hyperplasia.

PHYLLODES TUMOR

Phyllodes tumors (formerly cystosarcoma phyllodes) are uncommon fibroepithelial breast tumors that were first described in 1883 by Johannes Muller.[45] The histopathologic feature that characterizes the phyllodes tumor is the cellular periductal stroma, which is more cellular than that of a usual fibroadenoma. Because this tumor may exhibit either benign or malignant behavior, the preferred nomenclature is to drop the term *cystosarcoma* and use the phrase *phyllodes tumor*. Neither the size of the tumor nor its gross appearance is a prerequisite to making the diagnosis. A leaflike appearance ("phylloda") on cut section is not a constant feature.[47] The incidence of phyllodes tumor is approximately eight cases in 50,000 examinations,[37] or 2.5% of biopsy-proven fibroepithelial tumors.[44]

The age range has been reported to be 14 to 67 years, with an average age of 44.3 years.[48] Other reports agree that the average age is somewhere in the mid-forties, in general, 10 years older than the average age for women with fibroadenomas.[44,47]

The usual clinical history is that of a painless, mobile, firm mass increasing in size over weeks to years. Many masses are quite large at the time of clinical presentation (5 to 15 cm in diameter), but small tumors are also reported. A median size of 5 cm was recorded in one series, in which tumors ranged from 1 cm to 41 cm in diameter.[48] Bloody nipple discharge is uncommon.[49]

The gross appearance of the phyllodes tumor is usually described as lobulated, firm, and tan, gray, and/or yellow in color. Cystic and gelatinous areas are present in varying proportions. Large polypoid masses project into the cystic cavities, producing cleftlike spaces.[49] In fact, the presence of a cystic area or smooth fluid-filled clefts by ultrasonography in a large lobulated solid mass may suggest the diagnosis of phyllodes tumor.[34A,36,42] Ultrasonography differentiates this tumor as a solid lesion from multiple loculated cysts that may cause a similar mammographic appearance.[38] The principal imaging feature of phyllodes tumors is a well-circumscribed, lobular, smooth-marginated mass on mammography that is solid by ultrasonography with smooth walls, low-level internal echoes, and good through transmission of sound.[36] The differential diagnosis includes a non-calcified fibroadenoma and a well-circumscribed carcinoma.

Phyllodes tumors are difficult to classify by their histopathologic appearance as benign or malignant. A category of borderline malignant is important to include for these neoplasms. The features that suggest frank malignancy include high mitotic counts (more than 10 mitoses per 10 high-power fields) and frankly sarcomatous stroma. Of the malignant phyllodes tumors, only a small percentage (3% to 12%) actually metastasize by direct chest wall invasion or hematogenous dissemination.[43,46] More frequently, tumors recur locally, often multiple times, before metastasizing. Therefore any local excision should include a wide margin of normal tissue. Large or rapidly growing tumors may require simple mastectomy.[34]

Phyllodes tumors may rarely contain in situ carcinoma. The radiographic appearance is indistinguishable from that of benign phyllodes tumor.[36] It is the stromal component of the phyllodes tumors that metastasizes and not these uncommon incidental epithelial carcinomas.

It has been difficult to predict which phyllodes tumors will recur or metastasize.[39,40] Some authors stress that sarcomatous stromal overgrowth is a prerequisite for metastasis.[41,50] One group has reported that strong expression of carcinoembryonic antigen in the epithelial component of phyllodes tumor may be a predictor of local tumor recurrence. However, in this study, none of the 15 patients had metastatic disease.[33] In any case, adequate histopathologic sampling of the original tumor is encouraged to avoid overlooking a sarcomatous area and to facilitate accurate classification of the lesion into a benign, borderline, or malignant category.[41]

All phyllodes tumors are characterized by a proliferating cellular stroma. Many exhibit increased mitotic activity, stromal cellular atypia, heterologous stromal elements, and areas of stromal overgrowth with crowding out of epithelial elements. The problem for the surgical pathologist is to define which criteria warrant a diagnosis of malignant, benign, or borderline malignant tumor. Several studies have stressed the importance of high mitotic counts and stromal overgrowth in predicting metastatic disease.[41,50] A recent study of 77 cases from Sweden tabulated multiple histologic parameters and subjected them to multivariate analysis in an attempt to ascertain parameters most closely associated with malignant behavior. Although, by univariate analysis, factors such as mitotic activity and stromal overgrowth were significant, by multivariate analysis only the presence of tumor necrosis and heterologous stromal elements gave independent prognostic information. In this study, local recurrence was more frequent in cases treated by excision alone than in those treated by simple or radical mastectomy, reemphasizing the need for complete removal of tumor to control local disease.[35]

We may conclude from these published studies that phyllodes tumors exhibiting necrosis, heterologous (and malignant) stromal elements, areas of stromal overgrowth, and high mitotic counts (greater than 10 mitoses per 100 high-power field) should be classified as malignant and treated aggressively. Conversely, tumors lacking these parameters may be regarded as unlikely to exhibit malignant behavior. Tumors with one or more but not all of these features may be given a borderline malignant designation.

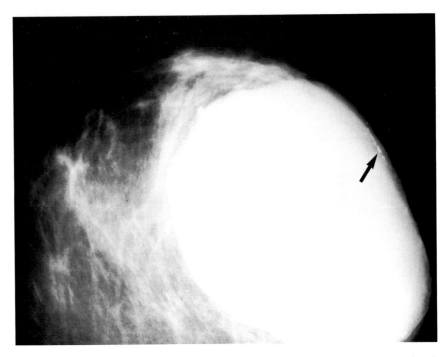

Fig. 9-9 Large oval high-density mass with circumscribed margins contains peripheral coarse benign calcifications (*arrow*). The pathologic diagnosis is phyllodes tumor. (Courtesy Dr. Terri Daniel, Corbin, Kentucky.)

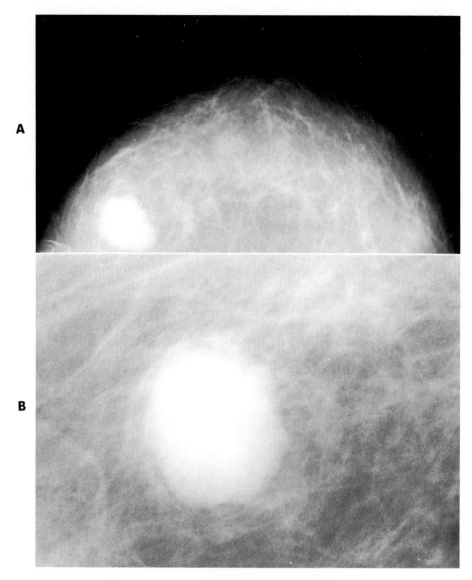

Fig. 9-10 Oval mass **(A)** demonstrated indistinct margins on close examination **(B).** Breast ultrasound examination confirmed a solid mass **(C)** with areas **(D)** of both hyperechogenicity and hypoechogenicity. The pathologic diagnosis is phyllodes tumor. (Courtesy Dr. Marie Lee, Seattle, Washington.)

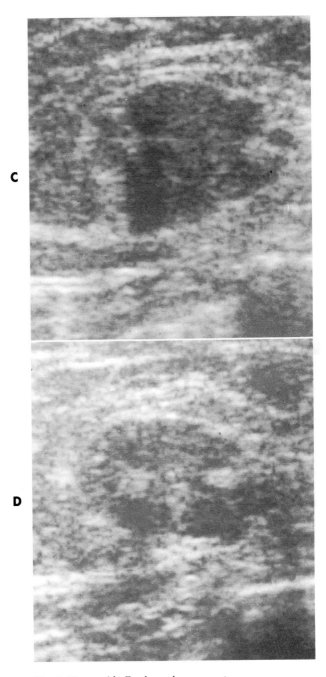

Fig. 9-10, cont'd. For legend see opposite page.

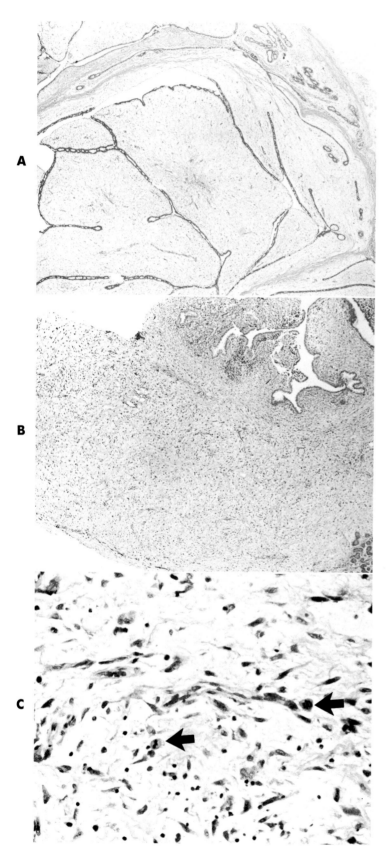

Fig. 9-11 The low-power photomicrograph (**A**) of a phyllodes tumor shows the leaflike protrusion of tumor into cystic spaces. In **B** and **C**, from another phyllodes tumor, stromal overgrowth is illustrated (**B**). The glandular elements are replaced or crowded out by the proliferating stroma, which at higher magnification (**C**) shows cellular atypia and several mitotic figures (*arrows*).

ADENOMA

Adenomas of the breast are unusual lesions, particularly when compared with the common fibroadenoma. Multiple types of adenomas can be seen in the breast, and these are listed in Box 9-2. Nipple adenomas are discussed in Chapter 10. Pleomorphic adenomas are uncommon.[56,57] Ductal adenomas may not represent a separate entity and are probably a group of lesions that include sclerotic papillomas, complex sclerosing lesions, or fibrosed tubular adenomas.[51,54] We have chosen to discuss the two most common types of these lesions, tubular adenomas and lactating adenomas.

BOX 9-2 BREAST ADENOMAS

Tubular adenoma
Lactating adenoma
Nipple adenoma
Ductal adenoma
Pleomorphic adenoma

Tubular adenoma

Tubular adenomas are one of the more common types of breast adenomas. A tubular adenoma is a circumscribed mass composed of closely packed ductules with minimal supporting stroma.[52,53,55] This lesion usually presents as a palpable mass in young women (16 to 40 years of age). There is no proven causal effect from birth control pills. Excision is therapeutic, and no recurrence has been reported.[11] If the lesion is infarcted, histologic diagnosis may be difficult. Caution must be exercised on frozen section because degenerating epithelial cells due to infarct can easily be misinterpreted as malignancy. This caveat holds true for infarcted fibroadenoma and other adenomas as well. A diagnosis of tubular adenoma confers no increased risk for malignancy.

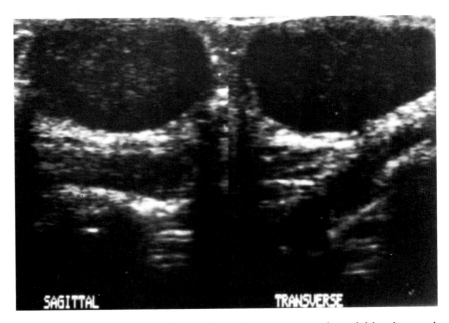

Fig. 9-12 Palpable mass in a 17-year-old female was not cystic but solid by ultrasound examination, with uniform low-level echoes throughout the oval circumscribed lesion. The pathologic diagnosis was tubular adenoma. (Courtesy Dr. Richard Bird, Charlotte, North Carolina.)

Histopathologically, the tubular adenoma consists of closely packed small tubular or glandular structures with an inconspicuous delicate fibrovascular stroma. There is not a true capsule surrounding the tumor, but the borders are smooth and well demarcated from the surrounding tissue. The tubules composing the tumor have both an epithelial and a myoepithelial layer, but the latter may be attenuated and difficult to identify.

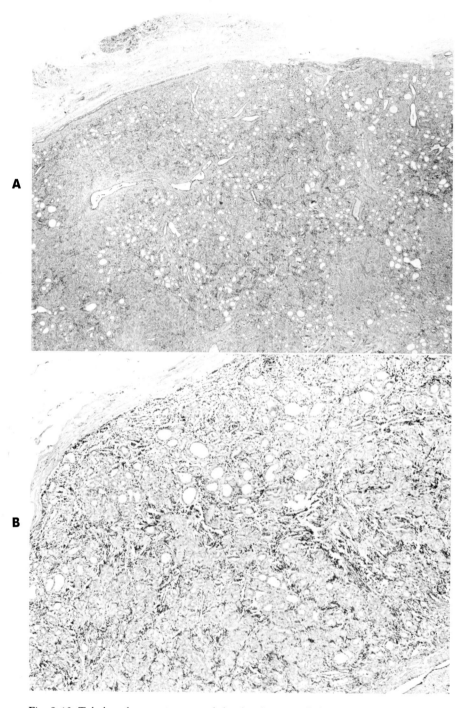

Fig. 9-13 Tubular adenoma is a smooth-bordered mass well demarcated from the surrounding breast parenchyma and composed of small, closely packed glands **(A).** At higher magnification some glands may appear solid and others have recognizable lumina. Stroma is sparse **(B).**

Lactating adenoma

Whether lactating adenoma represents a distinct entity is uncertain. Fibroadenomas removed during pregnancy or lactation may show secretory change in the epithelial component but do not lose the fibrous component. It is probable, therefore, that a lactating adenoma, defined as a closely packed grouping of ductules with secretory activity and no significant fibrous component, is in fact a preexisting tubular adenoma with the physiologic effect of pregnancy causing the secretory activity.[11,52] Other hypotheses are that lactating adenomas arise from small areas of a tubular adenoma contained within a fibroadenoma or are focal areas of lobular proliferation within breast parenchyma.

Similar secretory changes in fibroadenomas may be seen in young women using oral contraceptive pills. These lesions may be removed because of patient anxiety or because of fears of cancer when a lesion has appeared suddenly or increased in size during pregnancy. The mammographic appearance is identical to that of a benign fibroadenoma.

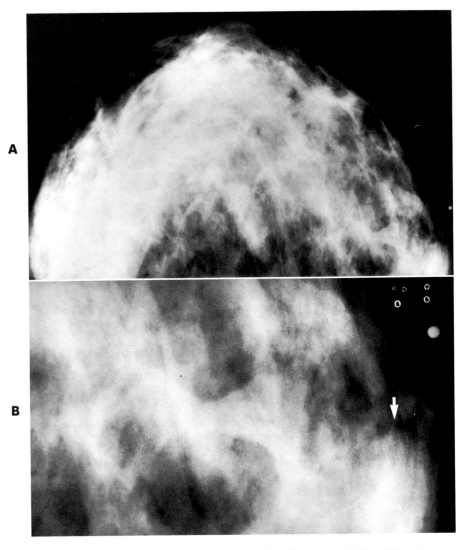

Fig. 9-14 Lactating 26-year-old woman with a palpable mass marked by a bb in the deep medial portion of the left breast **(A).** Inset **(B)** of this area shows an oval mass (*arrow*) with margins obscured by surrounding dense parenchyma. The pathologic diagnosis is lactating adenoma.

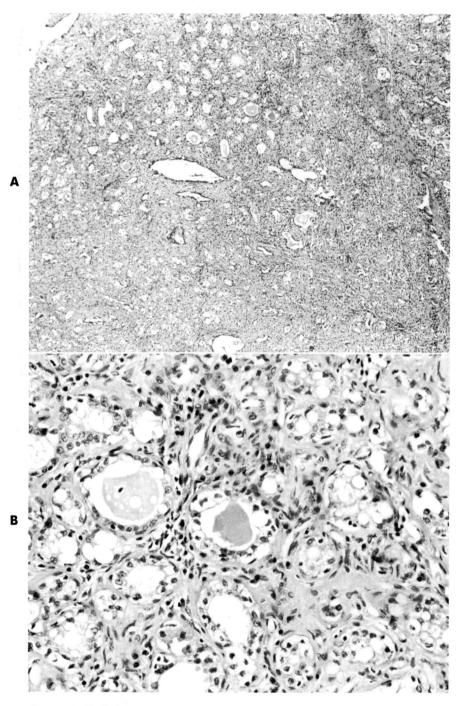

Fig. 9-15 The lactating adenoma, like the tubular adenoma, is composed of closely packed glands **(A).** The lining epithelium of these glands at higher magnification can be seen to be vacuolated, and the lumina frequently contain secretions **(B).**

LIPOMA

Lipoma of the breast is a benign encapsulated tumor of adipose tissue. Lipomas are common benign neoplasms of the chest wall and breast. They usually present in an older woman or man as a well-defined mass that is nontender, mobile, soft, and palpable and has been present for many years. Many of these patients have had other lipomas removed from the upper arm or chest wall. A mean age of 45 years and an average diameter of 2 cm have been reported.[60]

The role of mammography is to provide reassurance for the patient and referring physician. Mammograms often demonstrate a radiolucent fatty mass, sometimes surrounded by a visible thin fibrous capsule, displacing surrounding fibroglandular tissue. This classic mammographic appearance is sufficient to make a diagnosis, and usually a biopsy is not required.[62] Other fat-containing masses such as galactoceles and traumatic oil cysts may also give a characteristic appearance on mammography as radiolucent circumscribed masses, obviating excisional biopsy.

In some cases it may be difficult to distinguish a small lipoma from a normal fatty lobule that may be prominent on physical examination. When the palpable finding corresponds to predominately fatty tissue, a lipomatous pseudomass should be suggested.[61] Such clinical correlation is easily accomplished in a consultation or problem-solving mammography practice. The palpable area can be marked with a superficial radiodense marker, and a correlative physical examination can be performed after the mammogram. Lack of such correlation may lead to unnecessary breast biopsies for a prominent fatty lobule.

A lipoma is composed of mature adipose tissue, a delicate fibrovascular stroma, and a surrounding thin fibrous capsule. Rarely is the capsule observed histopathologically because it is most often ruptured during excision of the mass. A normal fatty lobule (prominent to palpation) has no such surrounding capsule. Rarely, a lipoma may calcify.[63]

Adenolipoma, a much less common entity, is also composed of mature adipose tissue but in addition contains small lobules and ducts. Characteristically, these are located within the fatty tissue, without a surrounding zone of fibrous connective tissue. It closely resembles the hamartoma and may perhaps be better classified as such.[11,58,59]

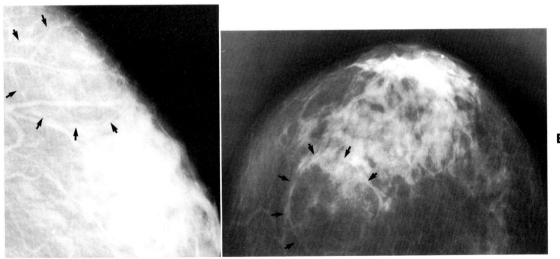

Fig. 9-16 Oval fat-density circumscribed mass is defined by a thin fibrous capsule (*arrows*) that outlined this palpable 6-cm mass on the lateral (**A**) and craniocaudal projections (**B**). The radiographic diagnosis is lipoma.

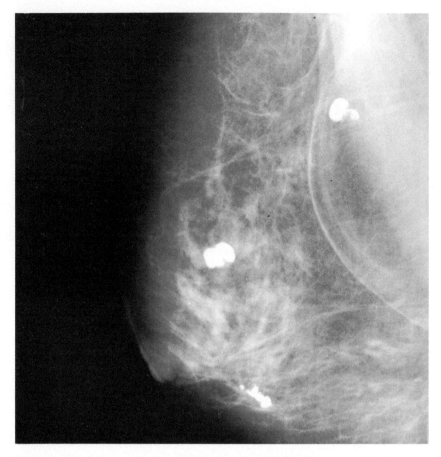

Fig. 9-17 Oval fat-containing circumscribed mass outlined by fibrous capsule. The radiographic diagnosis is lipoma. Note the multiple coarse calcifications indicating fibroadenomas.

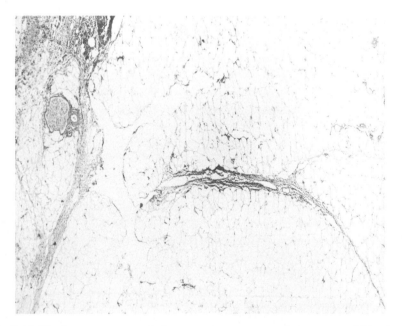

Fig. 9-18 The lipoma is composed of mature adipose tissue and contains small blood vessels. A portion of the fibrous capsule can be seen in this photomicrograph.

HAMARTOMA

Hamartoma, or fibroadenolipoma, is an unusual benign tumor that may have a characteristic mammographic appearance. It is a benign lesion composed of lobules set in a fibrofatty stroma producing a well-circumscribed mass.[66] As with a lipoma, the surrounding thin fibrous capsule, which may be imaged mammographically, is not usually seen grossly. It may in fact be a pseudocapsule of displaced breast trabeculae.[67] A frequency of 16 cases in 10,000 mammograms has been reported.[69] The hamartoma has been reported in women ranging from 15 to 88 years of age, with a mean age of 40 or 45 years.[67] It is usually 2 to 4 cm in diameter but may vary from 1 to 17 cm.

A breast hamartoma, usually painless, may be palpable as a relatively soft mass or thickening similar to normal breast tissue. Any difficulty in detecting the lesion by palpation is probably due to the fatty tissue component. Because of the increased numbers of screening mammograms being performed, more clinically occult hamartomas will undoubtedly be recognized.

Although the clinical presentation may not be impressive, the radiographic appearance is often characteristic because the admixture of fat and fibroglandular elements within the lesion produces a mottled pattern. This has been described as a "slice of sausage" appearance.[63] Calcification is not a usual feature but has been reported.[64,71] The ultrasonic appearance has been described as "sonolucent adenomatous tissue interspersed with echogenic septa of fat and fibrous tissue."[70]

Both the mammographic and ultrasonic appearance of hamartomas are inconsistent, reflecting the varying proportions of fat and fibroglandular tissue that may be present. When fatty tissue predominates, the lesion may closely resemble a lipoma. Conversely, when fatty elements are minimal, the lesion could be mistaken for a fibroadenoma. Synonyms in the literature include adenolipoma, fibroadenoma, and postlactational breast tumors.[65] If the pathologist is not aware of the presence of a capsule or of the mammographic diagnosis, a false interpretation of normal breast parenchyma or fibrocystic disease may be given. A close working relationship between radiologist and pathologist is essential for correct diagnosis.

Hamartoma may not be detected mammographically (e.g., small tumors in dense breasts). In a recent report, only two of 17 women with pathologically proven breast hamartoma had the typical pathognomonic mammographic features of a hamartoma. An additional five women had lesions with a classic mammographic appearance and did not receive a biopsy.[68] It has been hypothesized that the characteristic mammographic appearance may develop as the tumor enlarges over time.

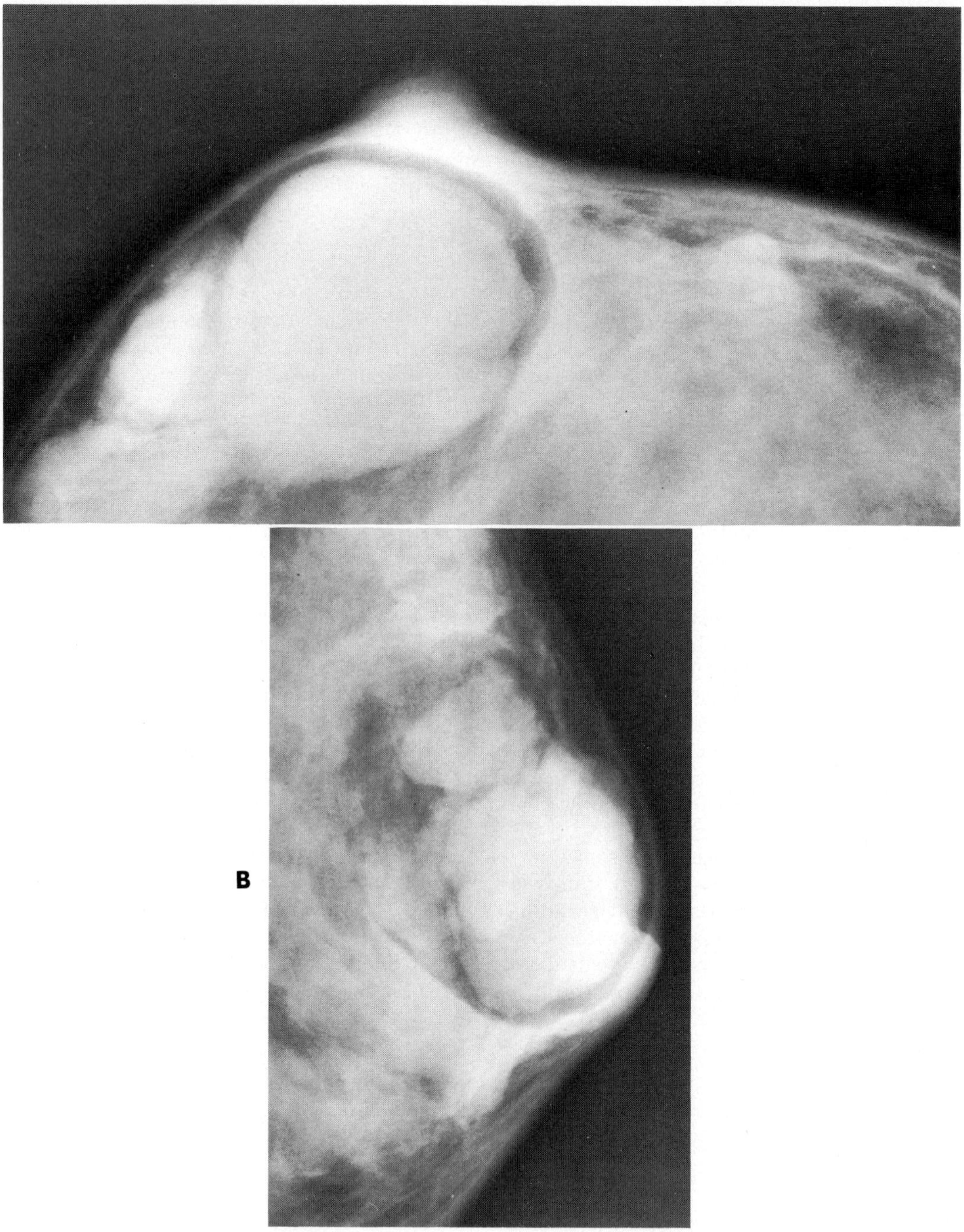

Fig. 9-19 Large oval mass of mixed fat and glandular tissue density demonstrates a circumscribed margin on both craniocaudal **(A)** and mediolateral oblique **(B)** projections.

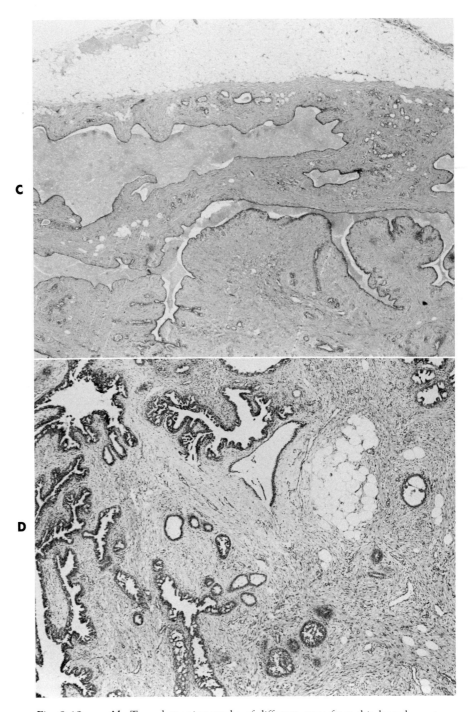

Fig. 9-19, cont'd. Two photomicrographs of different areas from this large hamartoma reveal glands that are markedly dilated and contain secretory material in **C**. Other areas (**D**) show glands with moderate hyperplasia as well as adipose tissue and smooth muscle, all within the tumor.

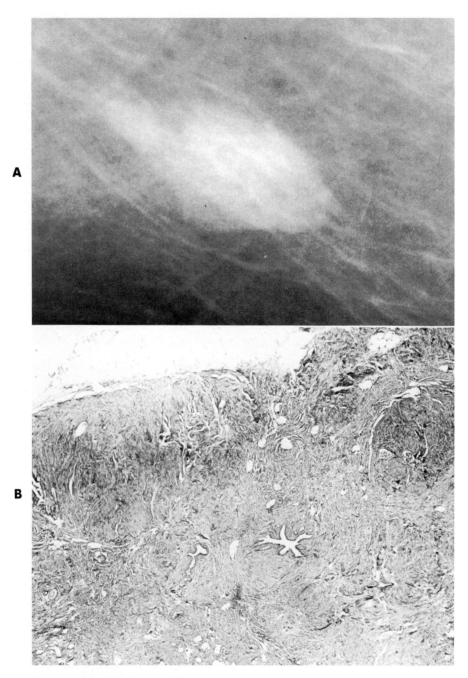

Fig. 9-20 (A) Ovoid low-density 2-cm mass with indistinct posterior margin was identified as a dominant lesion on a screening mammogram in a 49-year-old woman. This myoid hamartoma is composed of fibrous tissue, smooth muscle, and occasional glands. At low magnification **(B)**, the lesion is focally well circumscribed. In other areas **(C)**, strands of fibrous tissue and smooth muscle trail off into surrounding fat, giving the lesion a more irregular outline. The smooth muscle bundles stain more darkly in this trichrome stain. Immunohistochemistry for desmin **(D)**, which is an intermediate filament found in muscle cells, shows the prominent muscle component of this lesion.

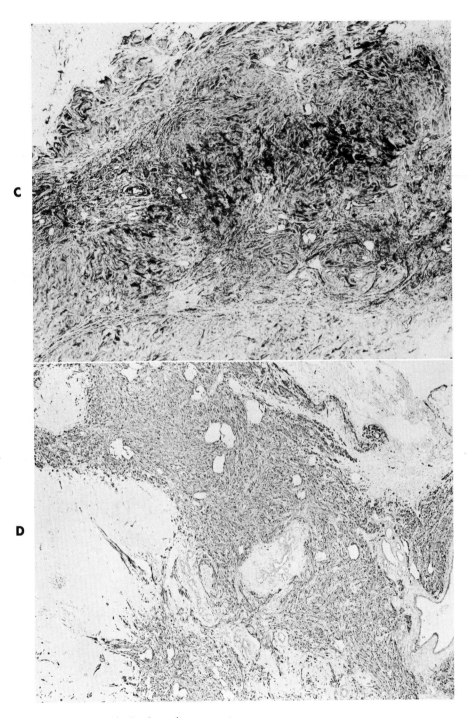

C

D

Fig. 9-20, cont'd. For legend see opposite page.

GALACTOCELE

Galactoceles are benign breast cysts containing milk. They are associated with lactation. They may be multiple, unilateral, or bilateral. The diagnosis is confirmed by aspiration of milklike liquid from the mass. No signs of inflammation or abscess occur in uncomplicated galactoceles.

Mammograms may show a well-circumscribed rounded mass. A horizontal-beam radiograph may demonstrate a fat–fluid level within the galactocele.[72-74] The radiolucent fat floats on top of the heavier water–protein component. Curdled milk may also be present within the cyst and can be demonstrated by pneumocystography.[72]

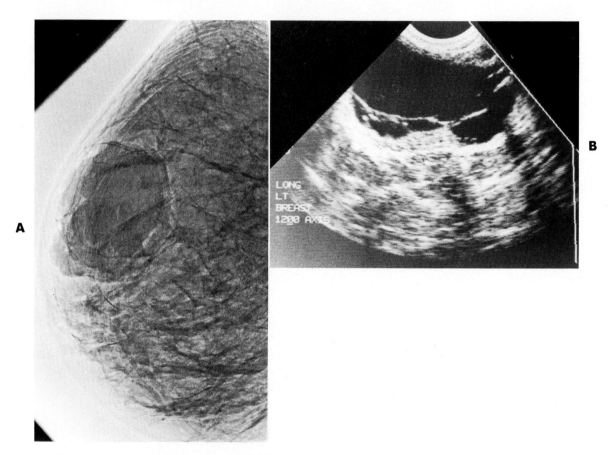

Fig. 9-21 Lobulated 7-cm mass in a 24-year-old lactating woman on xeromammogram **(A)** was anechoic with septations by ultrasound examination **(B).** Cyst aspiration confirmed a galactocele. (Courtesy Dr. Barbara Steinbach, Gainesville, Florida.)

REFERENCES

Fibroadenoma and variants

1. Baker KS, Monsees BS, Diaz NM, et al: Carcinoma within fibroadenomas: mammographic features, *Radiology* 176:371, 1990.
2. Bauer BS, Jones KM, Talbot CW: Mammary masses in the adolescent female, *Surg Gynecol Obstet* 165:63, 1987.
3. Black MM, Modan B, Lubin F, et al: A nationwide study of breast disease, *Cancer* 61:2547, 1988.
4. Brenner RJ, Sickles EA: Acceptability of periodic follow-up as an alternative to biopsy for mammographically detected lesions interpreted as probably benign, *Radiology* 171:645, 1989.
5. Buzanowski-Konakry K, Harrison EG Jr, Payne WS: Lobular carcinoma arising in fibroadenoma of the breast, *Cancer* 35:450, 1975.
6. Cole-Beuglet C, Soriano RZ, Kurtz AB, et al: Fibroadenoma of the breast: sonomammography correlated with pathology in 122 patients, *AJR Am J Roentgenol* 140:369, 1983.
7. Daniel WA Jr, Mathews MD: Tumors of the breast in adolescent females, *Pediatrics* 41:743, 1968.
8. Deschenes L, Jacobs S, Fabia J, et al: Beware of breast fibroadenomas in middle aged women, *Can J Surg* 28:372, 1985.
9. Dupont WD, Page DL, Parl FF: Breast cancer risk associated with fibroadenomas, *Mod Pathol* 3:28A, 1990.
10. Fechner RE: Fibroadenomas in patients receiving oral contraceptives: a clinical and pathologic study, *Am J Clin Pathol* 53:857, 1970.
11. Fechner RE: *Fibroadenoma and related lesions.* In Page DL, Anderson TJ, editors: *Diagnostic histopathology of the breast,* New York, 1987, Churchill Livingstone.
12. Gershon-Cohen J, Ingleby H: Roentgenography of fibroadenoma of the breast, *Radiology* 59:77, 1952.
13. Goodman ZD, Taxy JB: Fibroadenomas of the breast with prominent smooth muscle, *Am J Surg Pathol* 5:99, 1981.
14. Haagensen CD: *Diseases of the breast,* ed 3, Philadelphia, WB Saunders, 1986.
15. Heywang SH, Lipsit ER, Glassman LM, et al: Specificity of ultrasonography in the diagnosis of benign breast masses, *J Ultrasound Med* 3:453, 1984.
16. Jackson VP, Rothschild PA, Kreipke DL, et al: The spectrum of sonographic findings of fibroadenoma of the breast, *Invest Radiol* 21:34, 1986.
17. Kodlin D, Winger EE, Morgenstern NL, et al: Chronic mastopathy and breast cancer. A follow-up study, *Cancer* 39:2603, 1977.
18. Kudlickova Z, Svejda J: Calcified breast tumor eluding mammographic diagnosis: a case report, *Breast, Diseases of the Breast* 4:6, 1978.
19. Lanyi M: *Diagnosis and differential diagnosis of breast calcifications,* Berlin, 1986, Springer-Verlag.
20. LiVolsi VA, Stadel BV, Kelsey JL, Halford TR: Fibroadenoma in oral contraceptive users. A histopathologic evaluation of epithelial atypia, *Cancer* 44:1778, 1979.
21. McDivitt RW, Stewart FW, Farrow JH: Breast carcinoma arising in solitary fibroadenomas, *Surg Gynecol Obstet* 125:572, 1967.
22. Mies C, Rosen PP: Juvenile fibroadenomas with atypical epithelial hyperplasia, *Am J Surg Pathol* 11:184, 1987.
23. Morris JA, Kelly JF: Multiple bilateral breast adenomas in identical adolescent negro twins, *Histopathology* 6:539, 1982.
24. Moskowitz M, Gartside P, Wireman JA, McLaughlin C: Proliferative disorders of the breast as risk factors for breast cancer in a self-selected population: pathologic markers, *Radiology* 134:289, 1980.
25. Naraynsingh V, Raju GC: Familial bilateral multiple fibroadenomas of the breast, *Postgrad Med J* 61:439, 1985.
26. Oberman HA: Hormonal contraceptives and fibroadenomas of the breast, *N Engl J Med* 284:984, 1971.
27. Pike AM, Oberman HA: Juvenile (cellular) adenofibromas: a clinicopathologic study, *Am J Surg Pathol* 9:730, 1985.
28. Recabaren JA Jr, Albano WA, Organ CH Jr: Giant adenofibroma of youth: a case report, *Breast, Diseases of the Breast* 1:25, 1975.
29. Sickles EA: Breast masses: mammographic evaluation, *Radiology* 173:297, 1989.
30. Spagnolo DV, Shilkin KB: Breast neoplasms containing bone and cartilage, *Virchows Arch [A]* 400:287, 1983.
31. Troupin RH: *Mammographic-pathologic correlation.* In Feig SA, editor: *ARRS Breast Imaging Syllabus,* 1988, American Roentgen Ray Society.
32. Wolfe JN: *Xeroradiography of the breast,* Springfield, Ill, 1972, Charles C Thomas.

Phyllodes tumor

33. Alberti O Jr, Bretani MM, Goes JCS, et al: Carcinoembryonic antigen: a possible predictor of recurrence in cystosarcoma phyllodes, *Cancer* 57:1042, 1986.
34. Al-Jurf A, Hawk WA, Crile G, Jr, et al: Cystosarcoma phyllodes, *Surg Gynecol Obstet* 146:358, 1978.

34A. Buchberger W, Strasser K, Heim K, et al: Phyllodes tumor: findings on mammography, sonography, and aspiration in 10 cases. *AJR Am J Roentgerol* 157:715, 1991.

35. Cohn-Cedermark G, Rutquist LE, Rosendahl I, et al: Prognostic factors in cystosarcoma phyllodes: a clinicopathologic study of 77 patients, *Cancer* 68:2017, 1991.

36. Cole-Beuglet C, Soriano R, Kurtz AB, et al: Ultrasound, x-ray mammography and histopathology of cystosarcoma phylloides, *Radiology* 146:481, 1983.

37. D'Orsi CJ, Weissman BNW, Berkowitz DM, et al: Correlation of xeroradiography and histology of breast disease, *Crit Rev Diagn Imaging* 11:75, 1978.

38. Gershon-Cohen J, Moore L: Roentgenography of giant fibroadenoma of the breast (cystosarcoma phylloides), *Radiology* 74:619, 1960.

39. Grimes MM, Lattes R, Jaretzki A III: Cystosarcoma phyllodes: report of an unusual case, with death due to intraneural extension to the central nervous system, *Cancer* 56:1691, 1985.

40. Hajdu SI, Espinosa MH, Robbins GF: Recurrent cystosarcoma phyllodes: a clinicopathologic study of 32 cases, *Cancer* 38:1402, 1976.

41. Hart WR, Bauer RC, Oberman HA: Cystosarcoma phyllodes: a clinicopathologic study of twenty-six hypercellular periductal stromal tumors of the breast, *Am J Clin Pathol* 70:211, 1978.

42. Jellins J, Hughes C, Ryan J, et al: A comparative evaluation of a case of cystosarcoma phylloides: ultrasound, xeroradiography and thermography, *Radiology* 124:803, 1977.

43. Kessinger A, Foley JF, Lemon HM, et al: Metastatic cystosarcoma phyllodes: a case report and review of the literature, *J Surg Oncol* 4:131, 1972.

44. Lester J, Stout AP: Cystosarcoma phyllodes, *Cancer* 7:335, 1954.

45. Muller J: *Ueber den feinen Ban und die Formen der Krankhaften Geschwulste,* Berlin, 1883, G Reimer.

46. Norris HJ, Taylor HB: Relationship of histologic features to behavior of cystosarcoma phyllodes: analysis of ninety-four cases, *Cancer* 20:2090, 1967.

47. Oberman HA: Cystosarcoma phyllodes: a clinicopathologic study of hypercellular periductal stromal neoplasms of breast, *Cancer* 18:697, 1965.

48. Pietruszka M, Barnes L: Cystosarcoma phyllodes: a clinicopathologic analysis of 42 cases, *Cancer* 41:1974, 1978.

49. Treves N, Sunderland DA: Cystosarcoma phyllodes of the breast. A malignant and a benign tumor: a clinicopathological study of twenty-seven cases, *Cancer* 4:1286, 1951.

50. Ward RM, Evans HL: Cystosarcoma phyllodes: a clinicopathological study of 26 cases, *Cancer* 58:2282, 1986.

Adenoma

51. Azzopardi JG, Salm R: Ductal adenoma of the breast: a lesion which can mimic carcinoma, *J Pathol* 144:15, 1984.

52. Hertel BG, Zaloudek C, Kempson RL: Breast adenomas, *Cancer* 37:2891, 1976.

53. Moross T, Land AP, Mahoney L: Tubular adenoma of breast, *Arch Pathol Lab Med* 107:84, 1983.

54. Page DL, Anderson TJ: *Papilloma and related lesions.* In *Diagnostic histopathology of the breast,* New York, 1987, Churchill Livingstone, p 104.

55. Persaud V, Talerman A, Jordan RP: Pure adenoma of the breast, *Arch Pathol* 86:481, 1968.

56. Soreide JA, Anda O, Eriksen L, et al: Pleomorphic adenoma of the human breast with local recurrence, *Cancer* 61:997, 1988.

57. van der Walt JD, Rohlova B: Pleomorphic adenoma of the human breast: a report of a benign tumour closely mimicking a carcinoma clinically, *Clin Oncol* 8:361, 1982.

Lipoma

58. Brebner DM, Cosmann B, Shapiro J: Lipomata of the breast diagnosed by film and xeromammography, *S Afr Med J* 50:685, 688, 1976.

59. Dyreborg U, Starklint H: Adenolipoma mammae, *Acta Radiol* 16:362, 1975.

60. Haagensen CD: *Diseases of the breast,* ed 2, Philadelphia, 1971, WB Saunders.

61. Hall FM, Connolly JL, Love SM: Lipomatous pseudomass of the breast: diagnosis suggested by discordant palpatory and mammographic findings, *Radiology* 164:463, 1987.

62. Kopans DB, Meyer JE, Cohen AM, et al: Palpable breast masses: the importance of preoperative mammography, *JAMA* 246:2819, 1981.

63. Paulus DD: Benign diseases of the breast, *Radiol Clin North Am* 21:27, 1983.

Hamartoma

64. Abbitt PL, De Paredes ES, Sloop FB Jr: Breast hamartoma: a mammographic diagnosis, *South Med J* 81:167, 1988.
65. Andersson I, Hildell J, Linell F, et al: Mammary hamartomas, *Acta Radiol* 20:712, 1979.
66. Arrigoni MG, Dockerty MB, Judd ES: The identification and treatment of mammary hamartoma, *Surg Gynecol Obstet* 133:577, 1971.
67. Crothers JG, Butler NF, Fortt RW, et al: Fibroadenolipoma of the breast, *Br J Radiol* 58:191, 1985.
68. Helvie MA, Adler DD, Rebner M, et al: Breast hamartomas: variable mammographic appearance, *Radiology* 170:417, 1989.
69. Hessler C, Schnyder P, Ozzello L: Hamartoma of the breast: diagnostic observation of 16 cases, *Radiology* 126:95, 1978.
70. Kopans DB, Meyer JE, Proppe KH: Ultrasonographic, xeromammographic and histologic correlation of a fibroadenolipoma of the breast, *J Clin Ultrasound* 10:409, 1982.
71. Tabar L, Pentek Z: Fibroadenolipoma of the breast, *Radiologe* 15:77, 1975.

Galactocele

72. Gomez A, Mata JM, Donoso L, et al: Galactocele: three distinctive radiographic appearances, *Radiology* 158:43, 1986.
73. Salvador R, Salvador M, Jimenez JA, et al: Galactocele of the breast: radiologic and ultrasonographic findings, *Br J Radiol* 63:140, 1990.
74. Sickles EA, Vogelaar PW: Fluid level in a galactocele seen on lateral projection mammogram with horizontal beam, *Breast, Diseases of the Breast* 7:32, 1981.

CHAPTER 10

Papillary Lesions and Radial Scars

Carol B. Stelling
Deborah E. Powell

Solitary papilloma
Multiple papillomas
Papillomatosis
Complex sclerosing papillary lesion and radial scar
Papillary adenoma of the nipple
Juvenile papillomatosis
Intracystic papillary carcinoma

This chapter focuses on papillary breast lesions as defined by histopathologic criteria. Included in the discussion are both large duct and small duct peripheral lesions (Box 10-1). Methods of detection, characteristic radiographic appearance, and usual clinical presentation are reviewed, with special attention to those lesions that may present a diagnostic dilemma to the clinician, radiologist, or pathologist. Some of these papillary lesions may lead to an increased risk for subsequent development of breast cancer (Table 10-1).

The lesions discussed include solitary and multiple papillomas; papillomatosis, or epithelial hyperplasia; complex sclerosing lesion and radial scar; nipple adenoma; juvenile papillomatosis; and intracystic papillary carcinoma.

SOLITARY PAPILLOMA

The solitary intraductal papilloma is an uncommon benign tumor of large ducts arising usually within 1 to 2 cm of the nipple. The papilloma consists of epithelial cells arranged in a papillary pattern along fibrovascular fronds and attached to the wall of a dilated major lactiferous duct by a wide-based fibrovascular stalk. Its frequency is only one third that of breast cancer. This lesion may be diagnosed at any age but presents more commonly in the premenopausal years. Rare cases have been reported in males.[3]

The papilloma, usually solitary, is slow growing and, if not treated, has been reported to enlarge to considerable size (5 to 15 cm).[10] However, the solitary papilloma is most often small (less than 1 cm) and grows along the length of the duct, usually producing no mammographic findings. A distended duct or cyst created from accumulated secretions may occasionally be detected in a central location by breast self-examination or clinical physical examination, but most commonly no palpable mass is present.[11] More than 80% of patients present with spontaneous nipple discharge, most often serous or bloody in character.[1] Most women with spontaneous discharge have a solitary papilloma, with less than 10% found to have carcinoma.[8] A watery spontaneous unilateral discharge from a single duct should be considered more suspicious for a carcinoma than a papilloma.[4] In a case of spontaneous discharge and no palpable mass, detection of the depth and quadrant location of the papilloma may be achieved by careful physical examination. Focal pressure over the distended ductal system will elicit the discharge and assist in localizing the sector involved. Depth of the papilloma

BOX 10-1 PAPILLARY BREAST LESIONS

<u>Central (large duct) location</u>
Solitary intraductal papilloma
Nipple adenoma and florid nipple papillomatosis

<u>Peripheral (small duct) location</u>
Papillomatosis (epithelial hyperplasia)
Juvenile papillomatosis
Complex sclerosing lesion and radial scar
Multiple papillomas

<u>Variable location</u>
Intracystic papillary carcinoma

Table 10-1 **Risk for subsequent development of invasive breast cancer**

Lesion	Cancer risk
Complex sclerosing lesion and radial scar	Probably none
Solitary papilloma	None
Nipple adenoma	Unknown
Multiple papillomas	Moderate increase
Papillomatosis (epithelial hyperplasia)	Slight increase
Juvenile papillomatosis	Uncertain

relative to the nipple may be determined by radiography after contrast injection of the discharging duct—that is, galactography. The galactogram demonstrates only the location of the abnormality. A surgical biopsy is necessary to establish a pathologic diagnosis. The differential diagnosis of an intraluminal filling defect by galactography is listed in Box 10-2. Special surgical techniques of duct excision are required that differ from conventional breast biopsy[8] (see text in Chapter 5).

The role of cytology to evaluate nipple discharge is limited since a papilloma or carcinoma may be present with negative cytology. Hemoccult testing of discharge may be useful to confirm the presence of blood, which should support further intervention to establish a diagnosis.

The histopathology of a solitary intraductal papilloma is characterized by several features that differentiate this lesion from papillary carcinoma.[5] The key words for benign papillomas are *multiple* and *irregular*, with multiple referring to the fact that more than one epithelial cell type is present in the papilloma and irregular to the fact that the papillary and glandular growths are irregular in configuration. In contrast, papillary or intraductal carcinomas are characterized by a *uniform* proliferation of a single cell population. These lesions are also *regular* in their architecture. Apocrine metaplasia is common in papillomas but is not a component of papillary carcinomas. Likewise, myoepithelial cells are often part of the epithelial proliferation in papillomas. Solitary papillomas may undergo infarction either of the entire lesion or only in focal areas.[2] Partially infarcted papillomas are more likely to present with bloody nipple discharge. Areas of old hemorrhage and fibrosis, particularly at the base of a papilloma, may result in a "pseudoinfiltrative" appearance and cause diagnostic problems for the patholo-

BOX 10-2 DIFFERENTIAL DIAGNOSIS OF INTRALUMINAL FILLING DEFECTS ON GALACTOGRAM

Solitary papilloma
Papillomatosis
Multiple papillomas
Carcinoma (intraductal or papillary)
Blood clot
Inspissated secretions
Air bubble

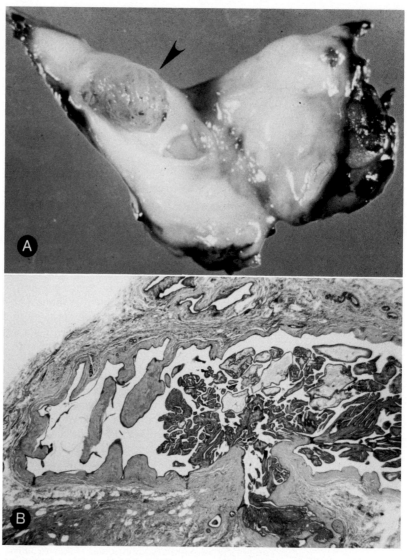

Fig. 10-1 A, Solitary intraductal papilloma protrudes into a large dilated duct (*arrowhead*). **B,** The solitary intraductal papilloma in this low-magnification photomicrograph demonstrates the characteristic papillary growth pattern and the central fibrovascular cores of the neoplasm. (From Golden A, Powell DE, Jennings CD: *Pathology: Understanding human disease*, Baltimore, 1985, Williams & Wilkins.)

gist. Glands and portions of papillary structures trapped within areas of fibrosis may simulate invasive tumor. Such areas are relatively common in larger papillomas. Some papillomas may ultimately become almost completely sclerotic, with resulting obliteration of the wall of the associated duct. These lesions may be difficult to recognize as an intraductal papilloma and have been classified by a variety of names.[10] They show varied histologic features of sclerotic papilloma, sclerosing adenosis, and complex sclerosing lesions.

Special handling of small lesions may be necessary to prevent loss. It is often helpful if the surgeon identifies the portion of the excised specimen closest to the nipple with a suture. Placing a small friable tumor in a "tea bag" during fixation will help to protect the specimen. Solitary papillomas are not associated with an increased risk for breast carcinoma (Table 10-1) or for recurrence.[6,7]

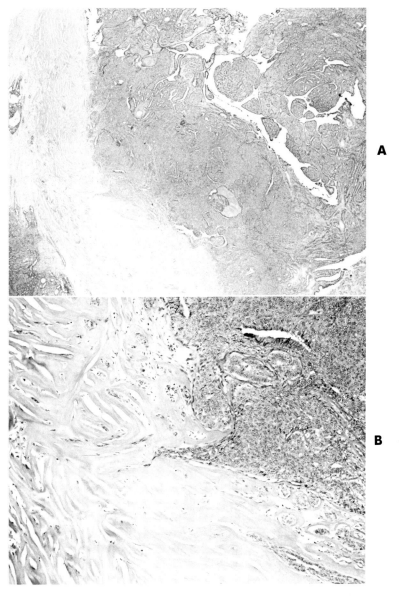

A

B

Fig. 10-2 A, Intraductal papilloma with extensive sclerosis. **B,** At high magnification the pseudoinfiltrative pattern of trapped epithelial cells in the dense reactive fibrous tissue can be seen.

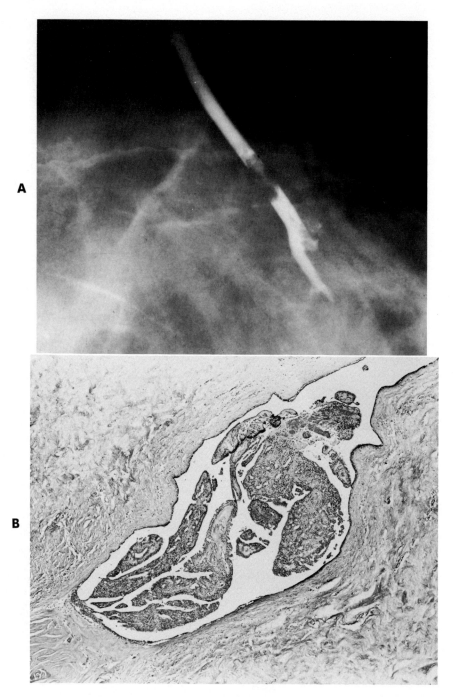

Fig. 10-3 A, Small intraductal mass located by galactography in a 22-year-old woman with spontaneous bloody nipple discharge. The pathologic diagnosis is intraductal papilloma. **B,** Intraductal papilloma from this patient almost completely fills the duct.

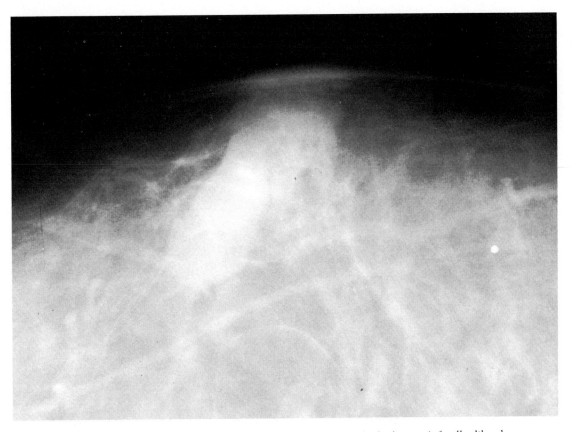

Fig. 10-4 A 56-year-old woman with spontaneous bloody nipple discharge. A focally dilated duct is visualized by mammography in this fatty breast. The pathologic diagnosis is intraductal papilloma.

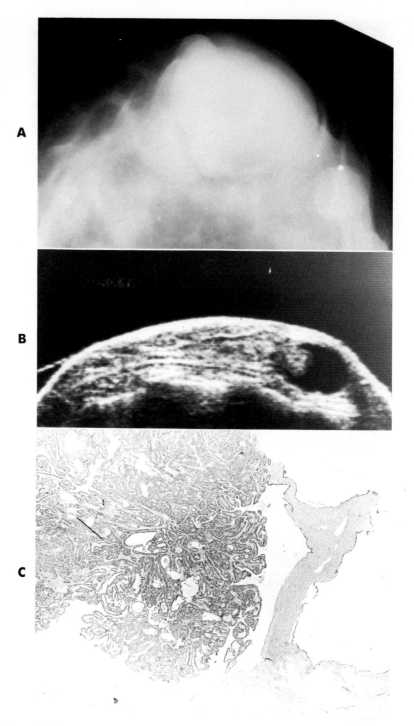

Fig. 10-5 A, Two well-circumscribed palpable masses in a young woman. The smaller mass (*bb* on skin), solid on ultrasound examination, was a fibroadenoma. The larger mass was cystic on ultrasound examination with a mural nodule **(B). C,** Pathologic examination of the biopsy from this patient shows a large papilloma within a cystically dilated duct.

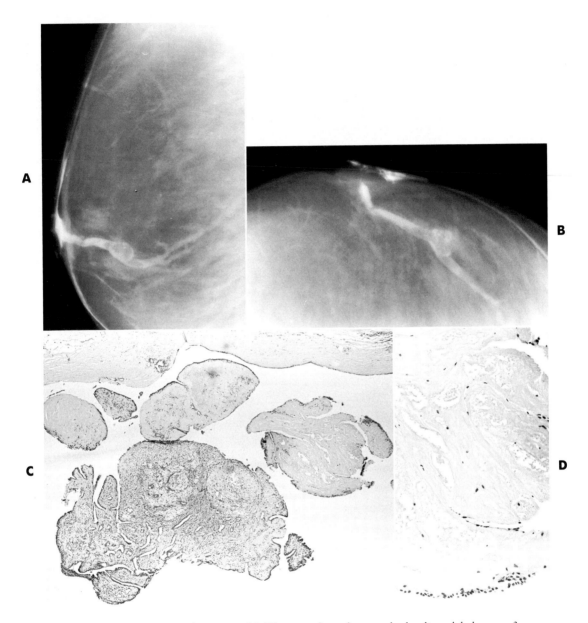

Fig. 10-6 Lateral (**A**) and craniocaudal (**B**) views after galactography localize a lobular mass 3 cm deep to the nipple in the 9:00 sector of the right breast. The pathologic diagnosis is intraductal papilloma with infarction. **C** and **D,** The partially infarcted papilloma from this patient is illustrated here. The low-magnification photomicrograph (**C**) demonstrates some residual viable areas as well as the acellular infarcted portion of the papilloma. At higher magnification (**D**) these infarcted areas show loss of cellularity and coagulative necrosis. (Courtesy Dr. Robert E. Fechner, Charlottesville, Virginia.)

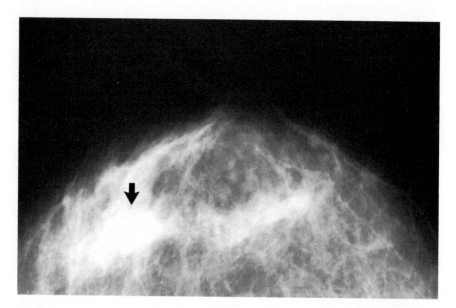

Fig. 10-7 Unusual presentation of a papilloma as a palpable mass *(arrow)*. The pathologic diagnosis was intraductal papilloma.

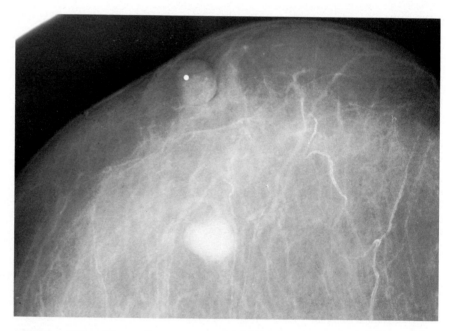

Fig. 10-8 Subareolar palpable well-circumscribed mass in an 84-year-old woman. Differential diagnosis included fibroadenoma, ductal carcinoma, intracystic papillary carcinoma, medullary or mucinous carcinoma, and papilloma. The pathologic diagnosis was intraductal papilloma.

MULTIPLE PAPILLOMAS

Multiple papillomas are a distinct histopathologic entity that should be differentiated from both solitary intraductal papilloma and papillomatosis.[12] This lesion is significant because it may be easily confused with papillary carcinoma histopathologically. Multiple papillomas are generally regarded as conferring more risk for subsequent development of breast cancer than papillary ductal epithelial hyperplasia without atypia, also known as papillomatosis.[13,15]

Unlike the papilloma, which involves a single major lactiferous duct, multiple papillomas are commonly lesions of more peripheral ducts. Meticulous reconstruction studies by Ohuchi and coworkers[15] have shown convincingly that multiple papillomas arise peripherally from the terminal ductal lobular units and are associated with epithelial hyperplasia (papillomatosis), which is frequently atypical. This latter finding is not as frequently associated with solitary papilloma and is probably the reason for the increased incidence of malignancy with multiple papillomas. Ohuchi prefers the designation *central and peripheral* to *single and multiple papillomas*.[16] The glandular pattern and secretory products are usually more exaggerated in multiple than in solitary intraductal papilloma, and the presence of cellular pleomorphism and associated apocrine change is expected. Multifocality is common, and recurrence or appearance of new lesions after local excision is frequent.[14] Malignant change has been described.[14]

Multiple papillomas may be very difficult to diagnose by frozen section and even present substantial difficulty for the pathologist on permanent sections (Table 10-2).

There are no specific clinical or radiographic features for multiple papillomas. They may be diagnosed as an incidental finding in a specimen removed for another reason or as a cause of spontaneous nipple discharge, positive galactogram, or clustered calcification.[14]

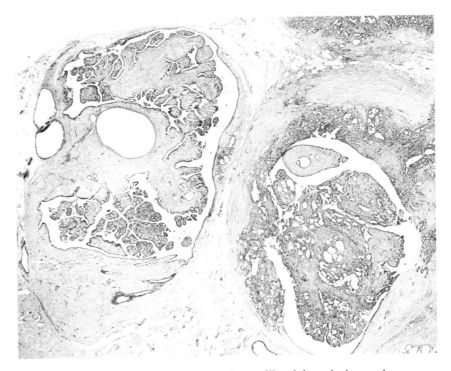

Fig. 10-9 Peripherally located multiple papillomas fill and distend adjacent ducts. There is periductal sclerosis, and associated papillomatosis (not illustrated) was present.

Table 10-2 **Benign papillary breast lesions: common diagnostic dilemmas**

Lesion	Differentiate from
Solitary papilloma with sclerosis	**Papillary carcinoma with invasion**
Epithelial cells "caught" in dense hyalinized fibrous tissue	Epithelial cells invade into desmoplastic stroma, are less sclerotic, more myxomatous and cellular
Internal lesion complex, multiple cell types	Internal lesion architecturally simple, one cell type
Infarcted papilloma	**Papillary carcinoma with necrosis**
Multiple cell types	Single cell type
Fibrous, hyalinized stroma	Delicate vascular stroma
DCIS absent	Cribriform DCIS may be present.
Multiple papillomas	**Papillomatosis**
Distinct fibrovascular stalks	No central fibrovascular stalk
Discrete lesions	Diffuse "field" change in multiple duct systems
Radial scar/complex sclerosing lesion	**Tubular carcinoma**
Low-power pattern—smooth border of distended ducts	Low-power pattern—infiltrating tubules trailing into tissue; irregular outlines
Central fibrosis with elastosis	Central fibrosis with elastosis
Glandular structures have basement membrane; double layer of epithelial cells	Glandular structures often lack basement membrane; have single layer of epithelial cells
DCIS absent; papillomatosis	DCIS present
Papillary adenoma of nipple	**Papillary carcinoma**
Characteristic location	Unusual in nipple
DCIS absent	Cribriform DCIS may be present.
Double epithelial layers of "infiltrating glands"	Single epithelial layer and cell type

DCIS = ductal carcinoma in situ.

PAPILLOMATOSIS

Papillomatosis is a benign condition of the small peripheral ducts characterized by an occasionally papillary hyperplasia (epitheliosis) of the epithelial cells. It is part of the spectrum of proliferative fibrocystic disease and is discussed in more detail in Chapter 11. When papillomatosis is associated with cellular atypia or an increasingly uniform growth pattern, a diagnosis of atypical hyperplasia may be given. Atypical hyperplasia is a high-risk lesion for the subsequent development of breast cancer.[17] Papillomatosis of varying degrees of severity is a common finding in breast biopsies containing other subtypes of fibrocystic change. It is estimated to occur in 15% to 20% of the population[18] and is found in approximately 25% of breast biopsy specimens.[17]

The diagnosis is most often an incidental finding in a breast biopsy specimen excised for a palpable thickening in the breast or a recurrent simple cyst. In recent years with the increased number of screening mammograms, papillomatosis may be detected as the cause of an isolated cluster of microcalcifications or an area of irregular mass density. Rarely are such focal areas of papillomatosis palpable.

Some authors use the terms *papillomatosis* and *focal papillomas* interchangeably. This practice should be avoided since the clinical significance of these two lesions differs considerably. Although both are considered hyperplastic lesions, the risk for subsequent development of breast cancer in an individual with the biopsy-proven diagnosis of papillomatosis is only slightly increased (1.5 to 2 times the normal population) as compared with multiple papillomas, for which the association of subsequent carcinoma may approach 40% (see Table 10-1).[13]

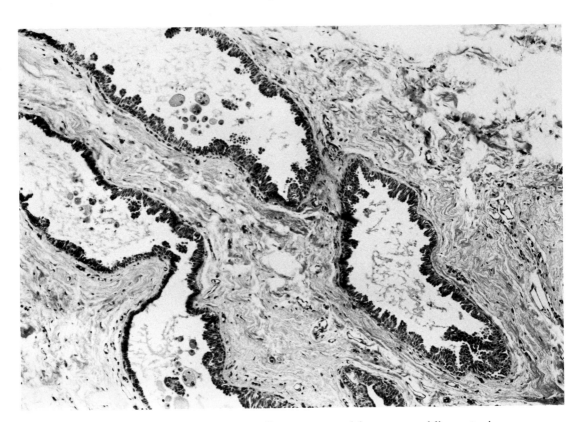

Fig. 10-10 Papillary hyperplasia, or papillomatosis, part of the spectrum of fibrocystic change, is illustrated here. The hyperplastic epithelial cells form varying-sized papillary projections. Central foam cells are seen within the ducts.

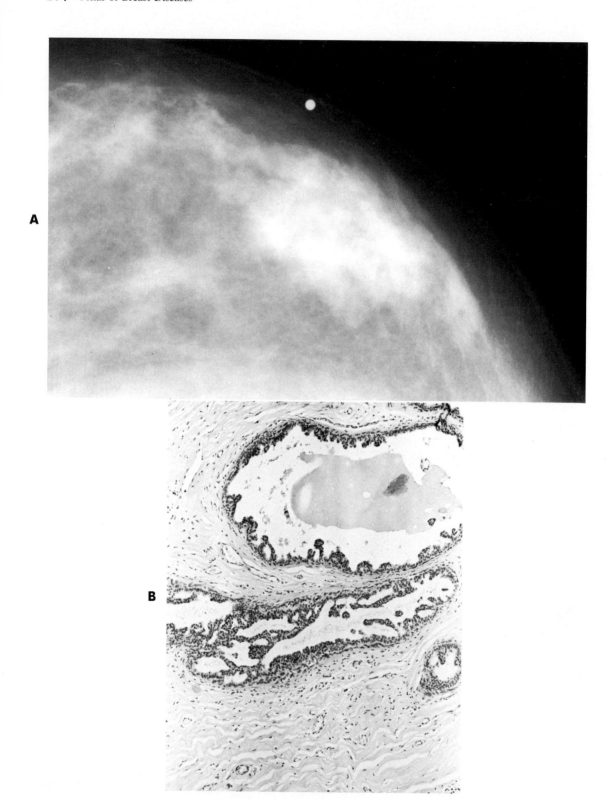

Fig. 10-11 A, Palpable (*bb* on skin) and painful focal asymmetric density in a 47-year-old woman. The pathologic diagnosis was extensive intraductal papillomatosis. **B,** In this patient, three adjacent ducts show papillary intraductal hyperplasia or papillomatosis. The proliferating epithelial cells protrude into and focally extend across the duct lumen.

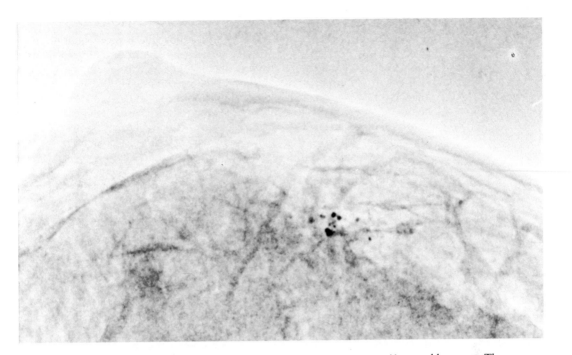

Fig. 10-12 Cluster of round calcifications on xeromammogram in a 41-year-old woman. The pathologic diagnosis was papillomatosis.

COMPLEX SCLEROSING PAPILLARY LESION AND RADIAL SCAR

These benign papillary proliferations, which have been given multiple names (Box 10-3), have been a diagnostic pitfall for surgical pathologists for many years.[20] The sclerosis and distortion that accompany this lesion lead to a pseudoinvasive pattern that may be mistaken for carcinoma. With the increased number of mammographic studies being performed, radiologists are now becoming more aware of this lesion, which is better known in the radiographic literature as radial scar or indurative mastopathy. It may likewise be mistaken for a spiculated carcinoma by mammography (Box 10-4).[27,28] Recently, Page and Anderson have proposed a simplified nomenclature for these lesions, suggesting that small lesions (less than 1 cm), usually identified histologically, be termed radial scars.[9] The larger lesions, more frequently identified mammographically, are called complex sclerosing lesions. Although not encompassing all of the histologic variability within the name, their suggestion has the decided merit of bringing together a group of lesions with probable similar pathogenesis and pathobiology, thus allowing for better communication between surgeons, pathologists, and radiologists.

The characteristic histopathologic feature of both radial scars and complex sclerosing lesions is a central area of fibrosis and elastosis surrounded by disordered ducts exhibiting degrees of papillary hyperplasia and microcystic change. This central area of scarring may engulf and trap fat and glandular elements, producing an area of parenchymal distortion on mammography that may have a fatty center.[30] This appearance has been coined the "black star" appearance as contrasted to the "white star" appearance of a dense center, most often seen in invasive breast cancer. Most mammography experts have agreed that although these trends hold true for many lesions, the appearance of the central area is not a reliable way to differentiate a radial scar from an invasive breast cancer.[19] Central calcifications may occur with either lesion. Biopsy is recommended for establishing a diagnosis for all of these spiculated lesions that have not developed at a biopsy site (i.e., known to be scar tissue).[27,28]

BOX 10-3 SYNONYMS FOR COMPLEX SCLEROSING LESION AND RADIAL SCAR

Complex sclerosing lesion and radial scar	Page and Anderson, 1987[9]
Radial scar	Anderson and Gram, 1984[21]
Indurative mastopathy	Rickert and others, 1981[29]
	Cohen and others, 1985[22]
Infiltrating epitheliosis	Azzopardi, 1979[12]
Nonencapsulated sclerosing lesion	Fisher, 1979[24]
Benign sclerosing ductal proliferation	Tremblay and others, 1977[31]
Sclerosing papillary proliferation	Fenoglio and Lattes, 1974[23]

Small radial scars are a frequent incidental finding in breast biopsy specimens.[26] These areas infrequently produce a palpable mass. Most often, if detected preoperatively, they produce a spiculated mass or area of parenchymal distortion that is mammographically suspicious for invasive breast cancer. These areas may or may not contain microcalcifications.[19,28] A preoperative localization procedure is usually performed to monitor excision of the area.

The significance of radial scar and complex sclerosing lesions with respect to risk for subsequent development of breast cancer is controversial. Although some authors have suggested that this lesion is a precursor of tubular carcinoma, most publications fail to confirm this association. To date, there is no definitive evidence for increased risk of subsequent carcinoma in these patients and the lesions should be considered benign.

In any case, the lesions may pose a diagnostic dilemma for radiologists (see Box 10-4) and surgical pathologists alike (see Table 10-2). For the latter, these lesions must be distinguished from tubular carcinoma by histologic criteria. These criteria for tubular carcinoma include the presence of in situ carcinoma in surrounding ducts, the absence of a recognizable myoepithelial cell layer and basement membrane in the trapped glands and tubules within the fibrotic area, and the overall low-power configuration of the lesion. The low-power appearance of tubular carcinoma has an infiltrative growth pattern of small tubules trailing into the surrounding stroma. In contrast, the low-power appearance of a radial scar has a more lobulated smooth outline of peripheral dilated ducts with a central area of scar formation and elastosis. No associated in situ carcinoma is found, although intraductal hyperplasia of the peripheral ducts is frequent in a radial scar. Finally, in a radial scar the glands within the central zone of fibrosis are frequently angulated and irregular, and in at least some, a distinct myoepithelial cell layer can be identified as well as a basement membrane, which may be demonstrated with periodic acid–Schiff stains.[25]

BOX 10-4 DIFFERENTIAL DIAGNOSIS OF SPICULATED RADIOGRAPHIC LESIONS

Invasive ductal or lobular cancer
Tubular carcinoma
Radial scar or complex sclerosing lesion
Fat necrosis
Fibrosis
Postbiopsy scar
Mammographic pseudomass
Granulomatous disease
Myoblastoma

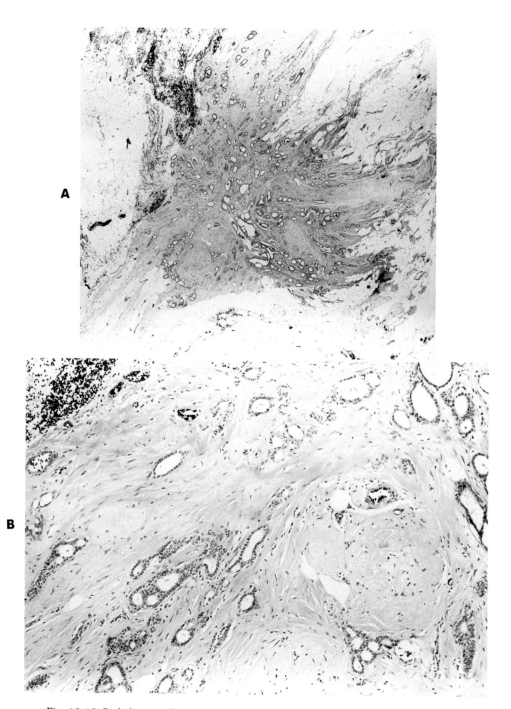

Fig. 10-13 Radial scar at low magnification demonstrates a stellate configuration with centrally located glands **(A).** These can be seen at higher magnification within the central core of fibrous and elastic tissue **(B).** Characteristically, these glands retain the double epithelial and myoepithelial lining.

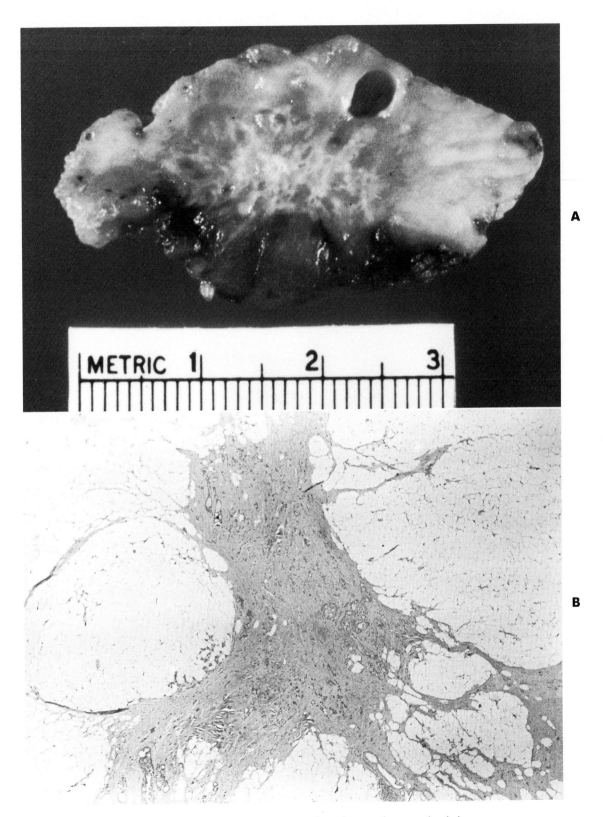

Fig. 10-14 A, The gross appearance of this complex sclerosing lesion and radial scar demonstrated the lack of circumscription and the variegated chalky white appearance of the fibroelastic tissue and trapped fat. (Courtesy Dr. Robert E. Fechner, Charlottesville, Virginia.) **B,** The trapping and incorporation of fat within a radial scar are illustrated in this photomicrograph.

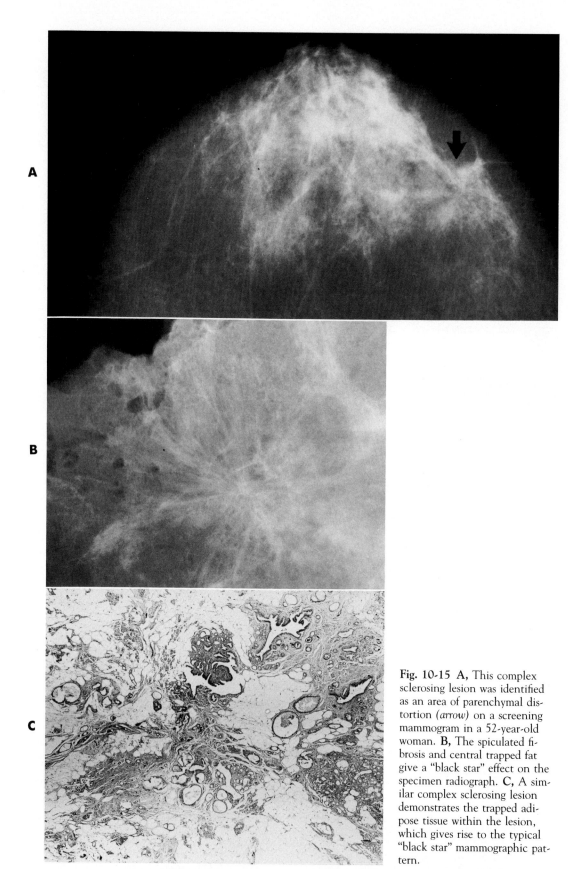

Fig. 10-15 A, This complex
sclerosing lesion was identified
as an area of parenchymal distortion *(arrow)* on a screening
mammogram in a 52-year-old
woman. **B,** The spiculated fibrosis and central trapped fat
give a "black star" effect on the
specimen radiograph. **C,** A similar complex sclerosing lesion
demonstrates the trapped adipose tissue within the lesion,
which gives rise to the typical
"black star" mammographic pattern.

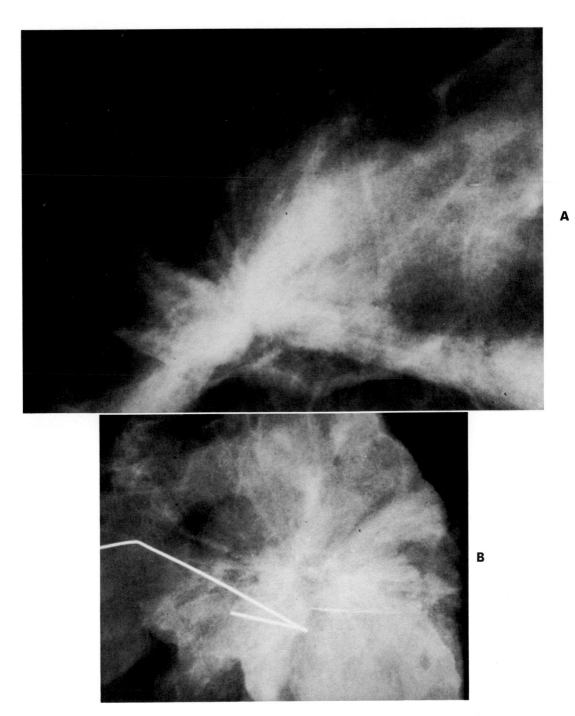

Fig. 10-16 This complex sclerosing lesion produced a misleading mammographic "white star" effect of a spiculated mass with a tent sign distorting the posterior parenchyma **(A).** Specimen radiograph showed faint central calcifications and trapped central fat **(B).** The pathologic diagnosis was complexing sclerosing lesion and radial scar.

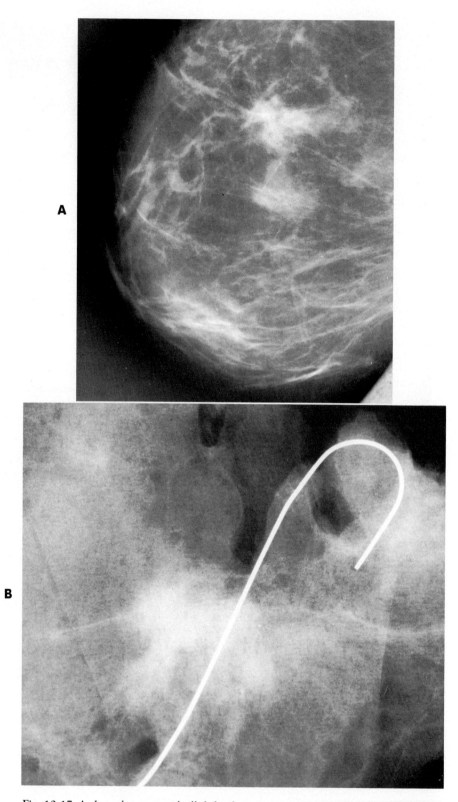

Fig. 10-17 A, Irregular mass with ill-defined margins in a fatty breast. **B,** Specimen radiograph better shows the spiculated margin of this mass. The pathologic diagnosis is complex sclerosing lesion and radial scar.

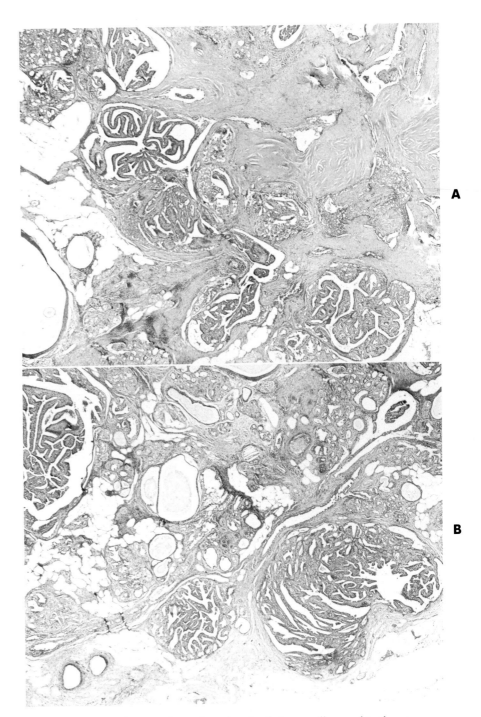

Fig. 10-18 Several features of complex sclerosing lesion are illustrated in these two photomicrographs from the same large lesion. In **A,** the peripheral papillomatosis and central fibroelastotic zone are well illustrated. In **B,** trapped fat, papillomatosis, and dilated ducts are present, all giving the lesion a variegated appearance.

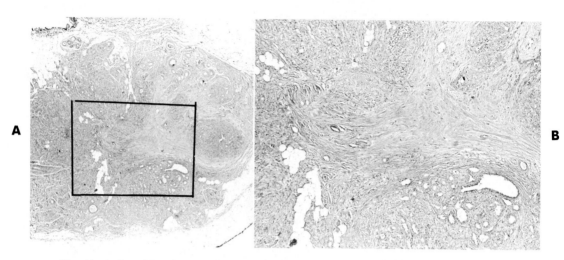

Fig. 10-19 **A** and **B,** The smooth peripheral outline of this complex sclerosing lesion is seen in this low-magnification photomicrograph. The peripheral ducts show extensive papillomatosis. The central area of scarring and elastosis with trapped glandular elements *(box)* is present and seen better in the higher magnification illustration **(B).**

Fig. 10-20 A biopsy of a focal cluster of granular calcifications **(A)** was taken with preoperative wire localization **(B)** in this woman who had a personal history of extensive comedocarcinoma in the contralateral breast. The pathologic diagnosis was complex sclerosing papillary lesion. **C** and **D,** Biopsy from this patient shows a complex sclerosing lesion with peripherally located dilated ducts, papillomatosis, and more centrally located fibrosis and elastosis seen better at higher magnification **(D).** Small calcifications seen mammographically are present in the illustrations.

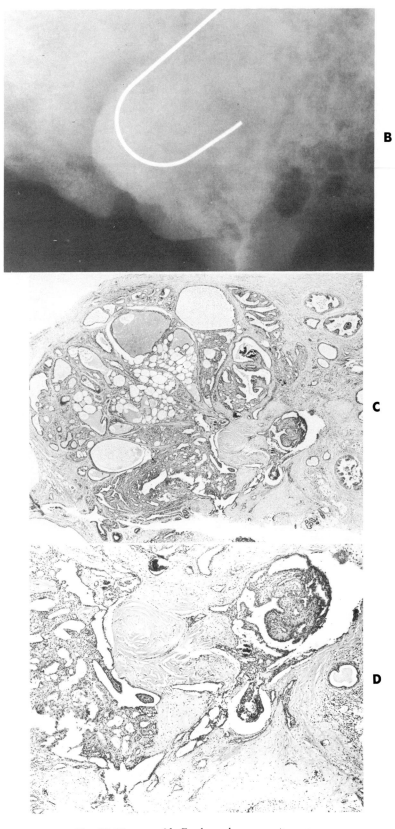

Fig. 10-20—cont'd. For legend see opposite page.

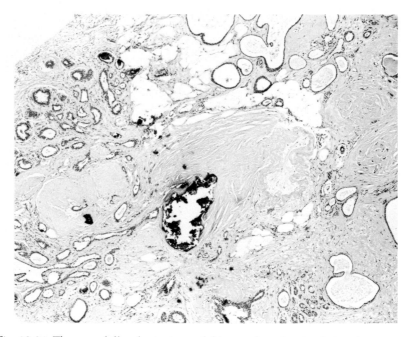

Fig. 10-21 The central fibroelastic tissue of this complex sclerosing lesion shows varying-sized calcifications.

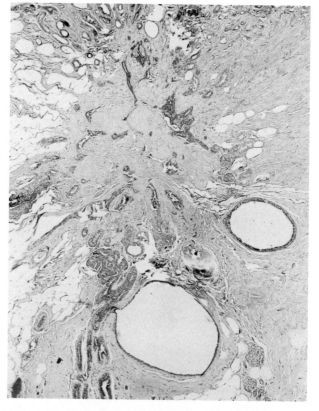

Fig. 10-22 This complex sclerosing lesion has a well-developed stellate fibrous core and peripheral dilated ducts.

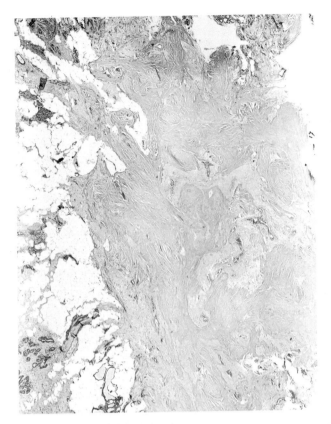

Fig. 10-23 This complex sclerosing lesion consists almost entirely of dense fibrosis and elastosis with some trapped glands and peripheral adipose tissue.

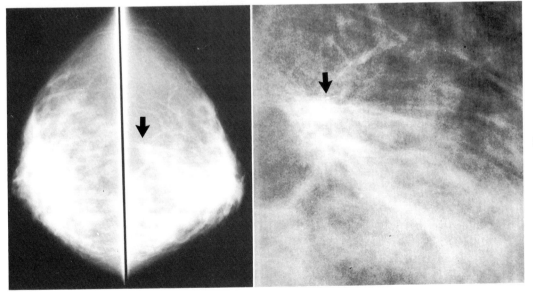

Fig. 10-24 Cancer mimicking a radial scar. **A,** Area of focal asymmetry with parenchymal distortion in posterior left breast (*arrow*). **B,** Photographic enlargement shows central trapped fat that could mimic a radial scar; however, the casting-type calcifications (*arrow*) indicate probable cancer. The pathologic diagnosis is infiltrating ductal cancer.

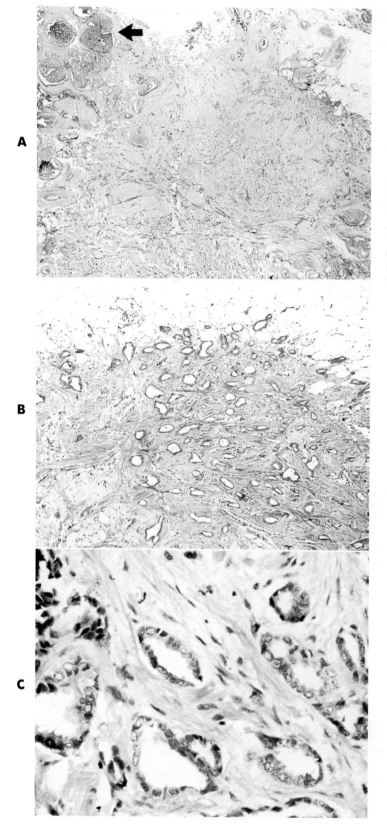

Fig. 10-25 Tubular carcinoma is an important differential diagnosis for complex sclerosing lesion and radial scar. Several differentiating features are illustrated in this case of tubular carcinoma. **A,** At low magnification the associated ductal carcinoma in situ is seen at the edge of the lesion (*arrow*). **B,** At slightly higher magnification the glands of the carcinoma extend beyond the area of fibrosis into surrounding fat. The glands are characteristically round or oval and regular in outline. **C,** At very high magnification the neoplastic glands show only a single epithelial cell layer, in contrast to the double cell layer configuration seen in normal ducts and in glands trapped in radial scars.

Fig. 10-26 In contrast to tubular carcinoma, this complex sclerosing lesion shows papillomatosis instead of ductal carcinoma in situ (**A**). The central fibroelastotic area traps and surrounds glandular elements, but the lesion is well circumscribed and no infiltration into the surrounding normal tissue is seen. In **B,** the irregular, often angulated trapped glands are seen within the fibroelastotic scar. As seen at higher magnification (**C**), these glands and cords of cells retain the double lining layers of normal ducts.

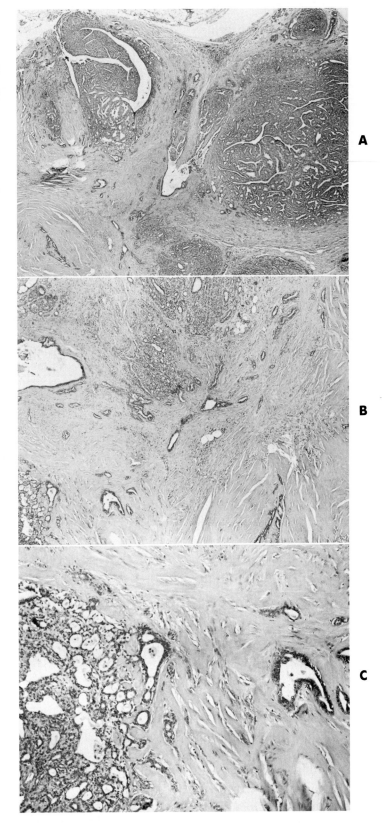

PAPILLARY ADENOMA OF THE NIPPLE

Papillary adenoma of the nipple is a rare benign lesion located within the nipple itself. It is characterized by a proliferation of small glands and tubules, occasionally exhibiting papillary epithelial hyperplasia, that grows into the stroma of the nipple, often displacing major ducts. These tubules are lined by two cell layers consisting of inner columnar epithelial and outer myoepithelial cells. Occasionally, squamous epithelial islands are seen. Some authors have characterized lesions with a tubular and solid configuration separately as syringomatous adenomas.[34,36] The lesion may ulcerate the skin of the nipple or may be covered by normal epidermis. Mitoses may be easily found, but cytologic atypia is rare. Instances of coexistent carcinoma have been reported, but the lesion is considered benign by most authors.

In addition to presenting as a mass lesion in or beneath the nipple, the lesion may alternatively present as a "blood-blister–like" lesion of the nipple, with nipple discharge, or as an excoriated or ulcerated nipple that may clinically mimic Paget's disease.[32] The latter finding may explain the synonym *erosive adenomatosis of the nipple*.[38] Palpation may elicit a discharge.[39] There are no described mammographic findings. Biopsy of the nipple is necessary for accurate diagnosis. Some writers refer to this lesion as florid papillomatosis of the nipple, while others believe that florid papillomatosis of the nipple and nipple adenoma are discrete entities.[33,37] There is an increased association of the lesion with a true intraductal papilloma involving the major lactiferous ducts.[35] It should be noted that rarely an intraductal papilloma can involve the most superficial portion of a lactiferous duct and actually extend onto the surface of the nipple. This should not be confused with papillary adenoma of the nipple.

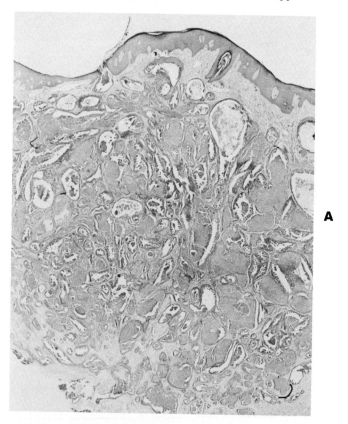

A

Fig. 10-27 Papillary adenoma of the nipple shows a complex arrangement of glands extending up to the intact skin of the nipple (**A**). The glands exhibit varying amounts of papillomatosis (**B**). At the base of the lesion (**C**) the glands are seen within the fibrous tissue and smooth muscle bundles of the nipple–areolar complex.

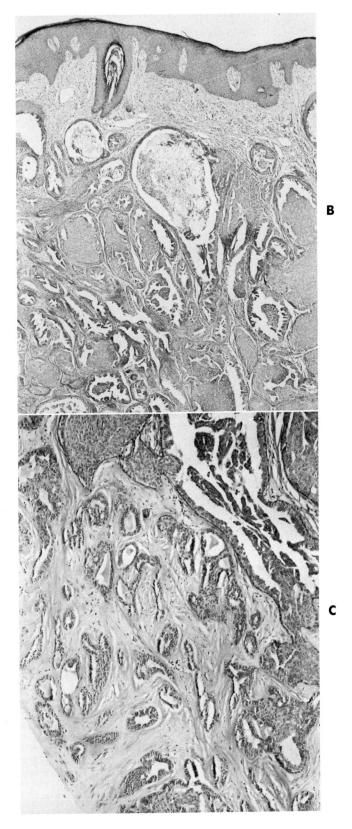

Fig. 10-27, cont'd. For legend see opposite page.

JUVENILE PAPILLOMATOSIS

Juvenile papillomatosis of the breast, also called Swiss cheese disease, is a very rare lesion of young women first described by Rosen in 1980.[43] Histopathologically, it is characterized by atypical papillary duct hyperplasia (papillomatosis) and numerous cysts, which are often clustered. Other components of fibrocystic change (apocrine metaplasia, sclerosing adenosis) are often seen. Subsequent findings based on the Juvenile Papillomatosis Registry indicate that juvenile papillomatosis not only is a marker for families at risk for breast cancer, but also may itself indicate that the patient herself is at jeopardy for coincident or subsequent carcinoma of the breast.[40,44,45]

The clinical presentation usually mimics that of fibroadenoma as a painless palpable mass in a young woman (mean age 23 years). The mass is most often single and discrete, ranging from 1 to 8 cm. Characteristically, all of the lesions contain cysts, most apparent grossly. This dominant histologic feature distinguishes this lesion from fibroadenoma and papillomatosis and explains its descriptive name of Swiss cheese disease of the breast.[42]

The marked papillary hyperplasia of duct epithelium (papillomatosis), which may show significant cytologic atypia, can be disturbing even in young women but does not justify a mastectomy.[44] However, female members of the immediate family should be evaluated as age dictates, and young patients with juvenile papillomatosis merit careful long-term follow-up.[40]

It can be predicted that the radiographic appearance of juvenile papillomatosis will add little to the preoperative evaluation. Because so many of these lesions occur before age 25, there is little experience with the mammographic findings. A palpable mass in this age group is usually treated by excisional biopsy without preoperative mammography. If ultrasound examination of the breast is performed, a cluster of cystic spaces may be detected, providing a clue to the correct pathologic diagnosis.[41]

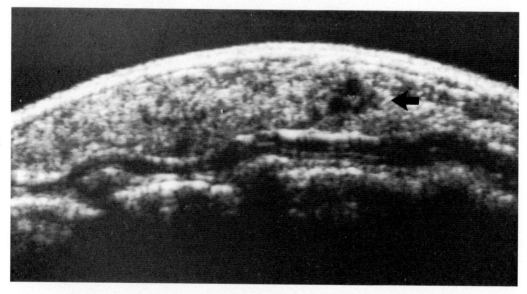

A

Fig. 10-28 An 18-year-old with a palpable mass for 2 years and a positive family history of breast cancer in her grandmother and aunt. Ultrasound examination **A** and **B** shows a complex mass (*arrow*) with multiple small hypoechoic spaces. The biopsy-proven diagnosis was juvenile papillomatosis. (Courtesy Dr. Phil Evans, Dallas.) **C,** Histopathology of juvenile papillomatosis. Juvenile papillomatosis is characterized by multiple cysts and associated epithelial hyperplasia or papillomatosis, which may be extensive. This biopsy of a mass from a 15-year-old girl shows a portion of the wall of a large cyst at left and several ducts with epithelial hyperplasia and papillomatosis at right.

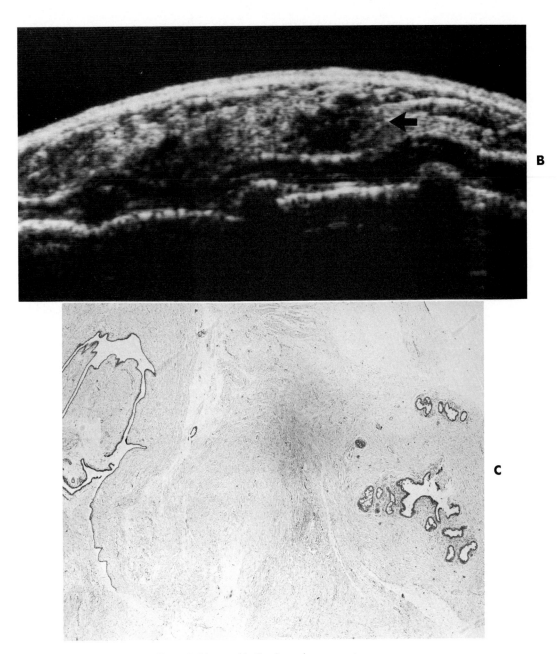

Fig. 10-28, cont'd. For legend see opposite page.

INTRACYSTIC PAPILLARY CARCINOMA

Intracystic papillary carcinoma must be distinguished from the more common papillary intraductal carcinoma (DCIS) and infiltrating ductal carcinoma with a papillary pattern.[46] The clinical presentation is frequently that of a solitary palpable or mammographically detected oval mass in an older obese patient (mean age of 63 years). Black women may have a higher incidence than white women.[47] The margins of the mass density may be well defined because of the slow growth of the lesion, allowing enlargement and distention of the involved ducts.[48] In some cases a large dilation or cystic space develops, frequently containing hemorrhagic fluid. The papillary cancer may be imaged as an irregularity or growth on the cyst wall by ultrasound examination or pneumocystography (Box 10-5).[50,51] The diagnosis of intracystic papillary carcinoma should be considered whenever hemorrhagic fluid is aspirated from a cystic mass, particularly in a postmenopausal woman. Fluid cytology is not reliable, and excisional biopsy is recommended for diagnosis. As with other carcinomas, the lesion may be detected when clinically occult by mammographic screening examination. A mass density with or without calcifications is the most likely radiographic finding.[47,48]

The prognosis for this uncommon subtype of breast cancer is very good. This carcinoma is reported to account for 0.5% to 2% of cases in extensive breast cancer series.[49] Despite a benign radiographic appearance, cancer should be suspected when a dominant mass occurs in a postmenopausal woman.

Histopathologic interpretation should await permanent sections because differentiation of papillary carcinoma from benign papillary lesions is hazardous by aspiration cytology or by frozen section. Characteristically, the intracystic papillary carcinoma manifests a papillary growth pattern characterized by neoplastic proliferation of a single cell type. This is in contrast to the intraductal papilloma, which characteristically exhibits a pleomorphic cellular pattern. The cells of the intracystic papillary carcinoma may be arrayed along fibrovascular cores or may be present as papillary epithelial growths. They customarily have rather regular nuclei, which in some tumors may be quite vesicular, giving a superficial resemblance to papillary thyroid neoplasms. Occasionally, the cells may be quite hyperchromatic. The most important features are architectural rigidity and cytologic uniformity. Hemorrhage and scarring in these tumors are common, as is also the case with intraductal papillomas. The fibrosis may extend to involve and obliterate the cyst wall and may trap small clusters of tumor cells, giving rise to a pseudoinfiltrative appearance.

BOX 10-5 IMAGING FEATURES OF PAPILLARY BREAST LESIONS

Lesion	Feature
Solitary papilloma	Normal mammogram usually and intraluminal defect on galactogram
Multiple papillomas	No specific features
Papillomatosis	No specific features
Complex sclerosing lesion and radial scar	Spiculated mass entrapping fat
Nipple adenoma	No specific features
Juvenile papillomatosis	Cluster of cystic spaces on ultrasound examination
Intracystic papillary carcinoma	Complex cyst by ultrasound examination

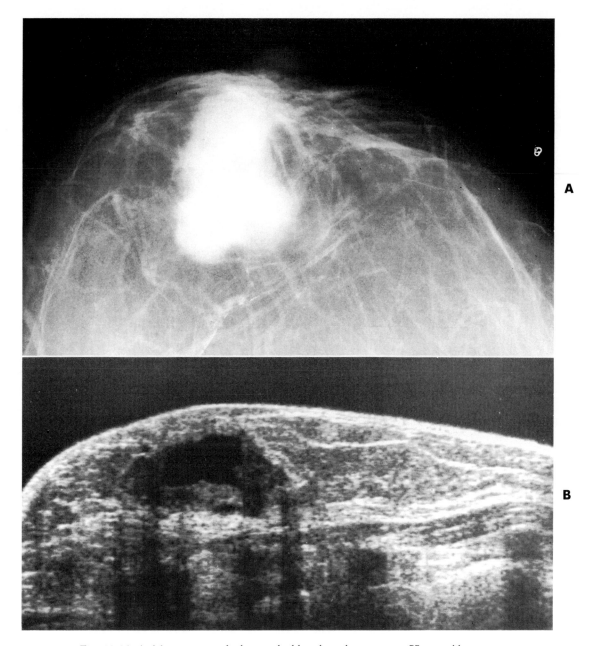

Fig. 10-29 A, Mammogram of a large palpable subareolar mass in a 77-year-old woman shows a lesion irregular in shape with indistinct margins, suspicious for malignancy. **B,** Breast ultrasound examination indicates an irregular wall lined with echogenic tissue and a central, irregular shaped cystic cavity. The pathologic diagnosis is intracystic papillary cancer. (Courtesy Dr. Phil Evans, Dallas.)

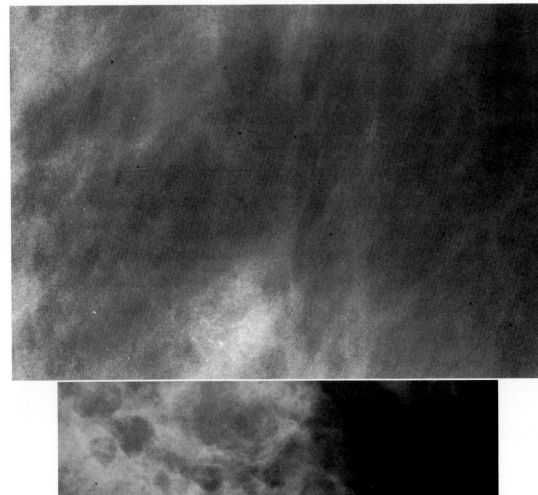

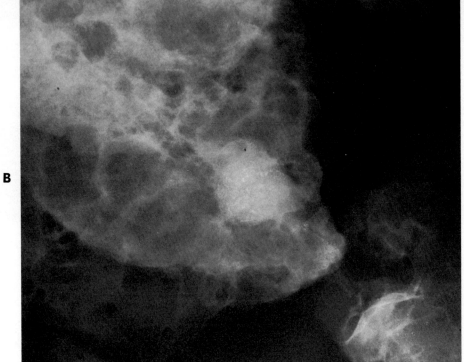

Fig. 10-30 Screening mammogram **(A)** shows a 1-cm mass with obscured margins and fine microcalcifications, which are better seen on the specimen radiograph **(B)**.

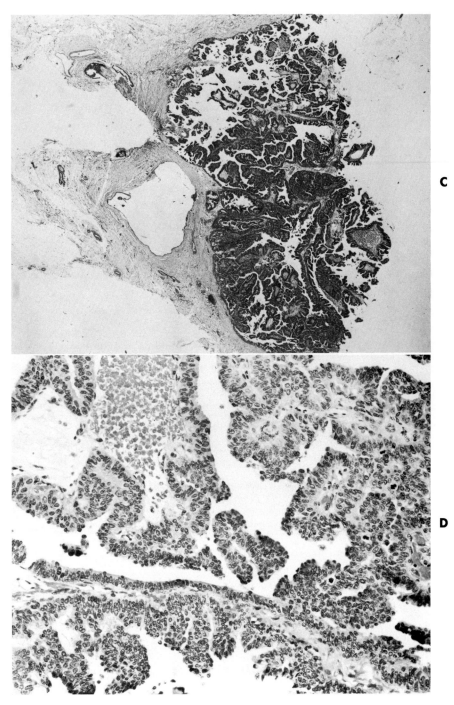

C

D

Fig. 10-30—cont'd The intracystic papillary carcinoma from this patient is illustrated in these photomicrographs. The papillary configuration is seen in the low-magnification photomicrograph **(C)**. Some of the papillary fronds exhibit a delicate fibrovascular core, whereas others are formed entirely of epithelial cells. At higher magnification **(D)**, the neoplastic epithelial cells have a monotonous appearance. The cells are small, regular, and somewhat hyperchromatic. The variation and multiplicity of cell types seen in intraductal papilloma are absent in this carcinoma.

REFERENCES
Solitary papilloma

1. Cardenosa G, Eklund GW: Benign papillary neoplasms of the breast: mammographic findings, *Radiology* 181:751, 1991.
2. Flint A, Oberman H: Infarction and squamous metaplasia of intraductal papilloma: a benign breast lesion that may simulate carcinoma, *Hum Pathol* 15:764, 1984.
3. Giltman L: Solitary intraductal papilloma of the male breast, *South Med J* 74:774, 1981.
4. Haagensen CD: *Diseases of the breast,* ed 3, Philadelphia, 1986, WB Saunders.
5. Kraus F, Neubecker R: The differential diagnosis of papillary tumors of the breast, *Cancer* 15:444, 1962.
6. Murad TM, Contesso G, Mouriesse H: Papillary tumors of large lactiferous ducts, *Cancer* 48:122, 1981.
7. Murad TM, Swaid S, Pritchett P: Malignant and benign papillary lesions of the breast, *Hum Pathol* 8:379, 1977.
8. Osuch J: Benign lesion of the breast other than fibrocystic change, *Obstet Gynecol Clin North Am* 14:703, 1987.
9. Page DL, Anderson TJ, editors: *Diagnostic histopathology of the breast,* New York, 1987, Churchill Livingstone, p 104.
10. Roy I, Meakins J, Tremblay G: Giant intraductal papilloma of the breast: a case report, *J Surg Oncol* 28:281, 1985.
11. Woods ER, Helvie MA, Ikeda DM, et al: Solitary breast papilloma: comparison of mammographic, galactographic and pathologic findings, *AJR Am J Roentgenol* 159:487, 1992.

Multiple papillomas

12. Azzopardi JG: *Problems in breast pathology,* vol, 11, in Major Problems in Pathology Series, Philadelphia, 1979, WB Saunders.
13. Haagenson CD: *Diseases of the breast,* ed 2, Philadelphia, 1971, WB Saunders.
14. Murad T, Contesso G, Mouriesse H: Papillary tumors of large lactiferous ducts, *Cancer* 48:122, 1981.
15. Ohuchi N, Abe R, Kasai M: Possible cancerous change in intraductal papillomas of the breast: a 3D reconstruction study of 25 cases, *Cancer* 54:605, 1984.
16. Ohuchi N, Abe R, Takahashi T, Tezuka F: Origin and extension of intraductal papillomas of the breast: a three-dimensional reconstruction study, *Breast Cancer Res Treat* 4:117, 1984.

Papillomatosis

17. Dupont WD, Page DL: Risk factors for breast cancer in women with proliferative breast disease, *N Engl J Med* 312:146, 1985.
18. Sloane JP: *Biopsy pathology of the breast,* New York, 1980, John Wiley.

Complex sclerosing papillary lesion and radial scar

19. Adler DO, Helvie MA, Oberman HA et al, Radial sclerosing lesion of the breast: mammographic features, *Radiology* 176:737, 1990.
20. Anderson JA, Carter D, Linell F: A symposium on sclerosing duct lesions of the breast, *Pathol Annu* 21:145, 1986.
21. Anderson J, Gram J: Radial scar in the female breast: a long-term follow-up study of 32 cases, *Cancer* 53:2557, 1984.
22. Cohen M, Matthies H, Mintzer R, et al: Indurative mastopathy: a cause of false-positive mammograms, *Radiology* 155:69, 1985.
23. Fenoglio C, Lattes R: Sclerosing papillary proliferations in the female breast, *Cancer* 33:691, 1974.
24. Fisher E, Palekar A, Kotwal N: A nonencapsulated sclerosing lesion of the breast, *Am J Clin Pathol* 71:240, 1979.
25. Flotte TJ, Bell DA, Greco MA: Tubular carcinoma and sclerosing adenosis: the use of basal lamina as a differential feature, *Am J Surg Pathol* 4:75, 1980.
26. Linell F, Ljungberg O: *Atlas of breast pathology,* Philadelphia, 1984, JB Lippincott, p 120.
27. Mitnick J, Vazquez M, Harris M, Roses D: Differentiation of radial scar from schirrhous carcinoma of the breast: mammographic pathologic correlation, *Radiology* 173:697, 1989.
28. Orel SG, Evers K, Yeh IT, Troupin RH: Radial scar with microcalcifications: radiologic-pathologic correlation, *Radiology* 183:479, 1992.
29. Rickert R, Kalisher L, Hutter R: Indurative mastopathy: a benign sclerosing lesion of breast with elastosis which may simulate carcinoma, *Cancer* 47:561, 1981.
30. Tabar L, Dean PB: *Teaching atlas of mammography,* New York, 1985, Thieme-Stratton, p 87.
31. Tremblay G, Buell R, Seemayer T: Elastosis in benign sclerosing ductal proliferation of the female breast, *Am J Surg Pathol* 1:155, 1977.

Papillary adenoma of the nipple

32. Brownstein M, Phelps R, Magnin P: Papillary adenoma of the nipple: analysis of fifteen new cases, *J Am Acad Dermatol* 12:707, 1985.

33. Doctor V, Sirsat M: Florid papillomatosis (adenoma) and other benign tumours of the nipple and areola, *Br J Cancer* 25:1, 1971.
34. Jones M, Norris H, Snyder R: Infiltrating syringomatous adenoma of the nipple: a clinical and pathological study of 11 cases, *Am J Surg Pathol* 13:197, 1989.
35. Perzin KH, Lattes R: Papillary adenoma of the nipple (florid papillomatosis, adenoma, adenomatosis), *Cancer* 29:996, 1972.
36. Rosen P: Syringomatous adenoma of the nipple, *Am J Surg Pathol* 7:739, 1983.
37. Rosen P, Caicco J: Florid papillomatosis of the nipple: a study of 51 patients, including nine with mammary carcinoma, *Am J Surg Pathol* 10:87, 1986.
38. Smith E, Kron S, Gross P: Erosive adenomatosis of the nipple, *Arch Dermatol* 102:330, 1970.
39. Waldo E, Sidhu G, Hu A: Florid papillomatosis of male nipple after diethylstilbestrol therapy, *Arch Pathol* 99:364, 1975.

Juvenile papillomatosis

40. Bazzocchi F, Santini D, Martinelli G, et al: Juvenile papillomatosis (epitheliosis) of the breast: a clinical and pathologic study of 13 cases, *Am J Clin Pathol* 86:745, 1986.
41. Kersschot E, Hermans M, Pauwels C, et al: Juvenile papillomatosis of the breast: sonographic appearance, *Radiology* 169:631, 1988.
42. Rosen P: Papillary duct hyperplasia of the breast in children and young adults, *Cancer* 56:1611, 1985.
43. Rosen P, Cantrell B, Mullen D, DePalo A: Juvenile papillomatosis (Swiss cheese disease) of the breast, *Am J Surg Pathol* 4:3, 1980.
44. Rosen PP, Holmes G, Lesser M, et al: Juvenile papillomatosis and breast carcinoma, *Cancer* 55:1345, 1985.
45. Rosen PP, Lyngholm B, Kinne DW, Bentsic EJ: Juvenile papillomatosis of the breast and family history of breast carcinoma, *Cancer* 49:2591, 1982.

Intracystic papillary carcinoma

46. Carter D, Orr S, Merino J: Intracystic papillary carcinoma of the breast: after mastectomy, radiotherapy or excisional biopsy alone, *Cancer* 52:14, 1983.
47. Czernobilsky B: Intracystic carcinoma of the female breast, *Surg Gynecol Obstet* 124:93, 1967.
48. Kalisher L: Intracystic carcinoma of the breast presenting as a benign-appearing mass, *Breast: Diseases of the Breast* 3:32, 1977.
49. McKittrick J, Doane W, Failing R: Intracystic papillary carcinoma of the breast, *Am Surg* 35:195, 1969.
50. Reuter K, D'Orsi C, Reale F: Intracystic carcinoma of the breast: the role of ultrasonography, *Radiology* 153:233, 1984.
51. Tabar L, Pentek Z, Dean P: The diagnostic and therapeutic value of breast cyst puncture and pneumocystography, *Radiology* 141:659, 1981.

Fibrocystic Breast Changes

Deborah E. Powell
Carol B. Stelling

DEFINITION

Fibrocystic disease is a term that encompasses a variety of histopathologic patterns. Because it represents a spectrum of morphologic changes and not a specific disease entity, the term *fibrocystic change* is preferred.[1,2] Some of the varying histopathologic entities encompassed by the term fibrocystic change are listed in Box 11-1.

The importance of fibrocystic change is that it is very common and that certain histopathologic patterns are associated with an increased risk of subsequent breast cancer. These high-risk patterns are uncommon but as yet cannot be distinguished from low- or no-risk patterns by either physical examination or imaging studies.

OVERVIEW OF FIBROCYSTIC CHANGES
Incidence

Although fibrocystic change has been reported to be very common, occurring in up to 80% of adult women in some autopsy series,[9,10] a careful forensic autopsy study[3] demonstrated gross or microscopic cystic change in only 13% and epithelial proliferation in only 25% of women over 14 years of age. This study compared rates of incidence for different patterns of fibrocystic change in three ethnic groups with different breast cancer risks: whites (high-risk), Hispanics (moderate-risk), and Native Americans (low-risk). The prevalence of moderate-to-marked cystic change and moderate-to-marked epithelial hyperplasia was higher in whites than in His-

BOX 11-1: SOME HISTOPATHOLOGIC PATTERNS INCLUDED IN FIBROCYSTIC CHANGE OF THE BREAST

Stromal fibrosis
Cysts
Sclerosing adenosis
Microglandular adenosis
Intraductal papillomatosis
Intraductal hyperplasia
Atypical ductal hyperplasia
Blunt duct adenosis
Lobular hyperplasia
Atypical lobular hyperplasia
Apocrine metaplasia
Papillary apocrine change
Apocrine hyperplasia
Sclerosing papillomatosis

panics or Native American women. The presence of several types of fibrocystic change (epithelial hyperplasia, sclerosing adenosis, lobular microcalcification) was more common than predicted in Hispanic women and was almost as common as that found in the higher risk white patients.

In contrast, a comparative study of Japanese and North American women[16] showed differences in the incidence of different patterns of fibrocystic change between the two populations. Solitary papillomas were more common in the Japanese population. Apocrine change (apocrine cysts and apocrine hyperplasia), sclerosing adenosis and intraductal hyperplasia, atypical lobular hyperplasia, and blunt duct hyperplasia were twice as common in the American patients. No difference was found in the incidence of cysts, periductal mastitis, or fibroadenomas.

Epidemiology

Epidemiologic risk factors for benign breast disease have been discussed in Chapter 1. As mentioned in that chapter, the term *benign breast disease* is very inclusive and encompasses benign tumors in addition to the numerous histopathologic changes of fibrocystic conditions. A few studies, however, have examined specific risk factors for fibrocystic disease and have even tried to look at individual histopathologic parameters. In a large study of women with biopsy-proven fibrocystic change, Berkowitz and associates[5] investigated risk factors associated with this diagnosis. In both premenopausal and postmenopausal women, a positive association was found with high socioeconomic status. For postmenopausal women, an association with late menopause was seen. In premenopausal women, there was an association with low parity and a history of breast cancer in a sister or mother as well as a low Quetelet index $[(weight/height^2) \times 10,000]$. A negative association between cigarette use and fibrocystic disease was found.

In another report, Berkowitz and colleagues[4] also examined the relation of oral contraceptive and exogenous estrogen use to the incidence of fibrocystic disease and to different histopathologic components of fibrocystic change. In contrast to a prior study carried out by one of the members of their group,[11] Berkowitz and colleagues found no decreased incidence of fibrocystic disease among oral contraceptive users. They also found no evidence of increased cases of marked ductal epithelial atypia in patients with either oral contraceptive or exogenous estrogen use. A positive association of exogenous estrogen use and fibrocystic change was found in postmenopausal patients, especially in patients with gross cysts, papillomatosis, and papillary hyperplasia. Numerous other studies have suggested a decreased incidence of fibrocystic change in oral contraceptive users. Berkowitz and colleagues[4] explain the differences in their study as possibly indicating that oral contraceptives decrease the symptoms but not the histopathologic features of fibrocystic change.

Other studies have investigated the relationship of caffeine and fibrocystic breast change with conflicting results. The same group of patients used for the previously discussed study on oral contraceptive and estrogen use was the subject of a report by Boyle and associates.[6] These authors found an increase in fibrocystic change in women who consumed caffeine, particularly marked in those consuming over 500 mg per day. There was a strong association of atypical lobular hyperplasia and sclerosing adenosis with papillary hyperplasia with caffeine intake. Conversely, a study by Schairer[15] failed to show an association between caffeine or any methylxanthine consumption and fibrocystic change or any of its specific histopathologic patterns.

Classification

As has been mentioned previously, the term fibrocystic change encompasses a large variety of histopathologic patterns. Although many studies indicated a slight overall risk to women with fibrocystic change for the subsequent development of breast cancer[2], the work of DuPont, Page, and others[7,8,12,13] was important in focusing attention on specific histopathologic patterns and breast cancer risk.[14] In a series of publications, this group reviewed and gathered follow-up information on more than 3000 women who collectively had over 10,000 breast biopsies. Median follow-up time for the group was 17 years. The authors determined that although some histologic patterns of fibrocystic change were associated with increased risk of breast cancer, others were not. The patterns associated with some increased cancer risk were characterized by epithelial hyperplasia.

When the data were analyzed, the fibrocystic patterns could be classified into three main groups: patterns associated with no statistically increased cancer risk or nonproliferative fibrocystic disease; patterns associated with a slight or minimally increased cancer risk or proliferative fibrocystic disease without atypia; and patterns associated with a more significant increased cancer risk or proliferative fibrocystic disease with atypia (atypical hyperplasia).[7]

When the prevalence of these categories in the study population was investigated, the authors found that nonproliferative disease was the most common problem, accounting for over 68% of biopsies. Proliferative lesions without atypia were the next most common, occurring in over 26% of the biopsies. The lesions showing the greatest increased cancer risk, the atypical hyperplasias, were the least common, occurring in only about 4% of all biopsies. Thus, most

Table 11-1 Prevalence of fibrocystic patterns

Type	Prevalence
Nonproliferative patterns (no increased cancer risk)	68%
Proliferative patterns without atypia (minimally increased cancer risk)	26%
Atypical hyperplasia (increased cancer risk)	4%
Carcinoma in situ (markedly increased cancer risk)	2%

Modified from Dupont WD, Page DL: Risk factors for breast cancer in women with proliferative breast disease, *N Engl J Med* 312:146, 1985.

women undergoing breast biopsy for fibrocystic disease are found to have changes that are not associated with a significantly increased breast cancer risk. A small number, however, are found to have lesions associated with an increased risk, and when these patterns are recognized the patients can be targeted for close follow-up care. A summary is presented in Table 11-1.

These same authors also identified that in all these categories the risk for subsequent breast cancer is increased in patients with a family history of breast cancer.[7] The additional effect of two risk factors is particularly significant for patients with atypical hyperplasia.

PATTERNS OF NO INCREASED CANCER RISK: NONPROLIFERATIVE FIBROCYSTIC CHANGE
Histopathology

Histopathologic changes in nonproliferative fibrocystic change were initially classified as epithelial cysts, epithelial-related calcification, mild hyperplasia of usual type, fibroadenoma, and papillary apocrine change.[7] As the result of subsequent studies, the latter two conditions have been removed from this category.[27,36] The lesions currently included in this category are listed in Box 11-2. Although stromal fibrosis is commonly seen in biopsies with fibrocystic change, it is not specifically included in this list because it was not identified separately in the studies cited.

Epithelial cysts are very common and can vary greatly in size, from less than 1 millimeter to several centimeters. Their walls can be lined by recognizable ductal epithelial cells, or the pressure of fluid within the cysts can cause the epithelium to undergo atrophy so that it is difficult to identify in histologic sections. The epithelium lining these cysts may show apocrine features (apocrine metaplasia). Apocrine change or apocrine metaplasia in cells is characterized by cellular enlargement and marked cytoplasmic eosinophilia. The atypical cytoplasm of these cells frequently exhibits a rounded protrusion or "apical snout."[30] There is also characteristically marked granularity to the cytoplasm. The nuclei of these epithelial cells are characteristically enlarged and exhibit prominent nucleoli. A specific glycoprotein, gross cystic disease fluid protein (GCDFP-15) has been found in apocrine cytoplasm and is considered by some to be a marker of apocrine change.[26]

Cysts are frequently surrounded by stromal fibrosis and occasionally by mononuclear cell infiltrates. The cyst contents can be varied as well, ranging from clear to cloudy fluid to blood-tinged or brown fluid due to the presence of hemoglobin breakdown products. Foam cells are frequently found. A large number of different biochemical components of breast cyst fluid have been identified, including polypeptide and steroid hormones, enzymes, immunoglobulins, and other proteins and electrolytes. The relation of these compounds to the etiology of fibrocystic change is uncertain or at best speculative.[35]

Studies by Wellings and associates[37] are convincing in identifying the site of origin of these epithelial cysts as the terminal ductal-lobular units (TDLU), rather than larger ducts. The TDLU may be obliterated during formation of the cysts, making the origin apparent only with painstaking subgross histopathologic studies.

BOX 11-2. FIBROCYSTIC PATTERNS OF NO INCREASED CANCER RISK

Epithelial cysts
Epithelial-related calcifications
Mild hyperplasia of usual type

Mild hyperplasia of usual type is characterized as a slight increase (three to four cell layers) in the number of epithelial cells lining a duct but without sufficient proliferation to bridge or cross the lumen of a duct.[7] Calcification may be found with or without epithelial hyperplasia, but its presence alone was not found to represent an increased cancer risk.

For patients with epithelial cysts, a family history of breast cancer was found to slightly increase the risk of subsequent cancer over that related to family history alone (3.0 to 2.5).[7]

Imaging

The imaging of nonproliferative fibrocystic change parallels the histopathologic descriptors and includes cyst formation (both microcystic and macrocystic), epithelial-related calcifications, and fibrosis. This section emphasizes the mammographic findings of these elements. The ancillary technique of ultrasonography and pneumocystography for diagnosis of simple macrocysts was discussed in Chapter 3. There is increasing use of either mammography- or ultrasound-directed aspiration of clinically occult breast cysts to confirm benignity when a cyst is suspected but the imaging features are atypical.[18,19,28] Cysts can be seen to collapse by real-time monitoring of ultrasound-guided aspiration.

Simple breast cysts may be microcystic or macrocystic. Haagensen and Mazoujian[22] define cysts 3 mm or smaller as microcysts and those larger than 3 mm in diameter as macrocysts. For many women with a fibrocystic condition on biopsy, the histologic cystic change is microcystic and, if not associated with sedimenting calcium, has no imaging correlate because these small cysts are obscured by surrounding stroma on mammography. Apocrine change may be present in many microcysts, but current imaging techniques do not differentiate apocrine microcysts from simple microcysts.

The macroscopic cyst classically causes a round or oval mass with well-circumscribed margins. Less frequently, the margins are lobulated. Microlobulation of the margin may be seen when apocrine cystic change is present. Surrounding parenchyma often obscures a portion of the margin, but spiculation is not a feature of a simple cyst and should raise suspicion of carcinoma. It is believed that cysts tend to be oriented along the directions of the breast segments or trabeculae. If cyst contents are under great pressure, pericystic inflammatory changes may be present and produce atypical mammographic features due to pericystic fibrosis.[24] The density of most cysts is isodense to breast parenchyma. Density may be increased by hemorrhagic fluid or hemosiderin.[21] Occasionally, eggshell calcifications are seen in the wall of a simple cyst.[33]

If palpable, a mass suspected of being a simple cyst should be aspirated. If not palpable, a single dominant mass suspected of being a cyst should be confirmed by ultrasonographic examination. Atypical sonographic features for a cyst may prompt aspiration by ultrasound guidance, a stereotactic fine-needle aspiration (FNA) or core biopsy, or a wire-directed biopsy, depending on the technology and expertise available. Clear and nonbloody cyst fluid is not customarily submitted for cytologic analysis. Turbid or bloody cyst fluid necessitates close follow-up or biopsy to exclude carcinoma.

It has been estimated that only 7% of the Western female population will develop a clinically aspirable cyst over a lifetime. As women age, the incidence of symptomatic breast cysts decreases. In an office-based gynecologic practice, only 6% of women over age 60 years had aspirable cysts compared with 15% in women less than 55 years of age.[17] Of the women over 55 years with aspirable cysts in this series, nearly 50% were taking a hormonal supplement. The increasingly widespread use of hormonal supplements in the postmenopausal woman may result in a widening of the age range during which aspirable breasts cysts present clinically.

Epithelial-related calcifications can be loosely grouped into lobular type calcification and milk of calcium within cysts. Another group of large round or oval

Table 11-2 **Spectrum of sedimented calcium in benign breast cysts in 287 women with bilateral mammograms**

Type	Prevalence
Milk of calcium in microcysts (<2 mm in diameter)	
Multiple, bilateral scattered, or clustered	60%
Unilateral, clustered, or scattered	29%
Solitary	4%
Milk of calcium in macrocysts	4%
Sand-like calcifications in cysts	2%

Modified from Linden SS, Sickles EA: Sedimented calcium in benign breast cysts: the full spectrum of mammographic presentations, *AJR Am J Roentgenol* 152:967, 1989.

benign calcifications are recognized mammographically, but their etiology is not known.[33] The lobular type calcifications are uniformly round, of similar size, and clustered.[34] These calcifications are characteristically seen in sclerosing adenosis and are discussed elsewhere in this chapter under that heading.

The milk of calcium condition, seen in about 4% of symptomatic women having mammography, is a mammographic manifestation of benign breast cysts, most often microcystic in size. The mammographic spectrum of this benign condition was reported by Linden and Sickles[25] in 1988 (Table 11-2). The mammographic hallmark is the fact that the calcium looks different on the craniocaudad projection from the lateral views. On the craniocaudad projection, the calcium has a smudge-like appearance with ill-defined edges. The horizontal beam lateral projection shows linear, crescentic, or teacup-shaped calcium layering in the bottom of a fluid-filled cyst.[32] Magnification views in the craniocaudad and true lateral projections are helpful to increase confidence in evaluating clustered amorphous or indistinct calcifications. Milk of calcium is a benign condition and does not require biopsy. Caution is necessary to avoid overlooking malignant microcalcifications within the same breast.

In spite of the widespread use of magnification mammography to characterize breast calcifications, a great deal is to be learned about differentiating calcifications associated with benign fibrocystic change from those associated with malignancy. Ultrastructure and microanalysis of breast calcifications have received little attention.[20] Nonsedimenting calcifications remain a common cause for biopsy. In a series of 500 consecutive needle localizations for nonpalpable breast lesions, microcalcifications without an associated mass were the reason for biopsy in 213 women (43%). Of these 213, the histologic results were benign in 165 (78%).[23] The histologic site of calcification in benign disease is variable and includes lumina of ducts, acini, areas of apocrine metaplasia, and stroma.[29] Spontaneous disappearance of round benign calcifications may occur.[31]

Focal compressed spot magnification views are the best current imaging tool to attempt to separate benign punctate uniform clustered microcalcifications from granular or casting-type calcifications considered suspicious for malignancy. Calcifications that are difficult to characterize even with magnification views are termed *amorphous* or *indistinct* under the American College of Radiology standard nomenclature. Decision to follow or perform a biopsy on such indeterminate calcifications is influenced by patient risk factors and interval change in number or pattern.

Focal stromal fibrosis should also be mentioned here with nonproliferative fibrocystic disease. Although not considered a significant histopathologic entity, focal fibrosis is a clinical entity that may lead to a biopsy procedure to evaluate either a palpable abnormality or a suspicious mammographic lesion.[24] The imaging correlate varies from a well-circumscribed solid mass to an irregularly shaped mass with ill-defined or spiculated margins. Particularly in a postmenopausal woman with fatty breasts, mammographic screening may detect focal areas, which, when biopsied, are areas of stromal fibrosis. The clinical entity of focal fibrous mastopathy of insulin-dependent diabetic patients is discussed in Chapter 13.

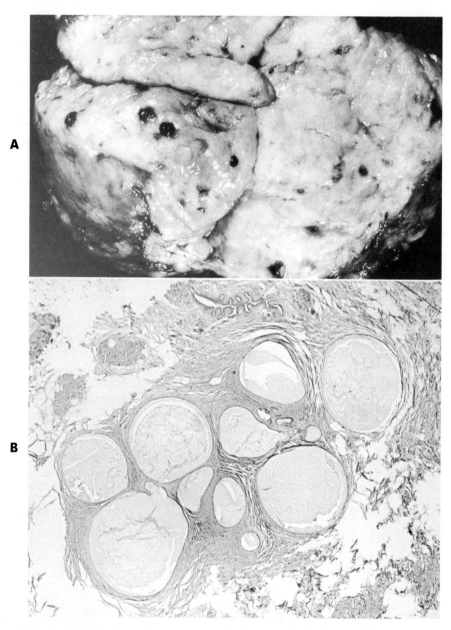

Fig. 11-1 (A) This breast biopsy specimen shows numerous cysts of varying size and dense mammary parenchyma. Some cysts appear dark due to the presence of blood within the cysts. (From Golden A, Powell DE, Jennings CD. *Pathology: Understanding disease,* ed, 2, Baltimore, 1985, Williams & Wilkins.) **(B)** Multiple cysts containing amorphous material and surrounded by dense fibrous stroma.

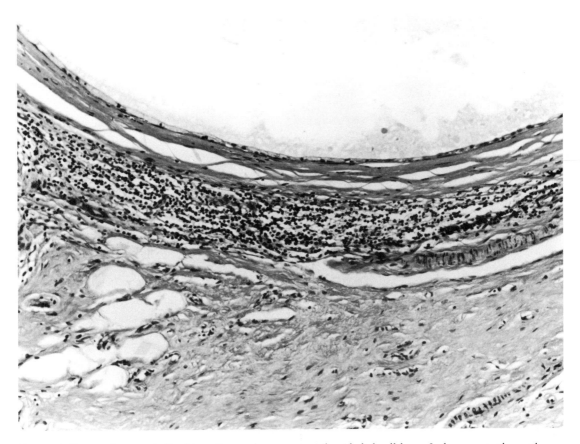

Fig. 11-2 Frequently a cyst is lined by a flattened or compressed epithelial cell layer. In larger cysts the epithelium may be quite inconspicuous, as in this example. A portion of the wall of this large cyst is illustrated in this photomicrograph. Fibrosis and an infiltrate of mononuclear inflammatory cells surround the cyst beneath the flattened epithelium.

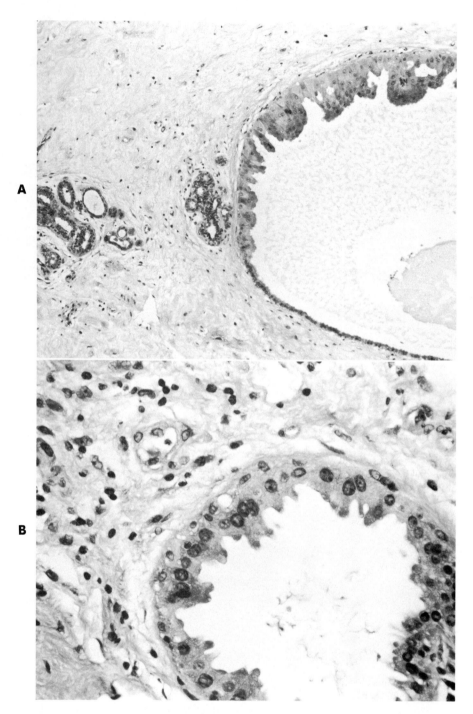

Fig. 11-3 (A) Frequently, the epithelial lining of the cysts shows apocrine features, often referred to as apocrine metaplasia. This is illustrated in the large cyst in this photomicrograph. In **B** the cytologic features are illustrated. These cells have large, somewhat pleomorphic nuclei and abundant granular cytoplasm with prominent apical cytoplasmic protrusions or "snouts."

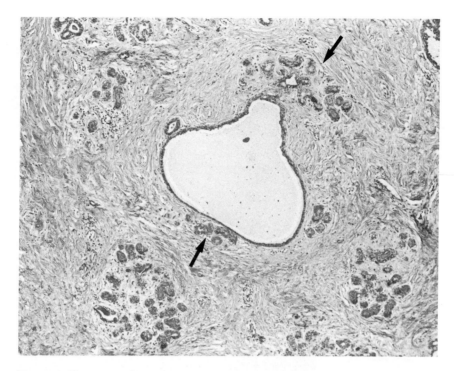

Fig. 11-4 The origin of cysts from the breast lobule is demonstrated by this photomicrograph. The residual lobular acini are seen above and below the forming cyst (*arrows*).

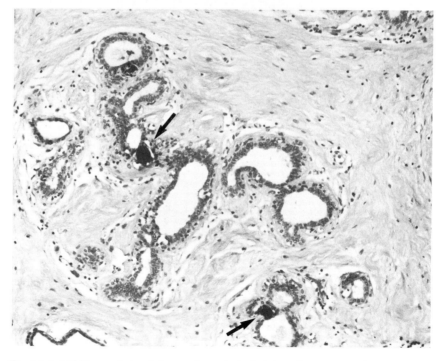

Fig. 11-5 Mild hyperplasia of the usual type is included in the category of "no increased risk" lesions. The epithelium is only minimally thickened (three to four cell layers rather than the usual two). Calcification within the epithelium may be found as illustrated here (*arrows*) but does not represent an increased cancer risk for the patient.

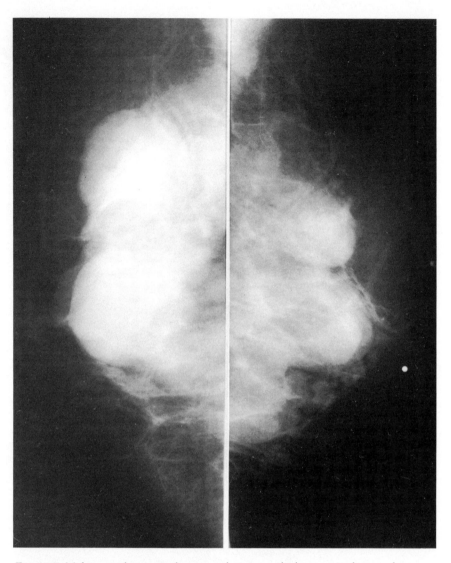

Fig. 11-6 Multicystic disease produces round circumscribed masses isodense to breast parenchyma in both breasts. Skin surface markers (bbs) over left breast denote symptomatic areas.

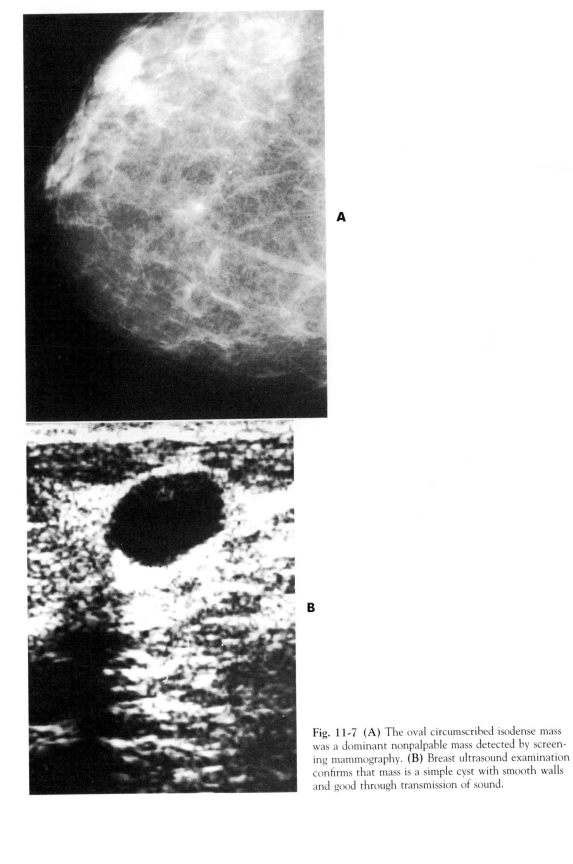

Fig. 11-7 **(A)** The oval circumscribed isodense mass was a dominant nonpalpable mass detected by screening mammography. **(B)** Breast ultrasound examination confirms that mass is a simple cyst with smooth walls and good through transmission of sound.

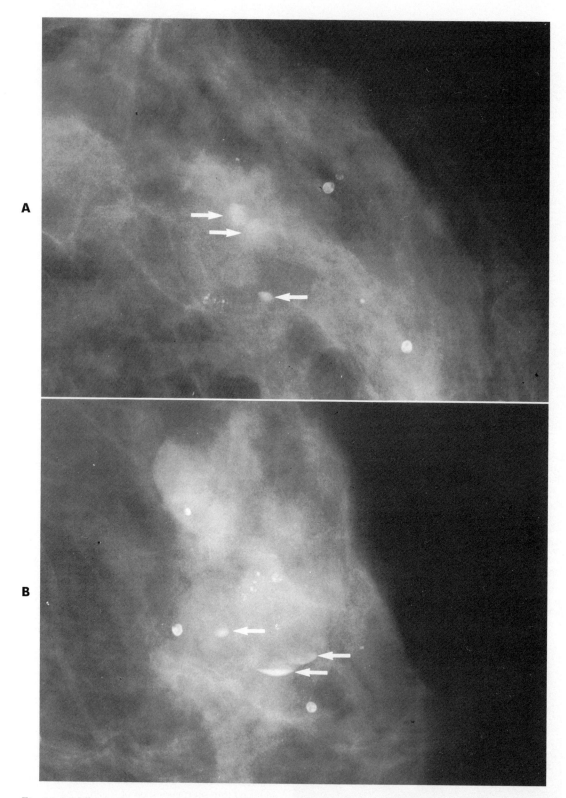

Fig. 11-8 Milk of calcium in macrocysts with background pattern of large, round, benign calcifications and a cluster of coarse and granular calcifications that were radiographically stable. The craniocaudad projection (**A**) shows milk of calcium to be three areas of hazy cloudlike opacity (*arrows*). The mediolateral projection (**B**) confirms layering of milk of calcium in macrocysts (*arrows*).

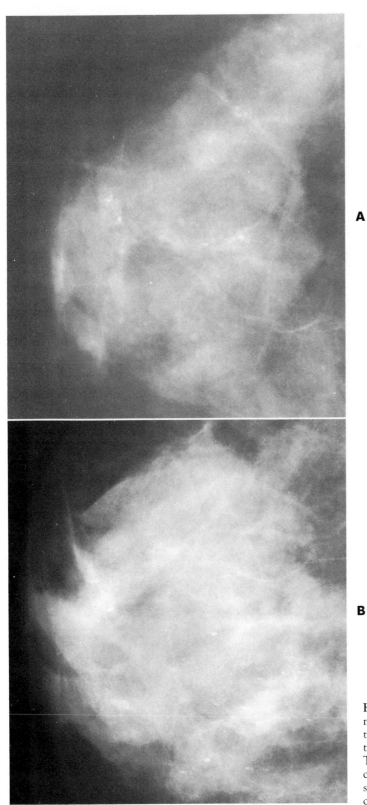

Fig. 11-9 Diffuse milk of calcium in microcysts. The craniocaudad projection **(A)** shows multiple hazy deposits throughout the breast parenchyma. The mediolateral projection **(B)** confirms milk of calcium in cysts smaller than 3 mm in diameter in the central and inferior breast.

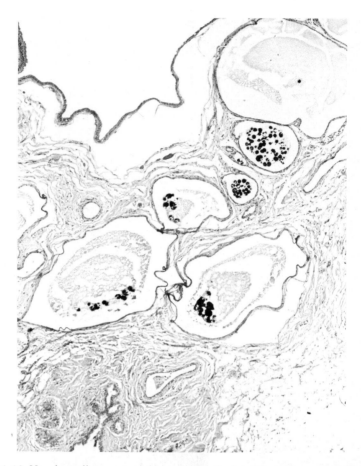

Fig. 11-10 Histologically, cases exhibiting "milk of calcium" mammographically may show amorphous calcified debris within cyst lumens, as illustrated in this photomicrograph.

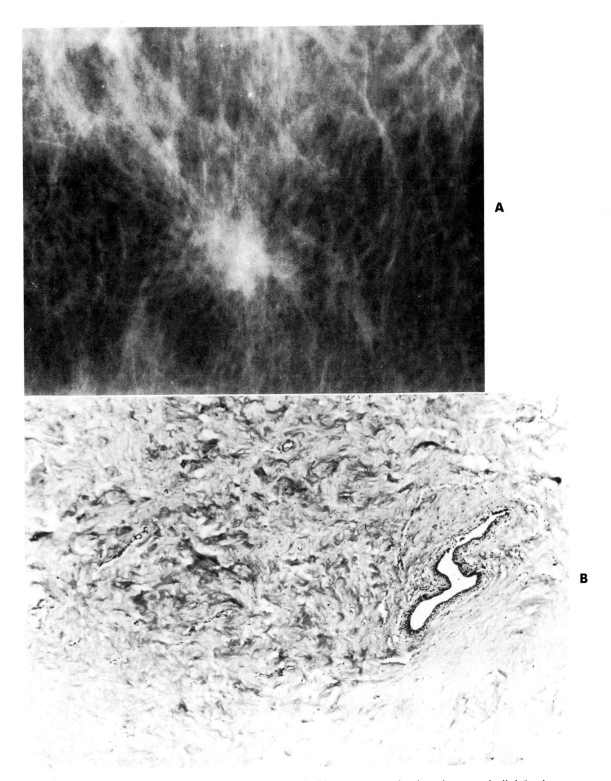

Fig. 11-11 (A) Photographic enlargement shows a nonpalpable, 1-cm, irregular-shaped mass with ill-defined margins in the retromammary fat. Histopathology was focal fibrosis with central calcification. **(B)** Focal stromal fibrosis is frequently not noted in pathology reports. This photomicrograph shows dense collagenous stroma replacing adipose tissue with a small duct trapped in the fibrous tissue.

PATTERNS OF MINIMALLY INCREASED CANCER RISK: PROLIFERATIVE FIBROCYSTIC CHANGE
Histopathology

Proliferative lesions in this category include hyperplasia of epithelial cells of both ducts and lobules, papillary apocrine change, fibroadenoma, and sclerosing adenosis (Box 11-3). Lesions in this category in general have a risk of subsequent invasive cancer of about 1.5 to 2 times that of the general population. Sclerosing adenosis is described later in this chapter and will not be discussed here. Fibroadenomas have been described in Chapter 9. They were originally included by Dupont and Page[7] in the group of nonproliferative or no increased risk lesions. Subsequent studies, however, have shown a slightly increased risk (1.7) for fibroadenoma alone or for fibroadenoma with associated hyperplasia in ducts or lobules elsewhere in the biopsy (3.7).[27] Other authors[42] have also reported similar increased risk; therefore, fibroadenomas are included in this category.

For more than 20 years, numerous papers have suggested an association of increased risk of subsequent breast cancer with particular patterns of fibrocystic changes.[38,39,40,43,44] Increased risk in all of these reports was associated with epithelial hyperplasia with varying degrees of cytologic and architectural atypia. Assessment of risk was determined by varying methodologies. In one study, patients determined to have atypical hyperplasia on breast biopsy were followed, and the incidence of subsequent cancer was compared with cancer incidence in the Third National Cancer Survey.[38] Another study[39] matched a group of Canadian women diagnosed with breast cancer after a previous benign breast biopsy with a control group of women with benign breast disease on biopsy who had not developed cancer in the study period. Fibrocystic changes in the biopsies were categorized. Other studies analyzed patterns of fibrocystic change in mastectomy or partial mastectomy specimens removed for breast cancer or benign disease.[43,44]

Some of the largest studies investigating this question were those from Vanderbilt University.[7,14] As previously mentioned, investigators from this institution have published a series of reports on a group of over 10,000 breast biopsies from over 3000 women with a median follow-up of 17 years. This large data base allowed investigators to determine relative risks for different patterns of epithelial hyperplasia including lesions such as atypical hyperplasia, which are found in a small percentage of biopsies for fibrocystic change. It is primarily from these studies that the categories of no risk, minimal risk, and increased risk have been derived.[7]

Common epithelial hyperplasia or hyperplasia without atypia is probably the most common change in this category of lesions. This lesion, also referred to as *papillomatosis* or *epitheliosis*, is found in about 25% of breast biopsies for benign disease.[7] To distinguish this type of hyperplasia from lesions of higher risk, it has been referred to as proliferative disease without atypia (PDWA).[7,12] Features of this pattern of hyperplasia, which usually occurs in terminal ducts, ductules, or both, have been well described.[12] PDWA is characterized by a lack of cellular uniformity and of architectural rigidity. Cells demonstrate variation in size both

---

BOX 11-3 FIBROCYSTIC PATTERNS OF MINIMALLY INCREASED CANCER RISK

Ductal epithelial hyperplasia without atypia
Papillary apocrine change
Sclerosing adenosis
Fibroadenoma

of the cell and of nuclei. The overall pattern of hyperplasia, although it may bridge across or fill ducts, has been described as streaming or swirling.

The proliferation may form secondary small lumina within the duct; these vary in size and shape and are often present at the periphery of the duct, close to the basement membrane. These described patterns of usual or nonatypical hyperplasia are found within ducts and small ductules. Usual or nonatypical hyperplasia of the acinar structure of lobules is difficult to recognize and distinguish from normal patterns on the one hand and atypical lobular hyperplasia on the other. Therefore, it is the practice of some experienced breast pathologists not to separately identify lobular hyperplasia without atypia.[30]

Although the presence of apocrine change in ductal epithelium does not increase risk for subsequent cancer, the finding of papillary apocrine change or papillary apocrine hyperplasia has been associated with a slightly increased cancer risk in the studies of Page and associates.[14] This risk was limited to women of perimenopausal and postmenopausal age groups in this study, and no increased cancer risk was found for premenopausal women with papillary apocrine change. This conclusion is also supported by Wellings and Alpers.[36] Papillary apocrine change refers to a papillary hyperplasia of cells exhibiting these apocrine features.

Imaging

The imaging features of proliferative fibrocystic disease without atypia are not specific. For the most part, the cellular hyperplasia is a microscopic change. Unless the presence of associated microcalcifications prompt a biopsy, there is no direct mammographic correlation in many cases. A history of having multiple breast cysts aspirated is a clinical marker of epithelial hyperplasia.[41] Seventy percent of women with a clinical diagnosis of multiple cysts have mild or florid epithelial hyperplasia.

In a series of wire-directed biopsies for mammographic abnormalities, proliferative fibrocystic disease is present as the most significant pathologic finding in 10% to 40% of cases.[45] Some studies have found papillomatosis (duct hyperplasia) present in about 40% of cases of biopsy-proven benign fibrocystic disease. This holds true for both premenopausal and postmenopausal women.[5] Nonpalpable mammographic abnormalities associated with the specific histologic diagnosis of papillomatosis are clustered microcalcifications, circumscribed or nodular mass, or mass with microcalcifications.[45] No radiographic feature is specific, but microcalcifications are a radiographic finding in over 50% (19 of 30) of biopsy-proven examples of papillomatosis excised because of mammographic abnormality. This observation reflects the fact that many biopsies for nonpalpable lesions are performed to evaluate suspicious clusters of microcalcifications. In a large retrospective series, calcification was seen histologically in about 20% (321 of 1693) of specimens diagnosed as proliferative fibrocystic change without atypia.[7]

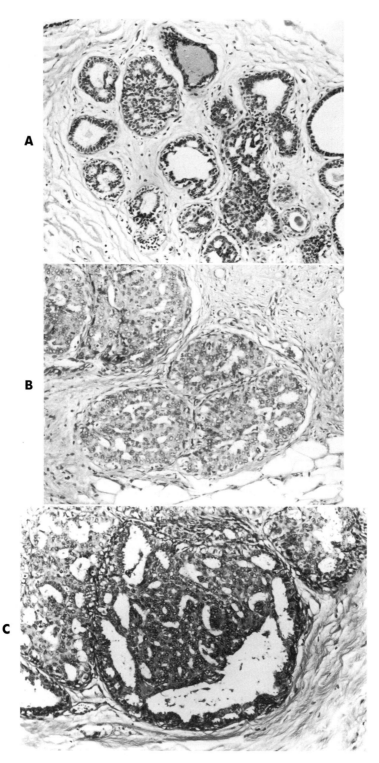

Fig. 11-12 Proliferative fibrocystic change (epithelial hyperplasia without atypia) is illustrated in these three photomicrographs. The low-magnification photomicrograph **(A)** illustrates the hyperplastic epithelium bridging across the ducts. Small lumens of varying size are formed within the epithelial proliferation. At higher magnification **(B),** the streaming or swirling nature of the hyperplasia is seen. The variable size of the secondary lumens can be better appreciated. The high-magnification photomicrograph **(C)** also shows the variable size of the secondary lumens, some of which are located close to the basement membrane. The variation in the size and morphology of the cells, which characterizes the epithelial proliferation, can be seen.

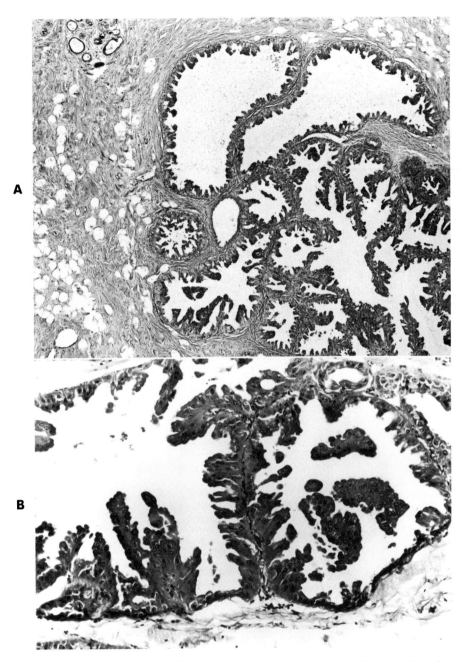

Fig. 11-13 Papillary apocrine hyperplasia is seen in these low-magnification (**A**) and high-magnification (**B**) photomicrographs. The papillary configuration of the epithelial proliferation is easily seen in **A** and the apocrine morphology of the hyperplastic cells is apparent at higher magnification (**B**). These cells exhibit abundant granular cytoplasm and large nuclei.

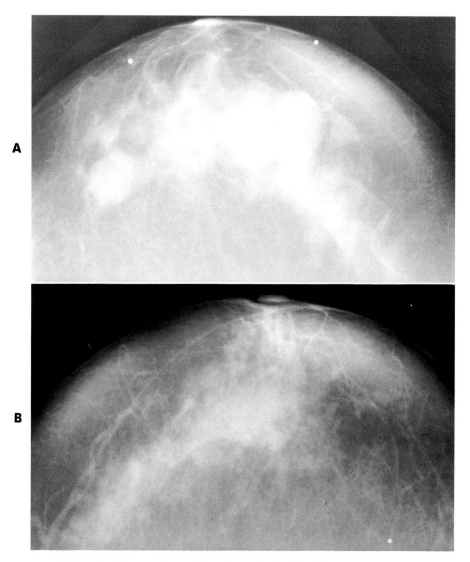

Fig. 11-14 Papillomatosis associated with multicystic disease. This postmenopausal woman had asymmetric multicystic disease in the right breast as seen in the cranio-caudad view **(B)** as compared with the same projection **(B)** of the left breast. Biopsy confirmed cystic disease with papillomatosis.

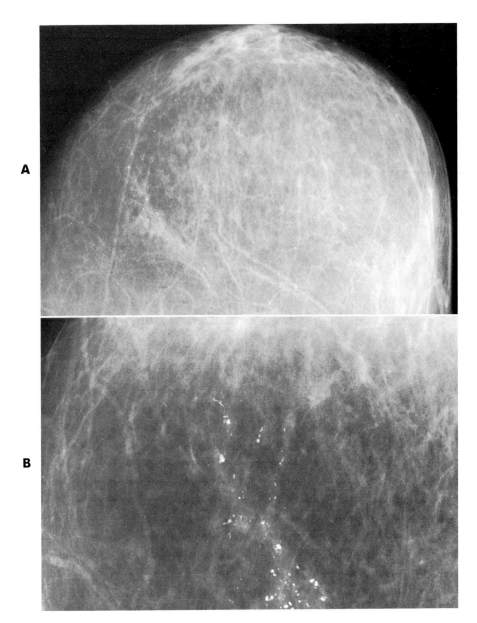

Fig. 11-15 Papillomatosis associated with suspicious microcalcifications. A segmental grouping of coarse and linear microcalcification **(A)** is associated with prominent ductal structures on magnification mammography **(B)**. Biopsy-proven papillomatosis. (Courtesy of Dr. A. Pollack, Brooklyn, N.Y.)

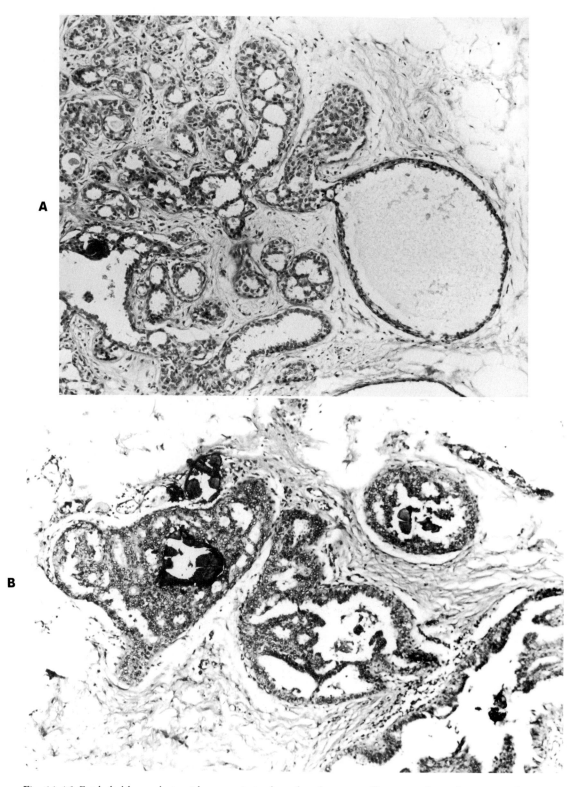

Fig. 11-16 Epithelial hyperplasia without atypia is also referred to as papillomatosis. It is often seen within or associated with cysts, as shown in **A.** The papillary appearance is apparent in **B.** Calcification, shown in both **A** and **B,** is frequently found both within epithelium and lumens in epithelial hyperplasia.

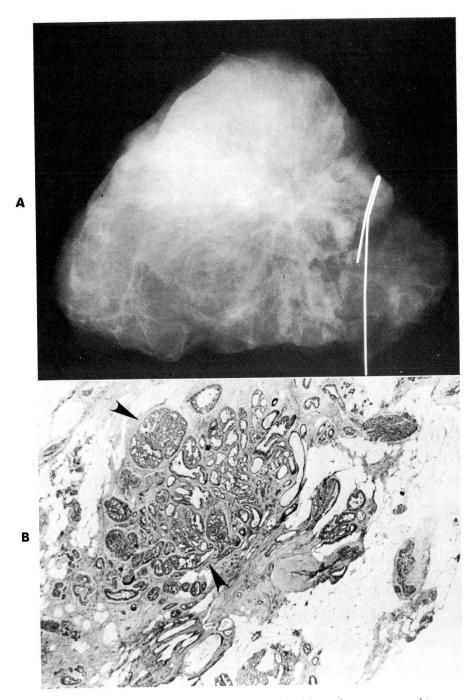

Fig. 11-17 Proliferative fibrocystic change with ductal hyperplasia was proven histopathologically in this specimen biopsied for an area of parenchymal distortion **(A)**. Very faint punctate calcifications seen in the specimen were below the resolving power of mammography. The photomicrograph **(B)** shows epithelial hyperplasia in the varying-sized cysts *(arrows)* and some fibrosis and elastosis. (From Golden A, Powell DE, Jennings CD. *Pathology: Understanding human disease*, ed 2, Baltimore, 1985, Williams & Wilkins.

PATTERNS OF INCREASED CANCER RISK: PROLIFERATIVE FIBROCYSTIC CHANGE WITH ATYPIA
Histopathology

Patterns of fibrocystic disease associated with increased cancer risk include atypical hyperplasia occurring either in ducts or lobules (Box 11-4). These lesions are uncommon, representing only 3.6% of benign lesions in the large biopsy study of Dupont and Page.[7] They represent a breast cancer risk that is about 50% of that of in situ carcinoma, about 4 to 5 times the general population risk.[12] Risk conveyed by atypical epithelial hyperplasia is increased significantly, however, (to 11 times normal) in patients with a positive family history of breast cancer.[7]

Atypical hyperplasia in simplest terms can be described as a cellular proliferation, either in ducts or in the acinar units of lobules, which comes close to but does not meet the criteria for carcinoma in situ (CIS). In some less common instances, the cellular proliferation may meet the criteria for CIS qualitatively but not quantitatively, and a diagnosis of atypical hyperplasia is made on quantitative criteria. Quantitative criteria are more commonly used in diagnosing atypical lobular hyperplasia (ALH) but may be used for atypical ductal hyperplasia (ADH) as well.

The qualitative criteria important in the diagnosis of both atypical hyperplasia and carcinoma in situ are (1) a uniform cell population, (2) a rigid architectural configuration, and (3) hyperchromatic nuclei. ADH can usually be distinguished from ductal carcinoma in situ (DCIS) because either the first or the second criterion is incompletely present within the cellular proliferation. Thus, ADH may be diagnosed if a duct shows regular, even intercellular spaces reminiscent of DCIS, but the cell population, although uniform in most of the lesion, still shows some variation in size and cellular orientation in a portion of the duct. Thus, ADH is a lesion, which on low power concerns the pathologist because of its similarity to DCIS. However, on higher power the lesion is seen to vary slightly from established DCIS patterns; hence, a diagnosis of ADH is made. It should be emphasized that nuclear hyperchromasia is a less important criterion than cellular uniformity and architectural rigidity. Also, cytologic atypia is not important as a criterion for the diagnosis of ADH. The marked cytologic atypia of comedo DCIS is usually associated with characteristic central necrosis or with complete filling of the ducts by a uniform markedly atypical cell population, as described in Chapter 12. Some degrees of cytologic atypia may be seen even in usual hyperplasia (hyperplasia without atypia), found in a setting of a pleomorphic cellular population.

Occasionally, a cellular proliferation meets all the qualitative criteria for DCIS but is only a small isolated focus. Page and colleagues[13] require a minimum of two duct spaces to meet the histologic criteria of a diagnosis of DCIS. If only a single duct in a biopsy specimen meets all the criteria for DCIS, they would diagnose the lesion as ADH. Tavassoli and Norris[54] differ somewhat on this point. Their quantitative criteria for ADH are that the ducts or ductules involved in the proliferative process measure less than 2 mm in aggregate diameter if all the qualitative criteria for DCIS are met. In other words, if a lesion

---

BOX 11-4 FIBROCYSTIC PATTERNS OF INCREASED CANCER RISK

Atypical ductal hyperplasia
Atypical lobular hyperplasia

meets all the qualitative criteria for DCIS and involves either a single or multiple ducts whose aggregate diameter is under 2 mm, a diagnosis of ADH is made. Conversely, according to their system,[54] if all qualitative criteria for DCIS are met and the lesion is greater than 2 mm in diameter, a diagnosis of DCIS is made even if only a single duct is involved. The qualitative criteria used by Page and colleagues[13] and by Tavassoli and Norris[54] are similar. Also, studies by both groups agree as to the clinical significance of ADH. Practicing pathologists need to be aware that in some unusual cases a diagnosis of ADH may be preferable to DCIS solely because of the extremely small size of the lesion.

Atypical lobular hyperplasia is a diagnosis in which quantitative criteria assume an important role. The cellular proliferation of ALH cytologically is identical with the cells of lobular carcinoma in situ (LCIS), described in Chapter 12. In LCIS, this population of small round regular cells fills and distends all or most of the acinar units of the involved lobule, obliterating the acinar lumina in the process. In ALH, a similar cellular population is present but less than 50% of the acinar structures of the lobule are involved by the proliferative process.[30] One point to remember is that the acinar units are small, and thick sections may give a false impression that the acinar lumina are obliterated. Remember that acinar distention should be present as well. Also, improper fixation may result in a swollen cytoplasm of the lobular epithelial cells and may give the impression of luminal obliteration. The diagnosis of ALH or LCIS should be made on thin, well-fixed histologic sections.

Involvement of ducts by cells of LCIS is discussed in Chapter 12. Page and colleagues[50] have described a similar process occurring with ALH. The presence of ductal involvement by ALH cells increases the relative risk of subsequent breast cancer to seven times that of the general population, midway between the risk for ALH alone and that for LCIS.

Finally, a word needs to be said about the problem of reproducibility in diagnosis of atypical hyperplasia and of CIS among pathologists. A study by Rosai[51] illustrated a significant lack of agreement among five experienced breast pathologists on the classification of proliferative ductal and lobular lesions. This led to the suggestion by the author that a more global terminology such as *mammary intraepithelial neoplasia* with a grading scheme (analogous to that used for lesions of the uterine cervix) be used. However, a subsequent study by Schnitt and associates[53] showed good interobserver diagnostic concordance among six experienced surgical pathologists reviewing a series of 24 proliferative lesions. Three of the participating pathologists also participated in the study by Rosai.[51] An important difference in the two reports however, was that all six participants in the study by Schnitt[53] were instructed in the use of standardized diagnostic criteria and were supplied with both written criteria and a set of diagnostic teaching slides. The conclusion of these authors was that when standardized criteria are taught and used, good interobserver concurrence can be obtained in the diagnosis of proliferative breast lesions. An inescapable conclusion from both of these and many other reports is that the interpretation of proliferative breast lesions is difficult and subjective. There is also a strong indication that education in and understanding of defined criteria may significantly improve diagnostic accuracy.

Imaging

Histopathologic recognition of proliferative fibrocystic change with atypia and its significance for risk of development of subsequent breast cancer has prompted a search for correlative clinical or mammographic findings. Neither clinical breast density nor nodularity on physical examination correlate with high-risk breast pathology assessed in lumpectomy tissue specimens.[47] The mammographic correlation is somewhat stronger but not specific.

Initial pathologic series reporting hyperplasia with atypia were reviews of specimens from biopsies for palpable masses or areas of mammographic abnormalities.[38,52] In most patients, the areas of hyperplasia with atypia constituted an incidental histopathologic finding, and details of mammographic pathologic correlation were not discussed. Changing areas considered suspicious for malignancy on mammograms have been shown to be associated with benign breast disease in 160 of 195 cases. Of these 160 benign biopsies for interval mammographic change, hyperplasia with atypia was present in 7% to 12%.[55] The increasing number of biopsies generated from screening mammography provides an opportunity to assess the specific radiographic-pathologic correlation of ADH and ALH for those cases free of associated carcinoma. A detailed radiologic pathologic correlation in 58 women with atypical hyperplasia and no synchronous ipsilateral breast cancer indicates that direct correlation with mammographic abnormality, if present, is observed much more frequently for ADH than for ALH.[48]

Like LCIS, ALH is most often an incidental pathologic finding. Direct correlation of ALH with a mammographic finding was observed in only 1 of 11 cases (9%), and this lesion was considered to have a low level of suspicion.[48] A higher direct correlation of mammographic findings with ADH was observed in 20 of 42 cases (48%). The remainder were mammographic lesions near or remote to the focus of atypical hyperplasia. The correlative mammographic findings are listed in Table 11-3. These abnormalities are similar in appearance to small cancers and represent the usual reasons for wire-directed biopsy. It is interesting that the microcalcifications associated with ADH in this series[48] were not associated with cell necrosis even though most were irregular (amorphous or granular) in form and linear forms were also observed. Fibrosis accounted for mammographic nodular opacity and distortion. It has been emphasized that the stronger mammographic correlation with ADH than ALH parallels the mammographic appearances of DCIS and LCIS (see Chapter 12).

Women with biopsy-proven hyperplasia with atypia, both ductal and lobular, should be followed carefully. Breast self-examination should be taught and encouraged. Physical examination twice a year is recommended by many experts. Certainly, yearly screening mammography is advocated in this group with elevated risk for developing breast carcinoma in either breast. The risk is especially high for women who are premenopausal at time of biopsy and those with a family history of breast cancer.[46,49]

Table 11-3 Mammographic abnormalities correlating directly with ductal hyperplasia with atypia (20 cases)

Microcalcifications	46%
Spiculated mass	21%
Nodular opacity	17%
Distortion or asymmetric opacity	12%
Nodule and microcalcifications	4%

Modified from Helvie MA, Hessler C, Frank TS, et al: Atypical hyperplasia of the breast: mammographic appearance and histologic correlation, *Radiology* 179:759, 1991.

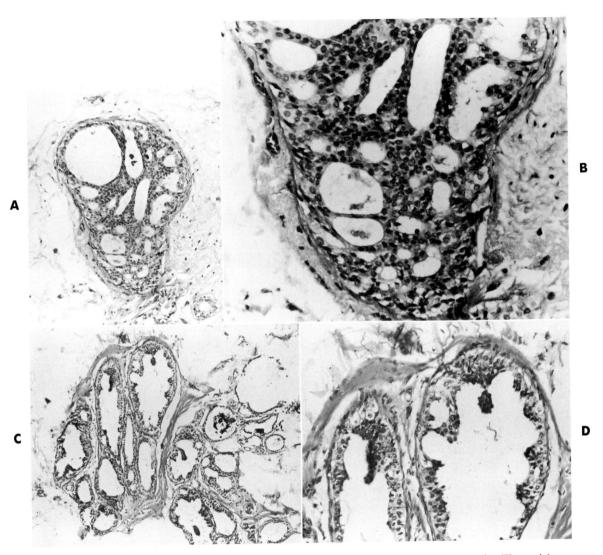

Fig. 11-18 Atypical ductal hyperplasia of varying degrees is illustrated in these photomicrographs. The proliferation seen in **A** and **B** is more rigid and regular than epithelial hyperplasia without atypia, illustrated in Fig. 11-12. Despite more architectural rigidity there is still considerable variation in the size of the secondary lumens, and some variation in cell type is seen in **B.** Smaller, darker cells are located more centrally, whereas those at the periphery are somewhat larger and paler. In **C** the hyperplastic epithelium has a more papillary pattern, which at low power is reminiscent of micropapillary carcinoma. At higher power **(D),** however, the variation in cell size and morphology can be seen.

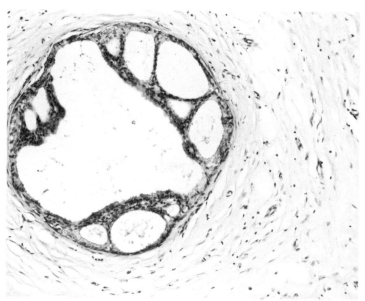

Fig. 11-19 This photomicrograph shows atypical ductal hyperplasia with histologic similarities to intraductal carcinoma. The proliferating epithelium forms rigid arches or palisades along the periphery of the duct. Only this single focus within the biopsy showed this degree of atypia and was therefore classified as atypical ductal hyperplasia.

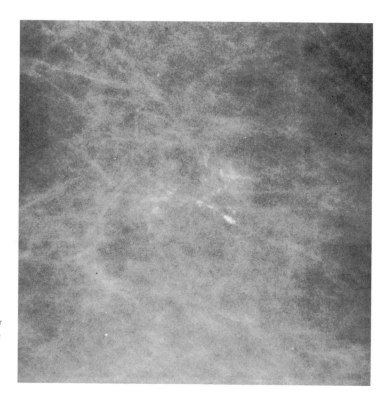

Fig. 11-20 Focal cluster of casting type microcalcifications on magnification mammography was biopsied due to high degree of suspicion for ductal carcinoma. Biopsy proved ductal hyperplasia with atypia.

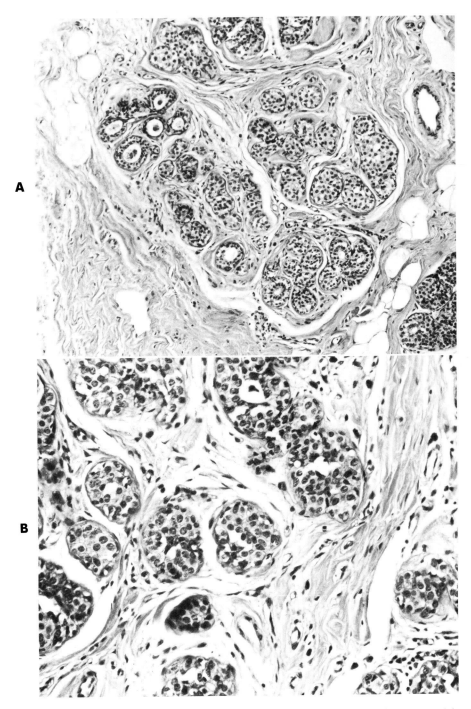

Fig. 11-21 Atypical lobular hyperplasia. In atypical lobular hyperplasia there is a proliferation of small regular cells in the terminal acinar units of the lobule. These cells are identical to those seen in lobular carcinoma in situ and fill and distend the lobular units, obliterating the lumens. In this lobule the proliferation has not yet obliterated the central lumen or distended more than half of the acini, and this lesion is diagnosed as atypical lobular hyperplasia. The morphology of the small cells of atypical lobular hyperplasia is seen in **B.** The cytoplasm is sparse, and the nuclei are small and regular.

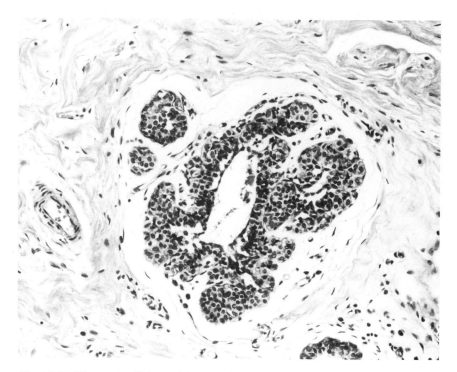

Fig. 11-22 The same cellular proliferation shown in Fig. 11-21 can also extend along the ducts, beneath the epithelium. This pattern of pagetoid spread can be seen with lobular carcinoma in situ as well as with atypical lobular hyperplasia.

SCLEROSING ADENOSIS AND MICROGLANDULAR ADENOSIS
Histopathology of Sclerosing Adenosis

Sclerosing adenosis (SA) is a component of fibrocystic change, which may clinically and pathologically simulate invasive breast cancer. In one large study,[65] the incidence of SA was found to be slightly higher than 5% of breast biopsies showing fibrocystic change. This same study showed that SA was most frequently identified in the perimenopausal age group (41 to 50 years) and was relatively infrequent in biopsies from women over age 50. Other studies have shown a somewhat higher incidence.[27]

Sclerosing adenosis is a proliferative lesion of the lobule, which expands the lobule with increased numbers of small, often compressed, ductules or tubules, myoepithelial cells, and intervening fibrous stroma. The lobulocentric growth of SA can be best appreciated on microscopic examination at low power where the whorled pattern of the compressed ductules can be identified. This lobulocentric expansible growth pattern can be extremely helpful in distinguishing SA from tubular carcinoma and microglandular adenosis.

Myoepithelial cells form an important component of SA. Although they may be difficult to identify in all cases on routine sections because of the marked distortion and compression of the ductules, immunohistochemical studies have readily identified myoepithelial cells surrounding each of the tubules and small ducts.[64] This is also a useful distinguishing characteristic, since the glandular structures of both tubular carcinoma and microglandular adenosis lack myoepithelial cells.[60,64]

Epithelial hyperplasia, apocrine change with or without atypia, and CIS all can occur within SA. Jensen and colleagues[65] reported an increased association of atypical lobular hyperplasia with SA. Apocrine change within SA, although uncommon, can present a difficult diagnostic problem, particularly when there is cytologic atypia. In a series of 60 cases of atypical apocrine metaplasia in sclerosing lesions, 4 had been called malignant or precancerous on initial interpretation resulting in mastectomy.[58] It is important for pathologists to recognize apocrine metaplasia within SA and not to overdiagnose those cases as malignant.

Carcinoma in situ can occur within SA, although it is uncommon.[61,70] Most frequently the in situ cancer is LCIS, although cases of DCIS have also been reported. The presence of more solid tubules in the central areas of SA may occasionally be confused with CIS, but usually in the peripheral, more dilated ducts the characteristic features of DCIS or LCIS can be recognized. It is important as well in cases of CIS occurring in SA not to overdiagnose invasive cancers. The sclerosis and small compressed tubules of SA may mimic invasive cancer, but unless true invasion is present the margins of the lesion should be smooth. Infiltration of small glands into adipose tissue is not seen in SA, but is seen in invasive cancer as well as microglandular adenosis, which is discussed later in this chapter. Whether CIS in areas of SA is more frequently found presenting as a palpable mass (adenosis tumor) is not known. However, it is interesting to point out that one third of cases of CIS presenting in SA reported by Oberman and Markey[70] were in palpable adenosis tumors. Of 27 cases of adenosis tumors reported by Nielsen,[68] 5 had associated CIS.

Adenosis tumor is an unusual presentation for SA. In the series reported by Nielsen,[68] most tumors presented as a clinically palpable mass. The mean diameter was 1.3 cm and in general the nodules had poorly defined borders.

Finally, because of the problem still presented by the differential diagnosis of SA from tubular carcinoma, O'Leary and colleagues[71] have suggested that neural networks may be of value in the differential diagnosis of these cases.

Histopathology of Microglandular Adenosis

Microglandular adenosis (MA) is a relatively uncommon glandular proliferation, which may be found incidentally in a setting of fibrocystic change or may be identified as the cause of a clinically and mammographically identified mass.[74,76] Characteristically, the glands of MA are small, round, and regular with open lumina containing eosinophilic secretory material, which occasionally may be calcified. These glands are surrounded by a basement membrane that may be identified by immunohistochemistry[60] or electron microscopy.[76] They characteristically lack a myoepithelial layer,[60,76] although one study has reported the immunohistochemical identification of myoepithelial cells in MA.[59]

The epithelial cells of MA are pale-staining and frequently have a characteristic vacuolated cytoplasm. They have been reported to be negative when stained for epithelial membrane antigen in contrast to the positive staining which occurs in normal mammary ductal epithelial cells.[60] MA infiltrates in an irregular fashion into fibrous and adipose tissue. Frequently, the infiltrating glands are associated with a fibrous stroma that is paucicellular. Although MA is usually readily distinguished from SA, it may be confused with tubular carcinoma. Differential features of these three entities and of the less common apocrine adenosis are listed in Table 11-4.

One important consideration is whether either SA or MA is associated with an increased risk of breast carcinoma. Studies by Jensen and associates[65] show a modestly increased risk (1.7 times) for subsequent breast cancer in women with SA, and they include SA as one of the lesions in the category termed proliferative fibrocystic disease without atypia. It is interesting that this same study also showed an increased association of ALH with SA. The authors found that ALH was present with SA almost three times more often than with other changes of fibrocystic disease. There has been at least one report suggesting that MA may have an increased association with breast carcinoma as well.[75] In this study, 25% of cases of MA were associated with carcinoma, a finding not reported by other authors.[76] All of the carcinomas in this report contained areas of clear cell change. The significance of this is not known, but it is of interest because clear cell change is unusual in ductal carcinomas and, as previously mentioned, cells of MA are characterized by clear, vacuolated cytoplasm. These same authors[75] describe features that they term *atypical microglandular adenosis* and suggest that these changes may predict an increased likelihood of coexisting carcinoma.

Imaging of Sclerosing and Microglandular Adenosis

The mammographic features of SA are better known than those of MA. Both may be associated with a cluster of lobular type or punctate microcalcifica-

Table 11-4 Differential features of microglandular adenosis, tubular carcinoma, sclerosing adenosis and apocrine adenosis

Features	MA	TC	SA	AA
Myoepithelial cells	−	−	+	+
GCDFP-15	−	−	±	+
EMA	−	+	+	+
Basal lamina	+	−	+	+
Apocrine "snouts"	−	+	±	+
Infiltrative margin	+	+	−	−
Intraluminal secretions	+	±	±	−

MA, microglandular adenosis; TC, tubular carcinoma; SA, sclerosing adenosis; AA, apocrine adenosis; EMA, epithelial membrane antigen; GCDFP-15, gross cystic disease fluid protein.

tions.[72] In addition, the mammographic features of SA include more diffuse bilateral microcalcifications or nodularity.[63] More rarely a focal mass, spiculated, ill-defined, or circumscribed is described.[66,67,69] It is the associated fibrosis in the SA that may produce a local mass with distortion. In summation, SA has a variable mammographic appearance and some patterns mimic malignancy mammographically (Box 11-5).

In series of benign biopsies for mammographic abnormalities, punctate clustered calcifications are often associated with SA.[62] Within a subset of benign biopsy results of mammographic abnormalities, over one third of the cases were blunt duct adenosis or SA and all cases of adenosis in this series were associated with focal microcalcifications.[56] The mammographic appearance of the lobular type of round and smooth calcifications tightly grouped has been well described and illustrated by Tabar and Dean.[34] Although the lobular pattern of microcalcification is certainly associated with sclerosing adenosis, it is in no way specific. Lobular-type microcalcifications are also associated with atypical lobular hyperplasia and LCIS[72] (Box 11-6).

Sclerosing adenosis may less commonly present as a mass or focal asymmetry, palpable or clinically occult. The mass may or may not contain punctate microcalcifications. Linear branching forms are not associated with SA and should suggest a diagnosis of malignancy.

Finally, it should be noted that the accuracy of frozen section in distinguishing SA from invasive ductal carcinoma is low.[45,73] The pseudoinfiltrative pattern caused by fibrous distortion of the ductules frequently requires use of paraffin sections for accurate histopathologic interpretation.

BOX 11-5 MAMMOGRAPHIC FEATURES ASSOCIATED WITH SCLEROSING ADENOSIS

Punctate (lobular) calcifications
   Diffuse and bilateral
   Focal cluster
Mass (circumscribed or ill-defined)
Focal asymmetry (with or without architectural distortion)

Modified from Breast Group of Royal College of Radiologists: Radiological nomenclature in benign breast change, *Clin Radiol* 40:374, 1990.

BOX 11-6 PATHOLOGIC CHANGES ASSOCIATED WITH LOBULAR CALCIFICATIONS

Microglandular adenosis
Adenosis
Sclerosing adenosis
Lobular hyperplasia
Lobular hyperplasia with atypia
Lobular carcinoma in situ

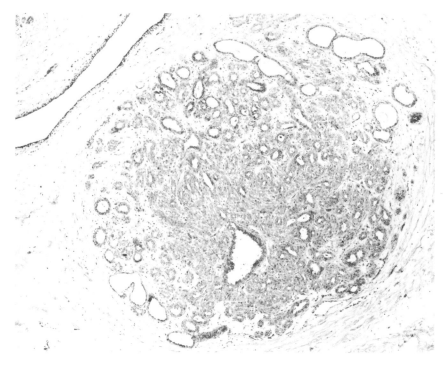

Fig. 11-23 Sclerosing adenosis is a lobulocentric proliferation that expands the lobule. The glands at the center of this focus of sclerosing adenosis are compressed, but the smooth, rounded outline is preserved.

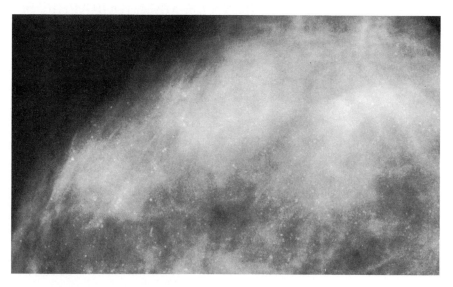

Fig. 11-24 Bilateral punctate diffuse microcalcifications are typical for the pattern classically described in sclerosing adenosis.

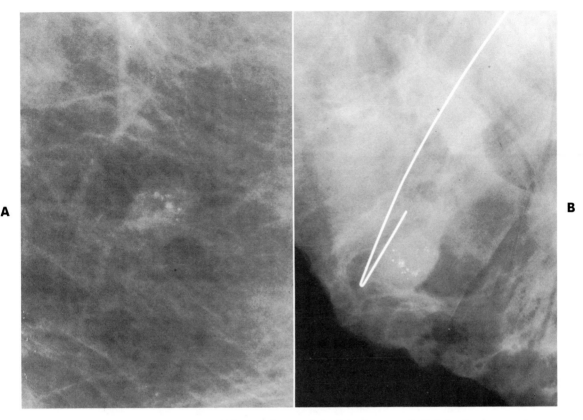

Fig. 11-25 Focal sclerosing adenosis caused this small, irregularly shaped mass with ill-defined margins and associated cluster of amorphous microcalcifications **(A).** The specimen radiograph shows that the microcalcifications are mostly lobular type **(B).**

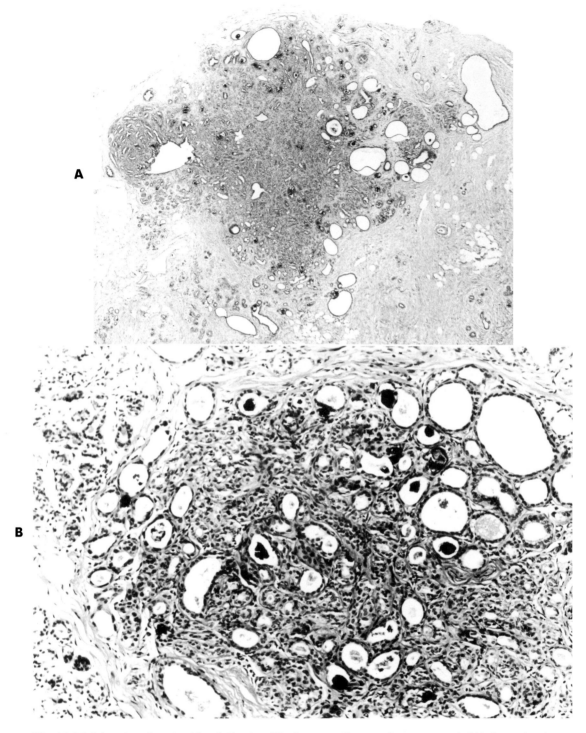

Fig. 11-26 Sclerosing adenosis with calcification. The low-magnification photomicrograph **(A)** shows the characteristic smooth peripheral contour of sclerosing adenosis. Microcyst formation is present, as are multiple small dark microcalcifications. These are seen better at higher magnification **(B).**

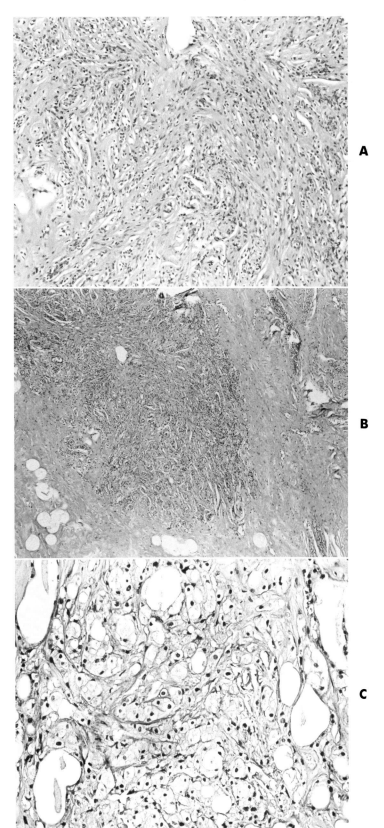

Fig. 11-27 Patterns of sclerosing adenosis may mimic carcinoma. The glands of sclerosing adenosis are often compressed by the surrounding stromal proliferation, giving a pseudoinfiltrative appearance (A). At low magnification (B), however, the smooth outline of the area of sclerosing adenosis can be appreciated. Occasionally apocrine change may be seen in sclerosing adenosis (C). The nuclear atypia associated with apocrine change should not be mistaken for carcinoma.

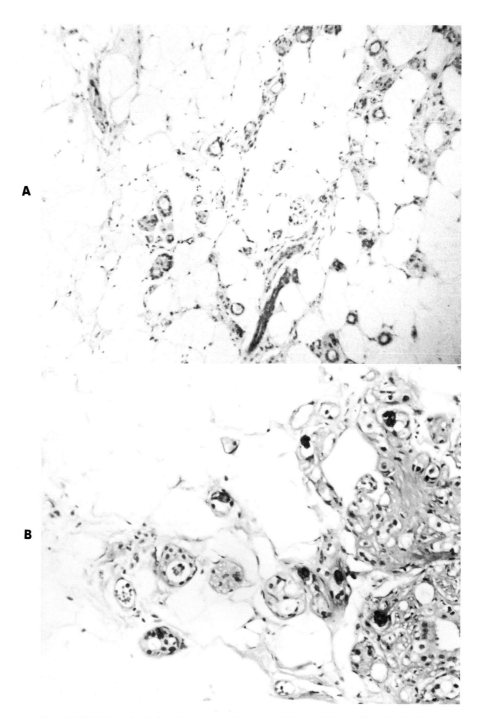

Fig. 11-28 Microglandular adenosis is characterized by small, rounded glands that frequently infiltrate into adipose tissue or fibrous stroma **(A)**. The proliferation does not have the characteristic lobulocentric growth pattern of sclerosing adenosis. The cells of microglandular adenosis are characteristically pale staining with a vacuolated cytoplasm and lack a myoepithelial layer **(B)**.

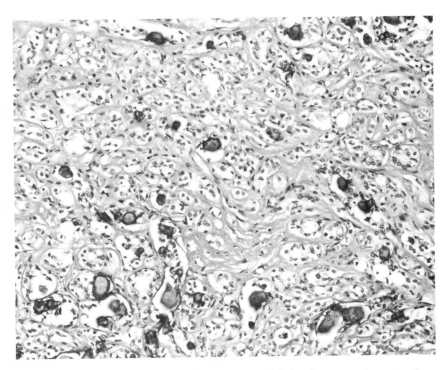

Fig. 11-29 Unlike microglandular adenosis, myoepithelial cells are prominent in sclerosing adenosis, as illustrated in this photomicrograph. Myoepithelial cells can be recognized by their clear vacuolated-appearing cytoplasm.

REFERENCES

Definition

1. Hutter RVP: Goodbye to "fibrocystic disease," *N Engl J Med* 312:179, 1985.
2. Love SM, Gelman RS, Silen W: Sounding board: fibrocystic "disease" of the breast: a nondisease? *N Engl J Med* 307:1010, 1982.

Overview of fibrocystic changes

3. Bartow SA, Pathak DR, Black WC, et al: Prevalence of benign, atypical and malignant breast lesions in populations at different risk for breast cancer: a forensic autopsy study, *Cancer* 60:2751, 1987.
4. Berkowitz GS, Kelsey JL, LiVolsi VA, et al: Exogenous hormone use and fibrocystic breast disease by histopathologic component, *Int J Cancer* 34:443, 1984.
5. Berkowitz GS, Kelsey JL, LiVolsi VA, et al: Risk factors for fibrocystic disease and its histopathologic components, *J Natl Cancer Inst* 75:43, 1985.
6. Boyle CA, Berkowitz GS, LiVolsi VA, et al: Caffeine consumption and fibrocystic breast disease: a case-control epidemiologic study, *J Natl Cancer Inst* 72:1015, 1984.
7. Dupont WD, Page DL: Risk factors for breast cancer in women with proliferative breast disease, *N Engl J Med* 312:146, 1985.
8. Dupont WD, Rogers LW, Vander Zwaag R, et al: The epidemiologic study of anatomic markers for increased risk of mammary cancer, *Pathol Res Pract* 166:471, 1980.
9. Frantz VK, Pickren JW, Melcher GW, et al: Incidence of chronic cystic disease in so-called "normal" breasts: a study based on 225 post mortem examinations, *Cancer* 4:762, 1951.
10. Kramer WM, Rush BF: Mammary duct proliferation in the elderly: a histopathologic study, *Cancer* 31:130, 1973.
11. LiVolsi VA, Stadel BV, Kelsey JL, et al: Fibrocystic breast disease in oral-contraceptive users: a histopathologic evaluation of epithelial atypia, *N Engl J Med* 299:381, 1978.
12. Page DL, Dupont WD: Anatomic markers of human premalignancy and risk of breast cancer, *Cancer* 66:1326, 1990.
13. Page DL, Dupont WD, Rogers LW, et al: Atypical hyperplastic lesions of the female breast: a long-term follow-up study, *Cancer* 55:2698, 1985.
14. Page DL, Vander Zwaag R, Rogers LW, et al: Relation between component parts of fibrocystic disease complex and breast cancer, *J Natl Cancer Inst* 61:1055, 1978.

15. Schairer C, Brinton LA, Hoover RN: Methylxanthines and benign breast disease, *Am J Epidemiol* 124:603, 1986.
16. Schuerch C, Rosen PP, Hirota T, et al: A pathologic study of benign breast disease in Tokyo and New York, *Cancer* 50:1899, 1982.

Patterns of no increased cancer risk

17. Devitt JE: Benign disorders of the breast in older women, *Surg Gynecol Obstet* 162:340, 1986.
18. Fornage BD, Faroux MJ, Simatos A: Breast masses: US-guided fine-needle aspiration biopsy, *Radiology* 162:409, 1987.
19. Fornage BD, Coan JD, David CL: Ultrasound-guided needle biopsy of the breast and other interventional procedures, *Radiol Clin North Am* 30:167, 1992.
20. Galkin BM, Feig SA, Patchefsky AS, et al: Ultrastructure and microanalysis of "benign" and "malignant" breast calcifications, *Radiology* 124:245, 1977.
21. Gershon-Cohen J, Ingleby H: Roentgenography of cysts of the breast, *Surg Gynec Obstet* 97:483, 1953.
22. Haagensen DE Jr, Mazoujian G: *Biochemistry and immunohistochemistry of fluid proteins of the breast in gross cystic disease*. In Haagensen CD, editor: *Diseases of the breast*, ed 3, Philadelphia, 1986:474, WB Saunders.
23. Homer MJ: Nonpalpable breast calcifications: frequency, management, and results of incisional biopsy, *Radiology* 185:411, 1992.
24. Kopans DB: *Pathologic, mammographic and sonographic correlation in breast imaging*, Philadelphia, 260, JB Lippincott.
25. Linden SS, Sickles EA: Sedimented calcium in benign breast cysts: the full spectrum of mammographic presentations, *AJR Am J Roentgenol* 152:967, 1989.
26. Mazoujian G, Pincus GS, Davis S, et al: Immunohistochemistry of a gross cystic disease fluid protein (GCDFP-15) of the breast: a marker of apocrine epithelium and breast carcinomas with apocrine features, *Am J Pathol* 110:105, 1983.
27. McDivitt RW, Stevens JA, Lee NC, et al: Histologic types of benign breast disease and the risk for breast cancer, *Cancer* 69:1408, 1992.
28. Meyer JE, Christian RL, Frenna TH, et al: Image-guided aspiration of solitary occult breast "cysts," *Arch Surg* 127:433, 1992.
29. Millis RR, Davis R, Stacey AJ: The detection and significance of calcifications in the breast: a radiological and pathological study, *Br J Radiol* 49:12, 1976.
30. Page DL, Anderson TJ: *Diagnostic histopathology of the breast*, Edinburgh, 1987, Churchill Livingstone.
31. Parker MD, Clark RL, McLelland R, et al: Disappearing breast calcifications, *Radiology* 172:677, 1989.
32. Sickles EA, Abele JS: Milk of calcium within tiny benign breast cysts, *Radiology* 141:655, 1981.
33. Sickles EA: Breast calcifications: mammographic evaluation, *Radiology* 160:289, 1986.
34. Tabar L, Dean PB: *Calcifications*. In *Teaching atlas of mammography*, New York, 1985:170, Thieme.
35. Wang DY, Fentiman IS: Epidemiology and endocrinology of benign breast disease, *Breast Cancer Res Treat* 6:5, 1985.
36. Wellings SR, Alpers CE. Apocrine cystic metaplasia: subgross pathology and prevalence in cancer-associated versus random autopsy breasts, *Hum Pathol* 18:381, 1987.
37. Wellings SR, Jensen HM, Marcum RG: An atlas of subgross pathology of the human breast with special reference to possible precancerous lesions, *J Natl Cancer Inst* 55:231, 1975.

Patterns of minimally increased cancer risk

38. Ashikari R, Huvos AG, Snyder RE, et al: A clinico-pathologic study of atypical lesions of the breast, *Cancer* 33:310, 1974.
39. Black MM, Barclay THC, Carter SJ, et al: Association of atypical characteristics of benign breast lesions with subsequent risk of breast cancer, *Cancer* 29:338, 1972.
40. Black MM, Chabon AB: *In situ* carcinoma of the breast, *Pathol Annu* 4:185, 1969.
41. Bundred NJ, West RR, Dowd JO, et al: Is there an increased risk of breast cancer in women who have had a breast cyst aspirated? *Br J Cancer* 64:953, 1991.
42. Carter CL, Corle DK, Micozzi MS, et al: A prospective study of the development of breast cancer in 16,692 women with benign breast disease, *Am J Epidemiol* 128:467, 1988.
43. Gallager HS, Martin JE: Early phases in the development of breast cancer, *Cancer* 24:1170, 1969.
44. Kern WH, Brooks RN: Atypical epithelial hyperplasia associated with breast cancer and fibrocystic disease, *Cancer* 24:668, 1969.
45. Tinnemans JGM, Wobbes T, Holland R, et al: Mammographic and histopathologic correlation of nonpalpable lesions of the breast and the reliability of frozen section diagnosis, *Surg Gynec Obstet* 165:523, 1987.

Patterns of increased cancer risk

46. Dupont WD, Page DL: Relative risk of breast cancer varies with time since diagnosis of atypical hyperplasia, *Hum Pathol* 20:723, 1989.
47. Goodson WH III, Miller TR, Sickles EA, et al: Lack of correlation of clinical breast examination with high-risk histopathology, *Am J Med* 89:752, 1990.
48. Helvie MA, Hessler C, Frank TS, et al: Atypical hyperplasia of the breast: mammographic appearance and histologic correlation, *Radiology* 179:759, 1991.
49. London MC, Connolly JL, Schnitt SJ, et al: A prospective study of benign breast disease and risk of breast cancer, *JAMA* 267:941, 1992.
50. Page DL, Dupont WD, Rogers LW: Ductal involvement by cells of atypical lobular hyperplasia in the breast: a long-term follow-up study of the cancer risk, *Hum Pathol* 19:201, 1988.
51. Rosai J: Borderline epithelial lesions of the breast, *Am J Surg Pathol* 15:209, 1992.
52. Rubin E, Visscher DW, Alexander RM, et al: Proliferative disease and atypia in biopsies performed for nonpalpable lesions detected mammographically, *Cancer* 61:2077, 1988.
53. Schnitt SJ, Connolly JL, Tavassoli FA, et al: Interobserver reproducibility in the diagnosis of ductal proliferative breast lesions using standardized criteria, *Am J Surg Pathol* 16:1133, 1992.
54. Tavassoli FA, Norris HJ: A comparison of the results of long-term follow-up for atypical intraductal hyperplasia and intraductal hyperplasia of the breast, *Cancer* 65:518, 1990.
55. Wilhelm MC, deParedes ES, Pope T, et al: The changing mammogram: a primary indication for needle localization biopsy, *Arch Surg* 121:1311, 1986.

Sclerosing adenosis and microglandular adenosis

56. Barnard NJ, George BD, Tucker AK, et al: Histopathology of benign non-palpable breast lesions identified by mammography, *J Clin Pathol* 41:26, 1988.
57. Breast Group of the Royal College of Radiologists: Radiological nomenclature in benign breast change, *Clin Radiol* 40:374, 1990.
58. Carter DJ, Rosen PP: Atypical apocrine metaplasia in sclerosing lesions of the breast: a study of 51 patients, *Mod Pathol* 4:1, 1991.
59. Diaz NM, McDivitt RW, Wick MR: Microglandular adenosis of the breast: an immunohistochemical comparison with tubular carcinoma, *Arch Pathol Lab Med* 115:578, 1991.
60. Eusebi V, Foschini MP, Betts CM, et al: Microglandular adenosis, apocrine adenosis and tubular carcinoma of the breast: an immunohistochemical comparison, *Am J Surg Pathol* 17:99, 1993.
61. Fechner RE: Lobular carcinoma *in situ* in sclerosing adenosis: a potential source of confusion with invasive carcinoma, *Am J Surg Pathol* 5:233, 1981.
62. Gisvold JJ, Martin JK Jr: Prebiopsy localization of nonpalpable breast lesions, *AJR Am J Roentgenol* 143:477, 1984.
63. Gold RH, Montgomery CK, Rambo ON: Significance of margination of benign and malignant infiltrative mammary lesions: roentgenographic-pathological correlation, *AJR Am J Roentgenol* 118:881, 1973.
64. Gottlieb C, Raju U, Greenwald K: Myoepithelial cells in the differential diagnosis of complex benign and malignant breast lesions: an immunohistochemical study, *Mod Pathol* 3:135, 1990.
65. Jensen RA, Page DL, DuPont WD, et al: Invasive breast cancer risk in women with sclerosing adenosis, *Cancer* 64:1977, 1989.
66. Keen ME, Murad TM, Cohen MI, et al: Benign breast lesions with malignant clinical and mammographic presentations, *Hum Pathol* 16:1147, 1985.
67. Marsteller LP, deParedes ES: Well defined masses in the breast, *RadioGraphics* 9:13, 1989.
68. Nielsen BB: Adenosis tumour of the breast: a clinicopathological investigation of 27 cases, *Histopathology* 11:1259, 1987.
69. Nielsen NSM, Nielsen BB: Mammographic features of sclerosing adenosis presenting as a tumor, *Clin Radiol* 37:371, 1986.
70. Oberman HA, Markey BA: Noninvasive carcinoma of the breast presenting in adenosis, *Mod Pathol* 4:31, 1991.
71. O'Leary TJ, Mikel UV, Becker RL: Computer-assisted image interpretation: use of a neural network to differentiate tubular carcinoma from sclerosing adenosis, *Mod Pathol* 5:402, 1992.
72. deParedes ES, Abbitt PL, Tabbarah S, et al: Mammographic and histologic correlations of microcalcifications, *RadioGraphics* 10:577, 1990.
73. Roos FD: Sclerosing adenosis: mammography, pathology correlations, *Breast Dis Breast* 4:28, 1978.
74. Rosen PP: Microglandular adenosis: a benign lesion simulating invasive mammary carcinoma, *Am J Surg Pathol* 7:137, 1983.
75. Rosenblum MK, Purrazzella R, Rosen PP: Is microglandular adenosis a precancerous disease? *Am J Surg Pathol* 10:237, 1986.
76. Tavassoli FA, Norris HJ: Microglandular adenosis of the breast: a clinicopathologic study of 11 cases with ultrastructural observations, *Am J Surg Pathol* 7:731, 1983.

CHAPTER 12.

Carcinoma of the Breast

Deborah E. Powell
Carol B. Stelling

INTRODUCTION

This chapter discusses and illustrates carcinoma of the breast in both in situ and invasive forms. Special types of breast cancer with specific features—pathologic, mammographic, or clinical—are mentioned separately and look-alike lesions and differential features are stressed.

Carcinoma of the breast currently affects 12% of U.S. women.[6] Moreover, 3.5% of U.S. women will die of breast cancer, placing this tumor second to lung cancer as a major cause of cancer deaths in women. The rates of breast cancer have been increasing steadily, particularly in postmenopausal women.[5,8] Overall, the age-adjusted mortality rates have been stable over time but different patterns emerge when different age groups and races are analyzed separately. For example, mortality rates have increased in the last 40 years for women aged 55 and older but have decreased for women under 45 years. In the past 15 years, rising breast cancer mortality rates for black women have surpassed breast cancer mortality rates for white women.[3] Breast cancer is a continuing major health problem for U.S. women.

Risk factors for breast carcinoma have already been discussed in Chapter 1. Some confer substantially increased risk; others, more modest predisposition. Genetic susceptibility is certainly a major risk factor, but hereditary breast cancer represents a small percentage of the total breast cancer cases.[7] Several syndromes of hereditary breast cancer have been identified, including hereditary site-specific breast cancer and the hereditary breast/ovarian cancer syndrome.[1] The putative gene or genes associated with the latter syndrome have recently been mapped to the long arm of chromosome 17.[4,9] The hereditary breast cancer syndromes may be recognized by early age at onset and a high rate of bilaterality. However, considerable interfamily heterogeneity may exist; in a recent study, the mean age at diagnosis in 217 family members was 44.9 years with a standard deviation of 12.5 years and a range of 22 to 83 years.[7]

A prior history of breast cancer increases the patient's risk of a second breast cancer.[2] The risk is higher for certain histologic subtypes, notably lobular carcinoma, as will be discussed later. Other important risk factors are age and a history of certain subtypes of fibrocystic disease, notably atypical ductal and lobular hyperplasia.

Carcinoma of the breast is traditionally classified as either *ductal* or *lobular*. This terminology is probably more important for emphasizing histologic features than for predicting specific sites of origin of the different varieties of breast cancer. In fact, considerable evidence shows that all epithelial tumors of the breast probably arise in or near the lobules from the terminal ductal lobular unit.[10,11]

The classification of cancers as ductal and lobular carcinoma is based on long-standing convention and conveys important information about behavior of specific tumor types. Eighty-five percent of all breast carcinomas are classified as ductal carcinomas. Although lobular carcinoma is less common, it has specific histologic features and clinical characteristics, particularly a high likelihood of multifocality and bilaterality, which provide important information and convey implications for treatment. Within the two broad categories of breast carcinoma, multiple special types of cancer exist, some of which are important to understand because of their prognostic implications for the patient.

In addition to the major classifications as lobular or ductal, breast cancer exists in either in situ or invasive forms. This distinction is important because in situ carcinoma, either ductal or lobular, is a marker of increased risk of subsequent invasive cancer. Therefore the patient in whom a diagnosis of in situ carcinoma is made must be treated definitively or followed carefully because of this increased risk.

The diagnosis of in situ carcinoma does not imply inevitable progress to invasive carcinoma in the same breast. Nevertheless, a small proportion of patients with in situ carcinoma, particularly ductal, will have concurrent lymph node metastases. This fact is probably due to unrecognized areas of invasion. Therefore, the diagnosis of ductal carcinoma in situ, usually conveys such significant risk that some type of definitive treatment is undertaken.

In the following sections, we will consider first the main features of in situ carcinoma, then invasive carcinoma with special attention to some distinct histologic types of invasive carcinoma and carcinoma with special clinical presentations.

IN SITU CARCINOMA
Ductal carcinoma in situ

Intraductal carcinoma or ductal carcinoma in situ (DCIS) can present clinically as either a palpable mass, an occult mammographic abnormality, or an incidental finding in a setting of proliferative fibrocystic disease. The finding of DCIS implies that the patient is at high risk for developing invasive ductal carcinoma. In fact, several studies have shown that an untreated patient has a 25% to 40%

chance of developing invasive ductal carcinoma close to the site of previously diagnosed DCIS.[14,30] Furthermore, a small percentage (2%) of patients with pure intraductal carcinoma have been shown to have metastatic disease in axillary lymph nodes.[31,37]

DCIS presents with a variety of different histologic patterns.[33] Whether these patterns have a different prognostic implication for the patient is unclear, since many studies have not classified distinct histopathologic subtypes. Nevertheless, evidence shows that the tumor cell biology and possibly, by implication, the invasive potential of these subtypes are different.[24]

Comedo type. The most readily recognized histologic subtype of DCIS is the comedo type, characterized by a central necrotic mass of amorphous debris and degenerating tumor cells, which is frequently calcified. This central necrosis and calcification may be visible mammographically and are characteristic in appearance. The comedo tumor frequently presents as a palpable mass of multiple involved ducts. In addition to the prominent central necrosis that may be visible even grossly and that gives rise to the term, *comedocarcinoma,* the histology of the malignant intraductal cellular proliferation is distinctive. Tumor cells of comedocarcinoma are large with eosinophilic, slightly granular cytoplasm and large pleomorphic nuclei with prominent nucleoli. Mitotic figures are common in this type of intraductal carcinoma. Biologically, intraductal comedocarcinomas have been characterized by high proliferative indices and have been reported to show overexpression of the c-*erb* B-2 oncogene.[25,27]

Other types. Other patterns of intraductal carcinoma are *cribriform* and *micropapillary.* These patterns are not characterized by distinct areas of necrosis or calcification, although microcalcification may occasionally be present in the malignant epithelium lining the ducts. The cytologic appearance of micropapillary and cribriform DCIS is much more bland than that of the comedo type, with smaller cells and more regular uniform nuclei. In fact, the features that characterize both micropapillary and cribriform intraductal carcinoma are a homogeneous cell population, regular nuclei, and a rigid architectural configuration.

In the micropapillary pattern, the tumor cells rim the periphery of the duct as small papillary ribbons of epithelial cells without any fibrovascular network. These epithelial papillae extend into the lumen of the duct with slightly bulbous protruding ends. The cribriform carcinoma is usually more solid, involving the entire duct in the neoplastic proliferation. However, the arrangement of tumor cells in the lumen of the duct forms small, regular, rounded spaces. The regularity of these spaces and the presence of one single epithelial cell type serve to differentiate these types of DCIS from atypical ductal hyperplasia (discussed in Chapter 11). When cribriform carcinoma does not extend across the diameter of the duct and involves only the periphery, it shows a considerable similarity to micropapillary carcinoma. In these instances, small regular spaces may be seen and the tumor cells may arch around the periphery of the duct giving the classic "Roman bridge" appearance.[13]

Microinvasion. The question of microinvasion in the setting of in situ carcinoma is an important one. Certainly, the unusual cases of DCIS with lymph node metastases are considered by most investigators to contain within the tumor occult foci of microinvasive cancer. Criteria for microinvasion in a setting of predominantly intraductal carcinoma are not well defined. Although most ducts are surrounded by a distinct basement membrane that can be visualized with special histochemical or immunohistochemical stains, distortion of the duct by proliferating tumor cells or surrounding fibrosis or inflammation may attenuate or otherwise alter the histologic appearance of this structure. This is particularly true when the intraductal component is arising in smaller, more peripheral ducts. Page and Anderson note that in a definitive diagnosis of microinvasion, invasive tumor cells are expected to be seen beyond the confines of the duct and into the interlobular stroma beyond the specialized lobular connective tissue.[29a] The concept of microinvasive and minimal breast cancer is discussed later in this chapter.

Imaging. The incidence of DCIS in reported series varies depending on the method of detection. Before the use of screening mammography, DCIS presented clinically as a palpable mass, as spontaneous nipple discharge, or as Paget's disease of the nipple.[12,18] In these early series, DCIS accounted for approximately 5% of the total number of cancers diagnosed.[33] In addition to these clinical presenting signs, DCIS is now frequently detected by screening mammography.[17,21,34] DCIS accounts for 25% to 35% of the cancers that are clinically occult.[19,26,34] Overall, the use of screening mammography has nearly doubled the incidence of DCIS diagnosed in a screening population (35 of 100,000) compared with a control population (20 of 100,000).[23]

The typical mammographic findings of DCIS consist of a cluster of suspicious microcalcifications with or without an associated soft tissue density. This pattern was observed in 83.5% of 85 clinically occult cases of DCIS reported by Meyer[27] in 1990 and in 84% of 100 clinically occult cases reported by Stomper and others[39] in 1989. A mass was the predominant feature in these two series in 16.5% and 10% of patients, respectively. In both series, 6% to 7% of cases of DCIS were an incidental pathologic finding with no mammographic correlate.

The microcalcifications associated with DCIS can be further categorized into morphologic forms: *casting type* and *granular type*. In the 100 consecutive cases of clinically occult DCIS reported by Stomper and others, 52% were manifested by granular calcifications, 35% by linear microcalcifications, and 13% by granular shapes with several casting forms.[39] There is increasing evidence that the fine granular calcifications are associated with the small cell subtypes of DCIS, such as micropapillary, cribriform, and clinging morphology.[38] It is well understood that large cell comedocarcinoma produces the characteristic thin linear and branching calcifications that are a "cast" of the luminal space within the ducts. However, considerable overlap in these types prevents an accurate prediction of DCIS subtype from the mammographic appearance.

In general, the calcifications associated with DCIS tend to be smaller and more asymmetric within a density than those seen in fibroadenomas, which DCIS may mimic.[28] With comedo type DCIS, the casting calcifications may be large, up to 1 mm wide. Rarely, macrocalcifications are associated with DCIS.[35] Occasionally, the calcifications of DCIS and those of a degenerating fibroadenoma produce patterns that are sufficiently similar to require excisional biopsy to establish a pathologic diagnosis.

The soft tissue component of DCIS that may be detected mammographically usually represents either a reactive fibrosis and elastosis of the parenchyma or ducts filled with tumor.[39] These findings may produce some of the atypical radiographic manifestations of DCIS.[22] In particular, a focal nodular pattern may be detected mammographically, including retroareolar dilated ducts, subareolar mass, ill-defined rounded mass, developing density, and area of asymmetry or parenchymal distortion. A tangle of ducts or prominent tubular shadows has also been described. A circumscribed mass is recognized as one of the atypical manifestations of DCIS. Moreover, DCIS is more common than the special types of medullary, mucinous, and intracystic papillary carcinoma, which also may produce a circumscribed mass. Therefore, the most common circumscribed carcinoma is DCIS.

As already mentioned, DCIS may be associated with areas of microinvasion.[32,34,41] Approximately 2% of women with DCIS demonstrate tumor in axillary lymph nodes, reflecting subclinical microinvasion not detected by routine histopathology.[37] Mammographic indications for probable invasion include associated soft tissue densities, particularly if they are accompanied by architectural distortion or spiculation. The presence of frank invasion lowers the prognosis to that of invasive ductal carcinoma of no special type.

The role of mammography in DCIS is not only to detect the calcifications and characterize them by magnification mammography but also to evaluate the extent of the process.[40] The distribution may be focal, in multiple clusters, or regional. Extension along the lines of a ductal system is commonly seen in comedocarcinoma. *Multifocal* lesions are separated by 2 cm of normal tissue and are within the same quadrant. If multiple areas are in different quadrants or, if subareolar, separated by 5 cm, lesions are considered *multicentric.*[34] It is possible that this multicentric involvement is really extensive unicentric disease extending along the duct system.[20] Because localized DCIS may be treated by lumpectomy with radiation therapy, it is important to carefully evaluate the remainder of the breast for evidence of multifocality or multicentricity.[15] Lesions can track down the ductal system and extend into the subareolar and nipple ductal tissues. Presence of calcifications of the casting or granular type in the subareolar tissues is a contraindication to breast-conserving therapy. Magnification mammography is recommended to characterize calcifications and evaluate extent of involvement. The extent of carcinoma does not correlate well with the mammogram for the noncomedo types of cribriform or micropapillary DCIS.[33]

The prognosis for persons with pure DCIS is good when adequate treatment is provided. It is known that DCIS increases the risk of developing invasive breast cancer to approximately 30% over a 6- to 10-year follow-up.[18]

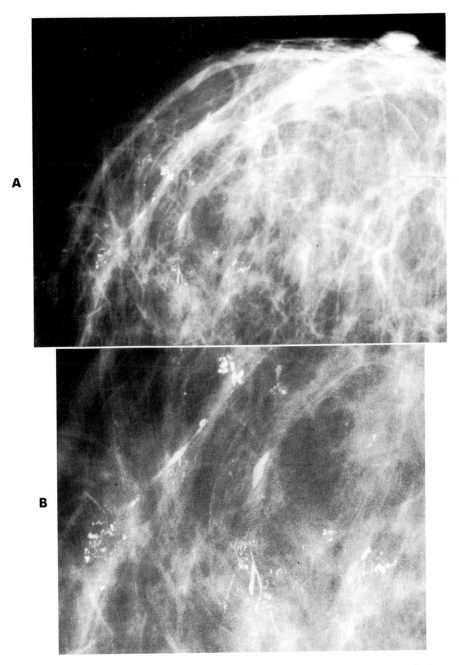

Fig. 12-1 Ductal carcinoma in situ. Classic comedo subtype with casting type calcifications distributed regionally and extending towards the nipple **(A)**. Close-up **(B)** shows branching and thin linear forms.

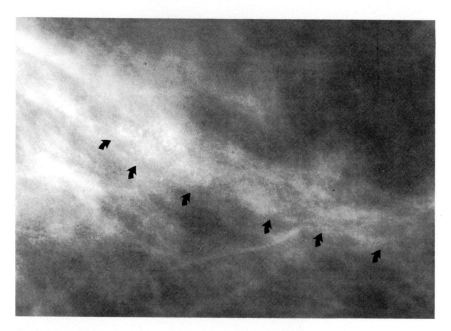

Fig. 12-2 Ductal carcinoma in situ. A cluster of granular and amorphous calcifications are focally grouped and extend along the ductal system *(arrows)*.

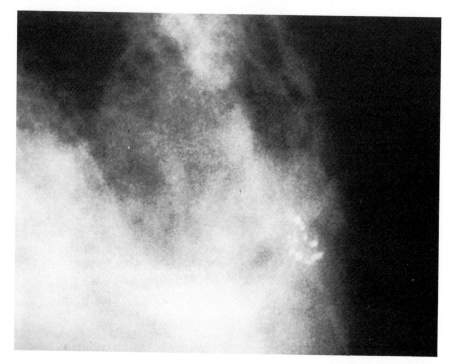

Fig. 12-3 Ductal carcinoma in situ. This cluster of heterogeneous coarse calcifications varies in size and shape.

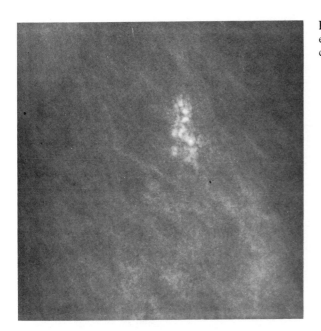

Fig. 12-4 Fibroadenoma. This small degenerating fibroadenoma mimics calcifications of comedo carcinoma.

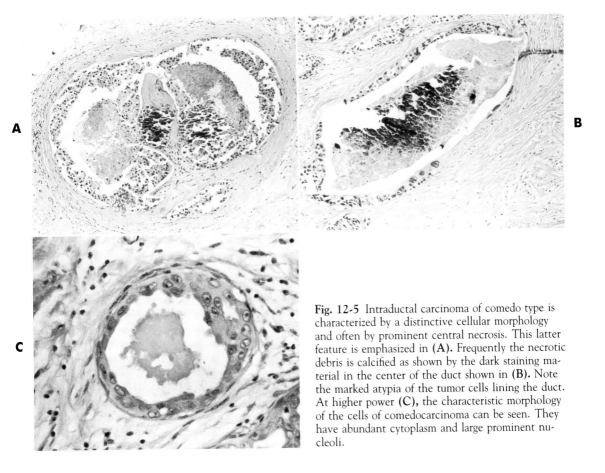

A

B

C

Fig. 12-5 Intraductal carcinoma of comedo type is characterized by a distinctive cellular morphology and often by prominent central necrosis. This latter feature is emphasized in **(A)**. Frequently the necrotic debris is calcified as shown by the dark staining material in the center of the duct shown in **(B)**. Note the marked atypia of the tumor cells lining the duct. At higher power **(C)**, the characteristic morphology of the cells of comedocarcinoma can be seen. They have abundant cytoplasm and large prominent nucleoli.

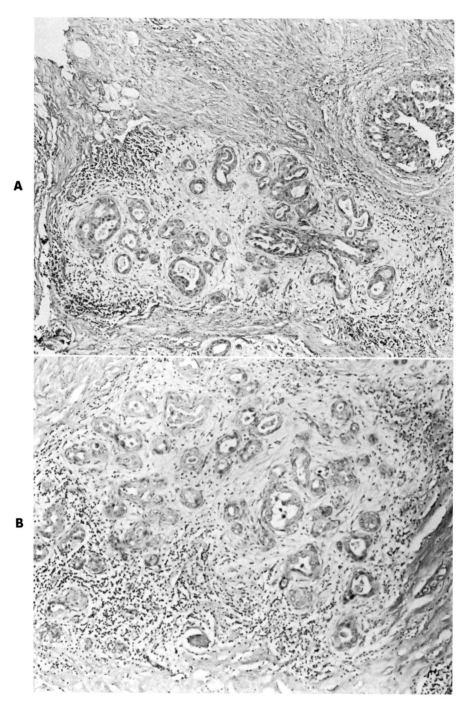

Fig. 12-6 Cancerization of the lobules by ductal carcinoma in situ. Cells of intraductal carcinoma of comedo type may extend into the small ductal and acinar units of the lobule **(A).** Their morphology is that of large cell ductal carcinoma in situ **(B).** This lobular extension does not constitute invasion.

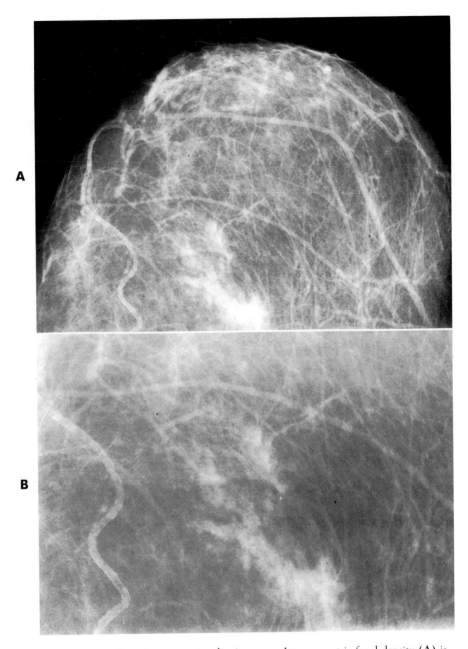

Fig. 12-7 Ductal carcinoma in situ clinging type. An asymmetric focal density (**A**) is shown to be a grouping of dilated ducts (**B**).

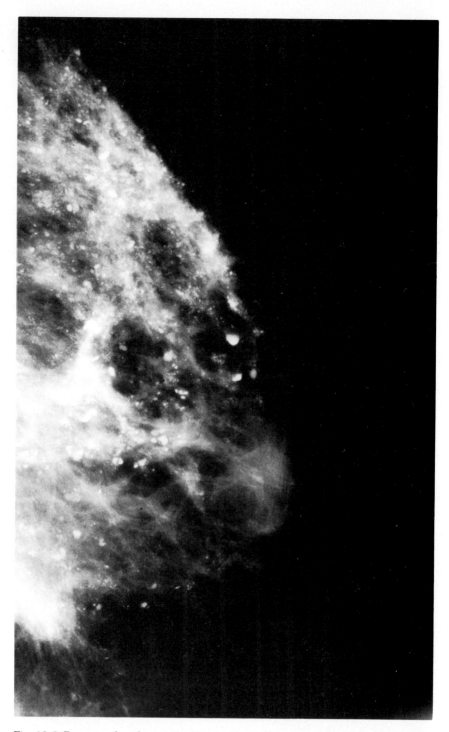

Fig. 12-8 Extensive ductal carcinoma in situ. Lateral projection shows granular, casting type and amorphous calcification diffusely distributed between larger collections of milk of calcium. (This unusual case courtesy of Dr. Susan Williams, Omaha, Nebraska.)

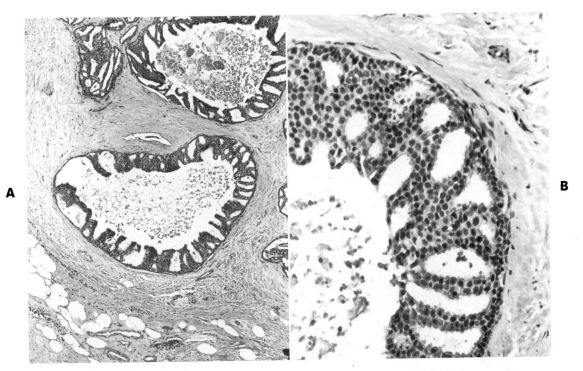

Fig. 12-9 Micropapillary and cribriform ductal carcinoma in situ (DCIS) are both characterized by less cytologic atypia than the comedo type. In this example of micropapillary DCIS, the cells form rigid papillary projections and arches that rim the periphery of the duct **(A).** At higher magnification **(B),** the tumor cells exhibit dark staining nuclei and represent a monomorphous cell population with little nuclear variation.

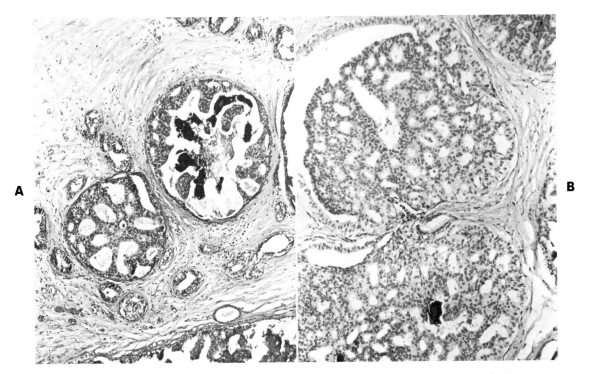

Fig. 12-10 While calcification is less common in ductal carcinoma in situ (DCIS) of cribriform and micropapillary types than in comedo DCIS, it is seen occasionally. The cribriform DCIS in **A** exhibits some central necrosis and dark staining areas of calcification. Smaller calcifications without necrosis are noted in **B.** The intraductal cellular proliferation in cribriform DCIS is monomorphous, and the small secondary lumens seen in **A** and **B** are regular in appearance.

Lobular carcinoma in situ

Histopathology. Lobular carcinoma in situ (LCIS) is a distinctive histologic lesion that is readily recognized by most surgical pathologists. First described by Foote and Stewart in the 1940s, its biologic significance became clearer in the late 1970s in two articles from two different institutions in New York City.[43] Based on more than 20 years' follow-up of patients with LCIS, LCIS was convincingly shown to be a lesion that predicts an increased risk for developing invasive cancer but is biologically distinct from DCIS[45,48,50] (Table 12-1). In these studies from Memorial Sloan-Kettering Cancer Center and Columbia University, it was shown that the risk of developing invasive cancer after 20 to 25 years was approximately 20% for patients with LCIS. Significantly, however, the likelihood of developing invasive cancer (ductal more frequently than lobular) was equal in both the ipsilateral breast containing the previously biopsied LCIS and in the contralateral breast. Therefore, the presence of LCIS predicts both an increased risk of subsequent development of invasive cancer and the likelihood of bilateral disease.[44,47] LCIS is now commonly grouped with benign high-risk lesions rather than with frankly malignant disease in outcome results.

Histologically, LCIS involves the terminal acini of the lobular unit. The cells of LCIS are small with a central small nucleus and a tiny nucleolus. Mitotic figures are infrequent and the nuclei themselves are histologically bland. Traditionally, virtually all of the acinar units in an affected lobule are involved by the neoplastic proliferation that distends each separate acinus. In addition to distending and involving uniformly the acini of a lobule, cells of LCIS characteristically may traverse along the terminal ducts, where they lie adjacent to the basement membrane and burrow beneath the duct-lining epithelium in a pattern that has been termed *pagetoid spread.* The finding of isolated pagetoid spread is a useful marker for the surgical pathologist and indicates the need to sample a biopsy further for the presence of LCIS or atypical lobular hyperplasia (ALH). The latter lesion is a proliferation of cells histologically similar to those of LCIS, but which does not involve the lobule as extensively as LCIS. ALH is discussed further in Chapter 11.

The cells of LCIS, in addition to their small size and characteristic nuclear and cytoplasmic features, may often be characterized by the presence of small cytoplasmic spaces. These are seen by electron microscopy to represent intracytoplasmic lumina and are fairly characteristic of cells of both in situ and invasive lobular carcinoma. This structure is mucin-positive with histochemical stains.

LCIS is not usually recognizable grossly or mammographically. It represents an unexpected finding in a biopsy that is usually performed for fibrocystic changes. The lesions of fibrocystic change that produce a detectable mass or palpable thickening characteristically have involved larger ducts or represent areas of sclerosing adenosis; the LCIS is discovered as an incidental finding. Occasionally, LCIS may show calcifications, but these are small and usually below the size of mammographic detection.

Table 12-1 **Relative risk for breast cancer**

Type	Risk
Lobular carcinoma in situ	8×
Lobular hyperplasia with atypia	4–5×
Ductal carcinoma in situ	10×
Ductal hyperplasia with atypia	4–5×

Imaging. Although a radiographic cluster of "stippled" calcifications was originally described as being associated with LCIS,[46,51] a review of the radiographic literature confirms that LCIS is rarely detected preoperatively.[42,49,52] Some reasons for biopsy in women in whom incidental LCIS is diagnosed histologically are a palpable mass, an empiric mirror image biopsy, and mammographic calcifications or opacities.[42,49] Review of histologic specimens show that the LCIS is a microscopic incidental finding.[42,49] Calcifications, if present, are usually either in adjacent ducts or lobules containing normal epithelial cells or in the stroma near normal ducts or lobules.[49] Calcifications may be up to 2 cm from the histologic focus of LCIS. It is now accepted that LCIS lacks distinctive mammographic features.

In general, breasts that contain LCIS tend to be mammographically dense (Wolfe's patterns P2 or Dy).[42,49] The rates of multifocality (70%) and bilaterality (50%) of LCIS support a thesis that LCIS patients have disease of the entire breast parenchyma.[42]

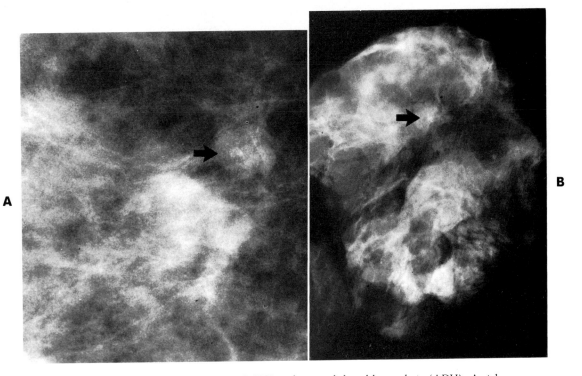

Fig. 12-11 Lobular carcinoma in situ (LCIS) and atypical ductal hyperplasia (ADH). A tight cluster *(arrow)* of amorphous calcifications **(A)** was biopsied with preoperative wire localization procedure. Specimen radiograph **(B)** confirms cluster *(arrow)* was excised. Pathologic diagnosis included incidental foci of LCIS and ADH.

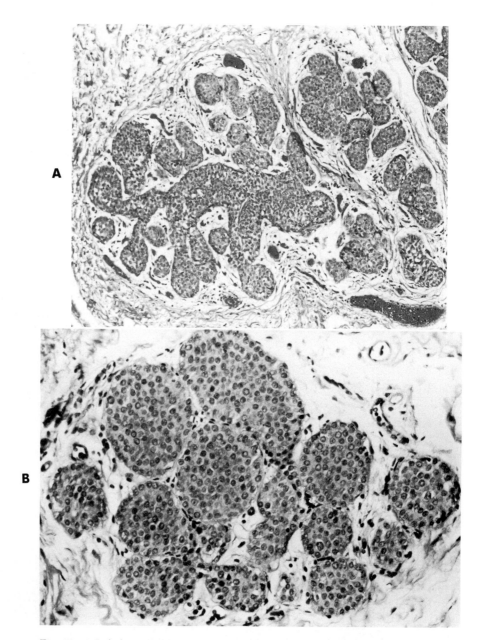

Fig. 12-12 Lobular carcinoma in situ is characterized by a cellular proliferation that fills and distends all of the ductules and acini of the lobule **(A).** The neoplastic cells are round and regular with small nuclei **(B).** (B is from Golden A, Powell DE, Jennings CD: *Pathology: Understanding human disease*, ed 2, 1985, Baltimore, Williams and Wilkins.)

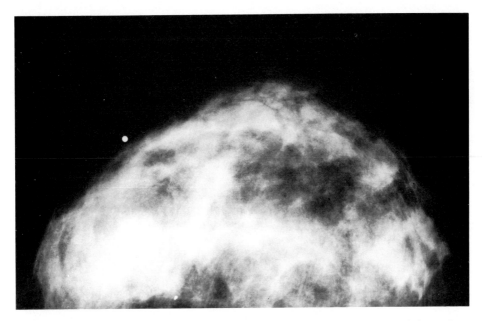

Fig. 12-13 Lobular carcinoma in situ (LCIS). Palpable left breast mass corresponded to radiographically dense parenchyma or craniocaudad view. Pathologic findings were proliferative fibrocystic disease and two sites of incidental LCIS.

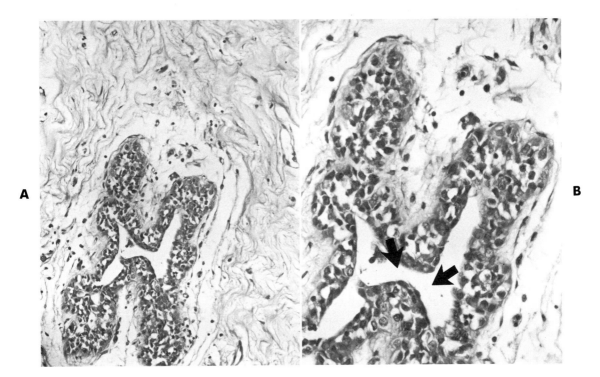

Fig. 12-14 Lobular carcinoma in situ can extend along larger ducts between the epithelium and the myoepithelial cells in a pattern known as "pagetoid spread" **(A).** The cytology of the neoplastic cells that are small with round, regular nuclei can be seen in **B.** Also note the attenuated normal epithelial cells *(arrows)*.

INVASIVE CARCINOMA
Invasive ductal carcinoma

Histopathology. Invasive ductal carcinoma (IDC) is the most common type of breast tumor. Unless characteristic histologic patterns make up the major portion of the tumor, these cancers are referred to as *ductal carcinomas of no special type*. Over 70% of invasive breast cancers fall into this category. Frequently, these tumors demonstrate an associated profound stromal fibrosis, giving rise to the older designation of scirrhous carcinoma. Ductal carcinomas of no special type are histologically more variable than invasive lobular cancer, showing considerable variation both in architectural growth patterns and in cellular morphology. Because these tumors are adenocarcinomas, they often show some attempt at gland or tubule formation or they at least aggregate in cohesive clusters of cells. Morphology of individual tumor cells can vary from relatively small cells with uniform nuclei and eosinophilic cytoplasm to cells with large vesicular nuclei and prominent large nucleoli with considerable pleomorphism of both cytoplasm and nuclei.

For ductal carcinomas of no special type, histologic grading is of considerable prognostic importance.[70,74] Many grading systems have been proposed for breast cancer[61]; probably the most commonly and widely used systems represent modifications of the system of Bloom and Richardson,[55] which combines assessment of architectural growth pattern, nuclear morphology, and proliferative activity as defined by mitotic count. Modifications suggested recently have sought to look more critically at the assessment of proliferative activity by examining criteria for interpreting mitoses[53,81] and more accurate quantification of mitotic activity.[65,76]

Although many studies have demonstrated the value and importance of histologic grading as a prognostic indicator for breast cancer, lack of reproducibility of grading among pathologists has been cited as a negative factor for relying on this information.[77] Recent data have shown that grading systems can be used in a reproducible fashion by pathologists, and other large studies are needed to substantiate the validity of histopathologic grading.[54,60,69]

A widely used grading system that represents a modification of the Bloom and Richardson schema proposed by Elston is illustrated in Table 12-2.[59] Some other modifications proposed by Simpson and Le Doussal are incorporated in Box 12-1.[69,76]

Assessment of extent of disease is important in determining optimal management and ultimate prognosis for the patient with breast cancer. In addition to careful staging, other important ancillary studies that may affect outcome often need to be performed at the time of initial diagnostic tissue examination.[73] Some of these studies are discussed in Chapter 8.

Careful staging is imperative in the evaluation of a patient with breast cancer. Axillary lymph node status with respect to number of nodes involved by metastatic tumor and other features (size of nodal metastases, extracapsular spread of metastatic tumor) is the single most important factor for predicting prognosis.[58] Tumor size is less important, but may be extremely important in determining prognosis in node-negative patients.[70] It also correlates directly with the incidence of lymph node metastases. Tumor size must be measured accurately by the pathologist in biopsy specimens. If a mastectomy is subsequently performed, the size or volume of residual tumor should be estimated.

The concept of minimal breast cancer relates to the factor of tumor size. As originally proposed, minimal breast cancer (MBC) was defined as all in situ carcinomas (both DCIS and LCIS) and all invasive carcinomas measuring 5 mm or less in greater dimension.[63] In 1984, Hartman expanded the definition to conform to that of the American College of Surgeons (Box 12-2), characterizing any invasive cancer of 1 cm or less in diameter as MBC.[64]

Table 12-2 **Histologic grading of invasive breast cancer**

Feature	Score (points)
I. Tubule formation	
Tubules with visible lumina are major component of tumor mass.	1
Tubules with visible lumina are moderate component of tumor mass.	2
Tubules with visible lumina are minor component of tumor mass.	3
II. Nuclear morphology	
Nuclei show little variation in size and shape.	1
Nuclei show moderate variation in size and shape.	2
Nuclei show marked variation in size and shape.	3
III. Mitotic rate	
<10 mitoses per 10 high-power fields	1
10–19 mitoses per 10 high-power fields	2
20 or more mitoses per 10 high-power fields	3
	TOTAL
Grade 1 (well differentiated)	3–5
Grade 2 (moderately differentiated)	6–7
Grade 3 (poorly differentiated)	8–9

Modified from Elston CW: *Grading of invasive carcinoma of the breast.* In Page DL, Anderson TJ, editors: *Diagnostic histopathology of the breast,* London, Churchill-Livingstone, p 303.
*Total represents score of I plus II plus III.

BOX 12-1 SUGGESTED MODIFICATIONS TO HISTOLOGIC GRADING SCHEMES

Modifications in mitotic counting
  Standardization of high-power field size[81]
  Mitoses per 1000 cells[76]

Modifications using nuclear and proliferative features (MSBR)
  Five grades rather than three[69]

Microinvasion in a predominantly in situ ductal tumor also is a concept that has less than total consensus among pathologists (referred to earlier in the section on DCIS). For some, identifiable tumor penetration through the basement membrane of a duct involved by DCIS constitutes microinvasion. Distortion due to fibrosis, elastosis, and inflammation may make recognition of such penetration difficult, and it is often difficult to determine whether small tumor glands represent invasion or merely DCIS involving more distal units of the lobule. Some clinicians regard the presence of a young fibroblastic tissue response as evidence of invasion. Although the biologic significance of MBC is known from studies of metastatic disease and survival in these patients, the same cannot be said for microinvasive breast cancer.[64] Certain more uniform criteria need to be adopted. Page and Anderson advocate as a minimum that more than a single focus of invasion be noted and that the cells characterized as microinvasion be in the interlobular tissue, that is, outside the lobular unit or periductal stroma.[72]

Accurate staging of breast cancer requires inclusion of relevant data about the tumor and lymph nodes in the pathology report. The most recent classification and staging systems for breast cancer are given in Tables 12-3 and 12-4.

BOX 12-2 MINIMAL BREAST CANCER

Noninvasive mammary carcinoma
Ductal (DCIS)
Lobular (LCIS)

Invasive mammary carcinoma
Equal to or less than 1 cm in greatest dimension
Ductal (IDC)
Lobular (ILC)

From Hartman WH: Minimal breast cancer: an update, *Cancer* 53:681-684, 1984.

Table 12-3 TNM classification and staging for breast cancer

Classification	Primary tumor (T)
TX	Primary tumor cannot be assessed
TO	No evidence of primary tumor
Tis	Carcinoma in situ (ductal or lobular or Paget's disease with no tumor)
T1	Tumor 2 cm or less in greatest dimension
T1a	0.5 cm or less in greatest dimension
T1b	More than 0.5 cm but not more than 1 cm in greatest dimension
T1c	More than 1 cm but not more than 2 cm in greatest dimension
T2	Tumor more than 2 cm but not more than 5 cm in greatest dimension
T3	Tumor more than 5 cm in greatest dimension
T4	Tumor of any size with direct extension to chest wall or skin
T4a	Extension to chest wall
T4b	Edema (including peau d'orange) or ulceration of skin of breast or satellite skin nodules confined to same breast
T4c	Both (T4a and T4b)
T4d	Inflammatory carcinoma

Table 12-3 **TNM classification and staging for breast cancer—cont'd**

Classification	Primary tumor (T)
	Regional lymph nodes (pathologic pN)
pNX	Regional nodes cannot be assessed
pNO	No regional node metastases
pN1	Metastases to movable ipsilateral axillary nodes
pN1a	Micrometastases only (none larger than 0.2 cm)
pN1b	Metastasis to node(s), any larger than 0.2 cm
pN1bi	Metastasis in 1 to 3 nodes, any more than 0.2 cm and all less than 2 cm in greatest dimension
pNbii	Metastasis to 4 or more nodes, any more than 0.2 cm and all less than 2 cm in greatest dimension
pNbiii	Extension of tumor beyond node capsule; metastasis less than 2 cm in greatest dimension
pNbiv	Metastasis greater than 2 cm in greatest dimension to a node
pN2	Metastasis to ipsilateral axillary nodes that are fixed to one another or to other structures
pN3	Metastasis to ipsilateral internal mammary nodes
	Distant metastasis (M)
MX	Presence of distant metastasis cannot be assessed
M0	No distant metastases
M1	Distant metastasis (includes metastasis to ipsilateral supraclavicular nodes)

From American Joint Committee on Cancer (AJCC) and International Union Against Cancer (UICC), 1992.

Imaging. The typical mammographic findings of IDC are those recognized as the classic or direct signs of breast cancer such as spiculated or ill-defined mass with or without associated casting or granular type calcifications (Box 12-3 and Table 12-5). Less frequently, IDC produces a focal area of asymmetric density or an area of parenchymal distortion.[71] An additional indirect sign of invasive breast cancer is the uncommon but highly sensitive sign of a developing density.[36] A single dilated duct may be an indirect sign of breast cancer, but is more often due to a benign process such as an intraductal papilloma or duct ectasia. If caused by cancer, a single dilated duct may be filled with DCIS with or without invasion. These subtle clues to the presence of breast cancer have been reported to be the mammographic signs leading to detection in as many as 20% of 300 consecutive cases of nonpalpable breast cancer[75] and are receiving greater emphasis in aggressive screening programs.

Table 12-4 **Stage grouping for breast cancer**

Stage 0	Tis	N0	M0
Stage I	T1	N0	M0
Stage IIA	T0	N1	M0
	T1	N1	M0
	T2	N0	M0
Stage IIB	T2	N1	M0
	T3	N0	M0
Stage IIIA	T0	N2	M0
	T1	N2	M0
	T2	N2	M0
	T3	N1	M0
	T3	N2	M0
Stage IIIB	T4	Any N	M0
	Any T	N3	M0
Stage IV	Any T	Any N	M1

From American Joint Committee on Cancer (AJCC) and International Union Against Cancer (UICC), 1992.

BOX 12-3 MAMMOGRAPHIC FEATURES OF BREAST CANCER

Direct signs
Clustered calcifications
    Casting type
    Granular type
Spiculated or ill-defined mass

Indirect signs
Single dilated duct
Architectural distortion
Focal asymmetric density[67]
Developing density

Modified from Sickles EA: Mammographic features of "early" cancer, *AJR Am J Roentgenol* 143:461, 1984.

In characterizing a mass within the breast, the radiographic density is compared with breast parenchyma and the margins of the mass are analyzed. High mammographic density is defined as density greater than an equal volume of parenchyma. High density in an IDC is believed to be a manifestation of the desmoplastic response of fibrosis and elastosis of the invaded tissues. A recent study has reported that not only was radiographic density difficult to reproducibly assess, but many malignant masses (52% of 40 cases) were classified as a density less than or equal to an approximately equal volume of normal paren-

Table 12-5 **Invasive breast cancer mammographic findings**

Features	Invasive ductal CA	Invasive lobular CA
Frequency	86.4%	13.6%
Mass as presenting sign	60.3%	68.5%
Asymmetric density/ architectural distortion	13.6%	57%
Malignant calcifications	47%	0%

From Newstead GM, Baute PB, Toth HK: Invasive lobular and ductal carcinoma: mammographic findings and stage at diagnosis, *Radiology* 184:623, 1992.

chyma.[66] Moreover, nearly all of these isodense or hypodense malignant tumors were infiltrating ductal carcinomas. Therefore, although many dense masses are likely to be malignant, visual assessment of radiographic density of a mass by mammography is not a reliable sign of IDC.

The margins of a mass can be characterized provided there is sufficient fat to visualize the interface of the cancer with the surrounding parenchyma. Most often infiltrating ductal carcinomas produce a mass with a spiculated or ill-defined or fuzzy margin. In a series of 20 noncalcified clinically occult breast cancers, 80% were found to have spiculated or indistinct margins on the specimen radiographs.[79] These observations have been long recognized in mammographic series as well. When marked, the spiculation may tether either Cooper's ligaments or the ductal system and result in the clinical findings of skin flattening, skin dimpling, or nipple retraction. These secondary skin and nipple changes may be accentuated by compression during mammographic imaging.

In a small percentage of cases (10%) of IDC, the margin of the mass is characterized as well defined or circumscribed.[79] Of course, the incidence of well-circumscribed IDC may vary with the series and the quality of the mammographic assessment, whether the assessment method is specimen radiography or magnification focal spot compression. Also, note that the halo sign—partial or complete—is not pathognomonic of a benign lesion but has been identified in malignant breast lesions.[80]

In any case, the numerous radiographic features of IDC overlap those of DCIS. It is not possible to distinguish IDC from DCIS based on the appearance of the mass features by mammography or specimen radiography. Both DCIS and IDC produce masses with either well-circumscribed or irregular margins.[79]

The malignant type of calcifications associated with IDC are identified mammographically in approximately 50% of palpable breast cancers. The subtypes of casting and granular morphology of these suspicious calcifications have already been discussed in the section on DCIS imaging. Note also that IDC is likely to be associated with an extensive intraductal component when calcifications (casting or granular) cover greater than a 3-cm area.[78] This is important because studies have shown that an extensive intraductal component (EIC) in women with IDC is associated with a 5-year local recurrence rate of 24% following lumpectomy and radiation therapy compared with 6% in patients without an EIC.[56]

As previously emphasized, IDC is commonly invasive at multiple sites within the breast. Whole organ sectioning was used by Gallager and Martin to correlate mammographic and histopathologic appearances in the mid-1960s.[62] Multicentric areas of invasion were identified in 47% of IDC. Most were examples of multiple nodules arising from ducts containing preexisting ductal carcinoma. Less frequently, the carcinoma spread by periductal lymphatics to a distant site. In a study reported by Lagios and colleagues, the overall incidence of multicentric cancers separated by at least 5 cm was 28%.[68] Of these multicentric lesions, 40% were separate invasive carcinomas and in the other cases there was a mixture of invasive and in situ lesions. The implication of these observations is that the mammographic assessment of breast cancer should include an aggressive evaluation of the breast with special views including magnification to identify areas of multifocal or multicentric cancer. The radiographic extent of malignancy may be an underestimate of the true extent of disease. Nevertheless, extent of disease is a significant factor in planning appropriate therapy.

A further word about the limitation of mammography seems appropriate. It is well recognized that 6% to 10% of breast cancers are not detected mammographically. These most often are palpable noncalcified masses in dense breasts. The margins of the mass are obscured by the surrounding parenchyma. A negative mammogram report in the presence of a palpable mass provides no additional information. These masses require further evaluation usually by fine needle aspiration cytology.[57]

Finally, considerable confusion exists concerning the definition and significance of the two descriptive terms: *focal asymmetric density* (a probable mass with obscured or ill-defined margins) and *asymmetric breast tissue* (a normal variant seen in 3% of a mixed population of symptomatic and asymptomatic women).[67] An asymmetric volume of breast tissue, asymmetrically dense tissue, or asymmetrically prominent ducts not associated with a palpable mass, thickening, calcifications, or distortion is probably a normal variation or is caused by contralateral surgical excision. However, such an area should be viewed with concern if a palpable mass or thickening is present which corresponds to the area of asymmetry. The more suspicious abnormality is called a focal asymmetric density, which warrants further investigation.

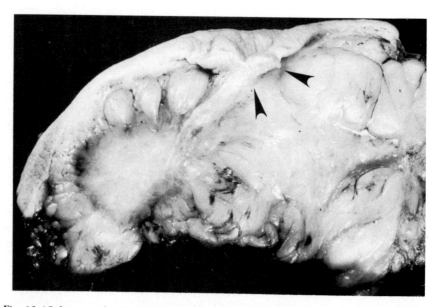

Fig. 12-15 Invasive ductal carcinoma. The large tumor, located in the lower left area of the mastectomy, has caused retraction of the overlying skin and nipple (*arrows*). (From Golden A, Powell DE, Jennings CD: *Pathology: Understanding human disease*, ed 2, 1985, Baltimore, Williams and Wilkins.)

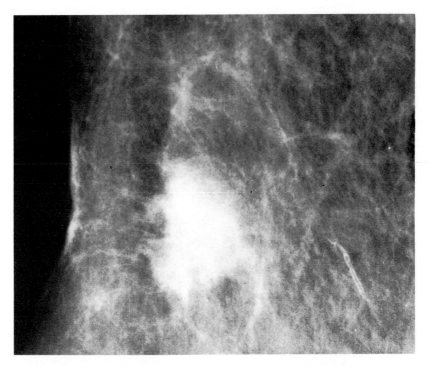

Fig. 12-16 Invasive ductal carcinoma. Irregularly shaped mass with ill-defined margins is superficial and associated with skin retraction. Breast compression accentuates skin dimpling when x-ray beam is positioned tangential to region of skin retraction.

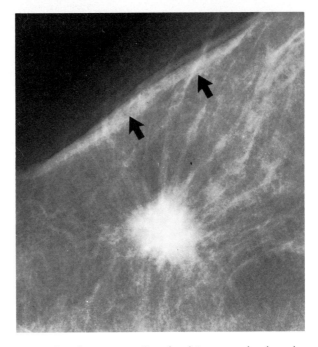

Fig. 12-17 Invasive ductal carcinoma. Spiculated 1-cm mass has long desmoplastic extensions into fatty tissue. Note skin retraction (*arrows*).

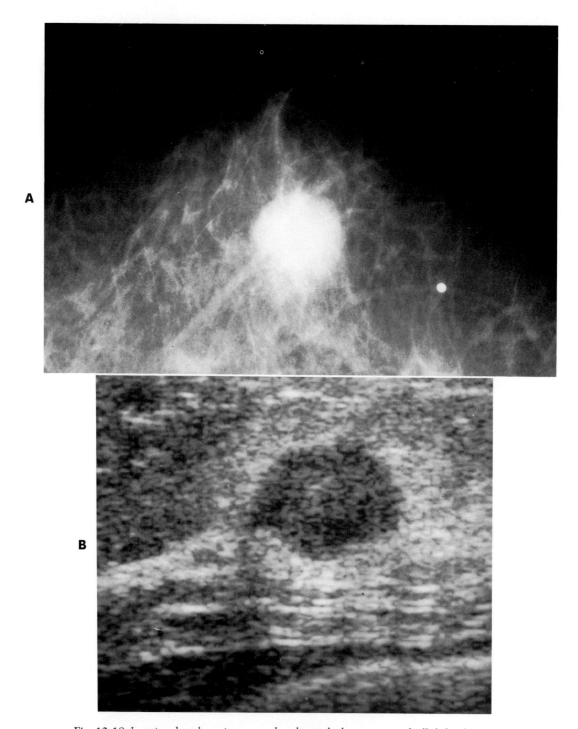

Fig. 12-18 Invasive ductal carcinoma produced round, dense mass with ill-defined posterior margin **(A)**, shown to be solid by ultrasound examination **(B).**

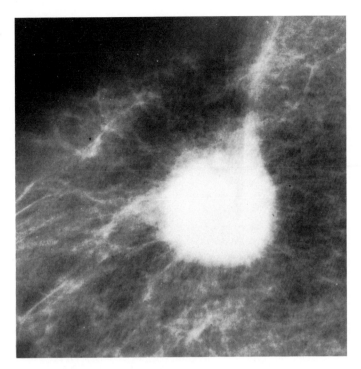

Fig. 12-19 Invasive ductal carcinoma. Round 2.5-cm spiralated mass has short desmoplastic extensions into surrounding fat.

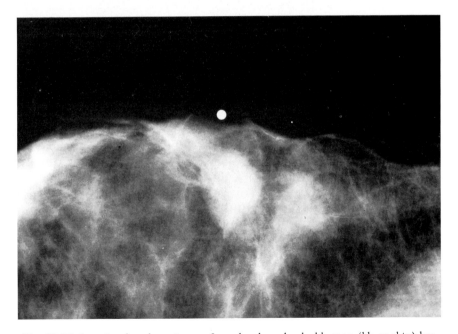

Fig. 12-20 Invasive ductal carcinoma. Irregular shaped palpable mass (bb on skin) has ill-defined margins.

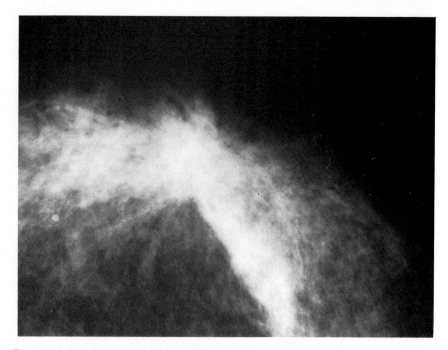

Fig. 12-21 Invasive ductal carcinoma. Focus of parenchymal distortion 2.5 cm in diameter causes tenting of posterior margin of parenchyma.

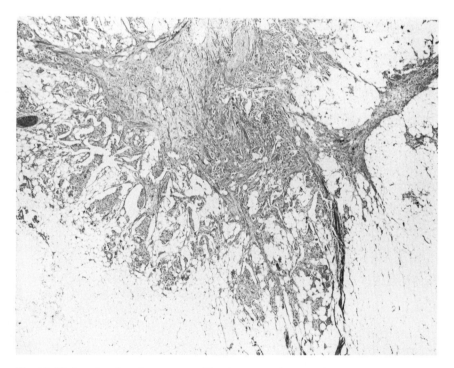

Fig. 12-22 Invasive ductal carcinoma. This low-magnification photomicrograph of a small invasive ductal carcinoma illustrates the irregular spiculated outline of the lesion with nests of tumor cells invading into adipose tissue.

Fig. 12-23 (A) Invasive ductal carcinoma (IDC). Mass irregular in shape with ill-defined margins is associated with casting type calcifications. **(B)** IDC. Atypical, coarse, dystrophic calcifications are a predominant feature of this 2.5-cm spiculated carcinoma. More subtle granular calcifications are regionally distributed in the same quadrant. **(C)** IDC and ductal carcinoma in situ. Palpable 1-cm mass with ill-defined margins is associated with granular calcifications of varying size, shape and density.

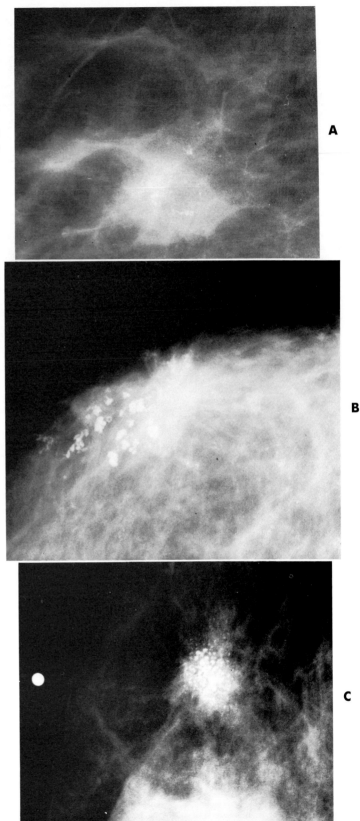

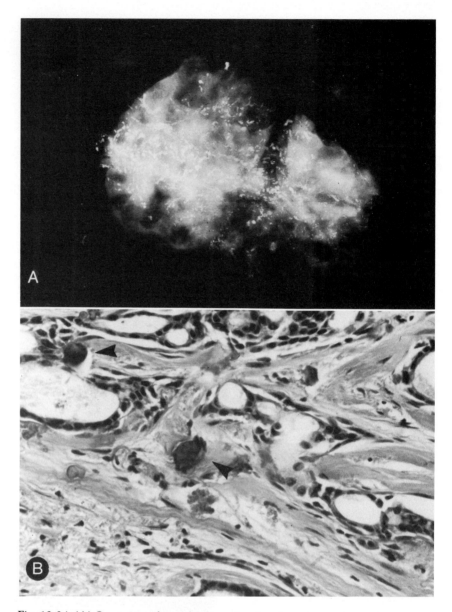

Fig. 12-24 **(A)** Specimen radiograph of invasive ductal carcinoma showing extensive calcification within the tumor. **(B)** High-magnification photomicrograph shows calcification *(arrows)* within epithelium and stoma of the invasive tumor. (From Golden A, Powell DE, Jennings CD: *Pathology: Understanding human disease,* ed 2, 1985, Baltimore, Williams & Wilkins.)

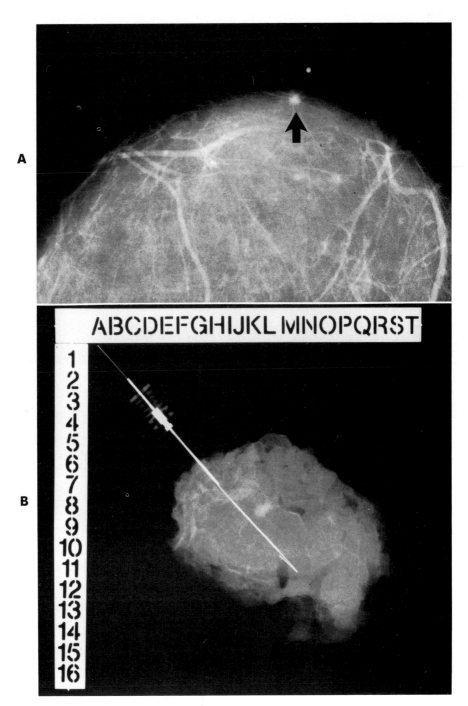

Fig. 12-25 Small 4-mm invasive ductal carcinoma caused dense spiculated mass (*arrows*) on screening mammogram (**A**) and in specimen radiograph (**B**).

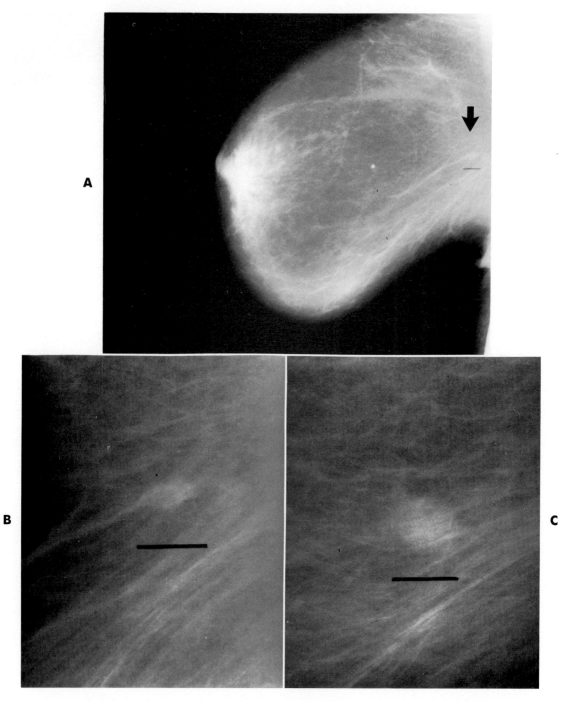

Fig. 12-26 Invasive ductal carcinoma. A small nodule *(arrow)* in a large fatty breast **(A)** was oval in shape with ill-defined margins **(B).** The nodule increased in size **(C)** over a 12-month interval interval. Black line represents 10-mm measure.

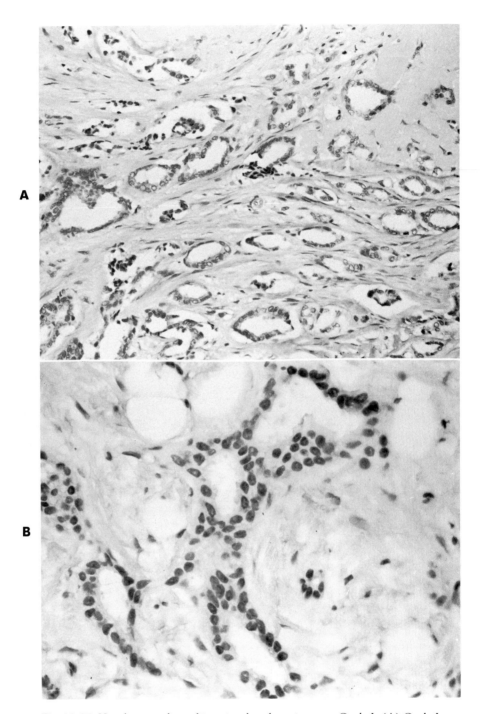

Fig. 12-27 Histologic grading of invasive ductal carcinoma—Grade I. **(A)** Grade I carcinomas show a pattern of infiltrating tubules with central open lumens in the major portion of the tumor. **(B)** The nuclei of Grade I carcinomas are characteristically regular with little pleomorphism. They are slightly larger than the nuclei of normal duct epithelial cells and lack prominent nucleoli. Mitoses are rare and absent.

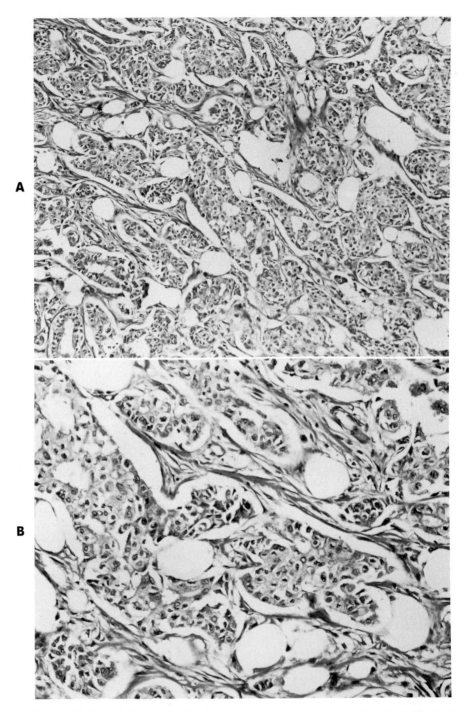

Fig. 12-28 Histologic grading of invasive ductal carcinoma—Grade II. **(A)** In Grade II carcinomas, generally a smaller number of the invasive tumor groups show well-defined tubular architecture. **(B)** The nuclei of Grade II carcinomas show some variation in size and show small nucleoli, and are generally larger than Grade I nuclei. Mitoses are not numerous, but may be seen.

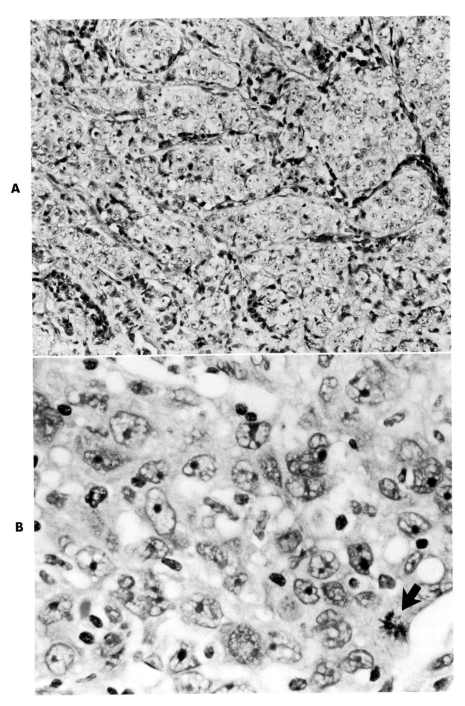

Fig. 12-29 Histologic grading of invasive ductal carcinoma—Grade III. **(A)** Grade III carcinomas infiltrate as solid masses of cells. There is little to no tubular formation. **(B)** Grade III nuclei are large and highly pleomorphic. They are often vesicular and usually have large prominent nucleoli. Mitoses *(arrow)* may be numerous.

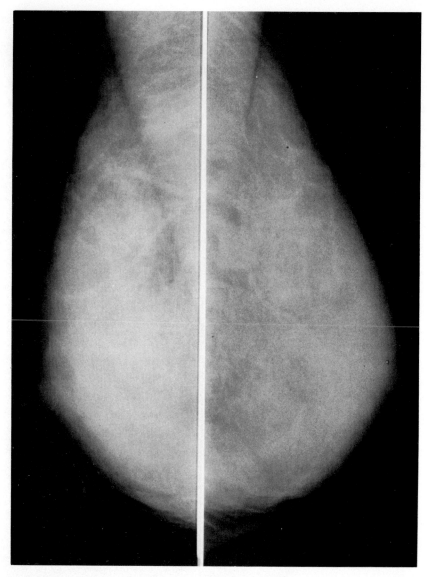

Fig. 12-30 Invasive ductal carcinoma. False-negative mammogram in a woman with very dense parenchyma. Palpable right lymphadenopathy was the presenting complaint.

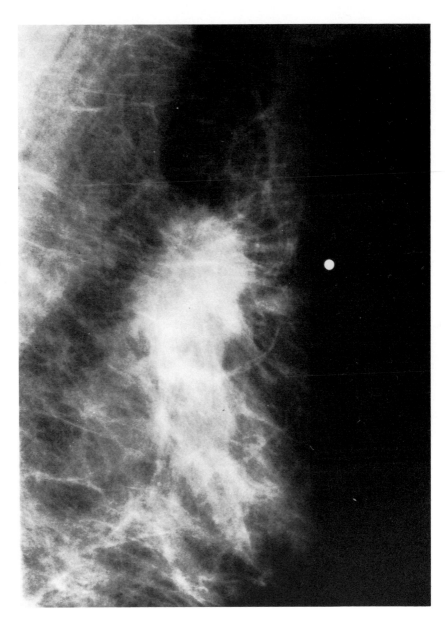

Fig. 12-31 Invasive ductal carcinoma. Palpable (skin bb) spiculated mass invades pec-toral muscle on this mediolateral oblique projection.

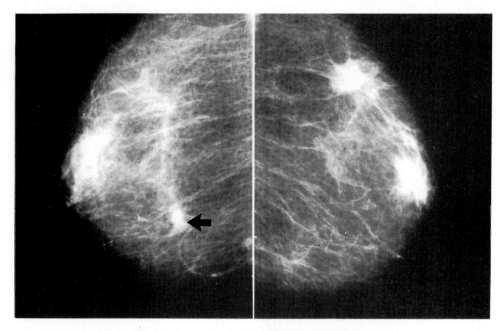

Fig. 12-32 Synchronous bilateral carcinoma: bilateral invasive ductal carcinoma. The larger left mass was palpable. The smaller right mass was clinically occult (*arrow*).

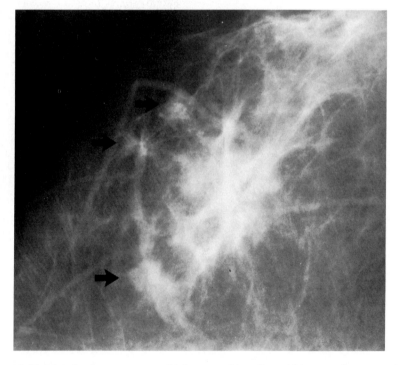

Fig. 12-33 Multifocal carcinoma: multiple areas of invasion within a quadrant are evident (*arrows*). Combined invasive lobular carcinoma and invasive ductal carcinoma.

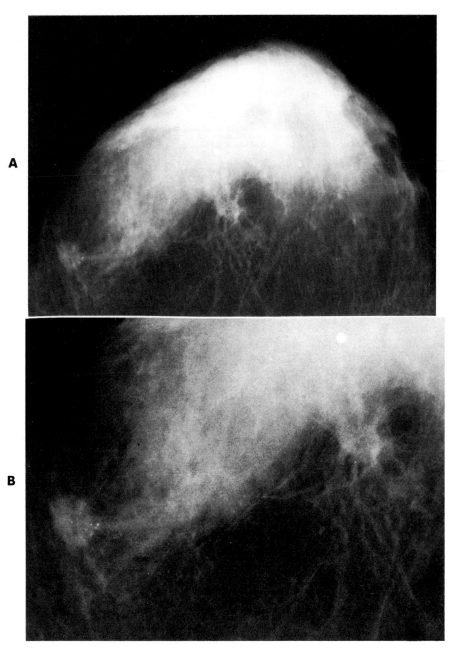

Fig. 12-34 Multicentric carcinoma. Multicentric spiculated masses were in separate quadrants separated by more than 5 cm **(A)** and close up **(B).**

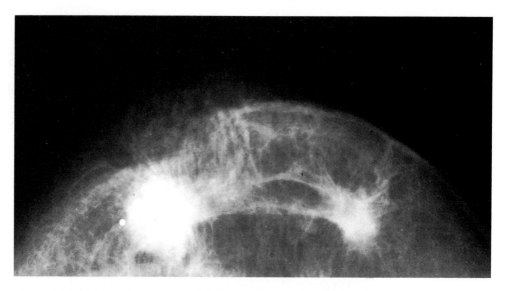

Fig. 12-35 Multicentric carcinoma of differing cell types. The larger palpable mass was invasive ductal carcinoma, and the smaller mass was invasive lobular carcinoma. Skin retraction and thickening was clinically apparent.

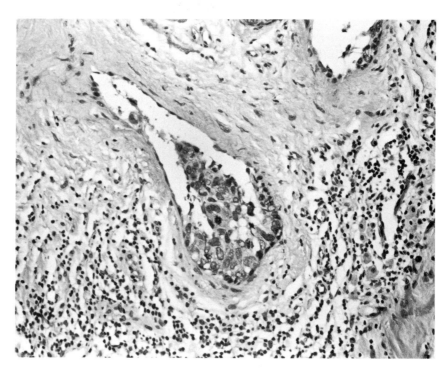

Fig. 12-36 Vascular invasion in breast cancer. Tumor invasion in breast carcinomas is a finding associated with unfavorable prognosis. Here tumor cells are present within an endothelial-lined space and are adherent to the wall.

Special types. Patterns of IDC associated with a special histologic appearance and frequently a more favorable prognosis have been recognized. The most common of these are tubular carcinoma, mucinous carcinoma, and medullary carcinoma. Invasive papillary carcinoma is less frequently seen but also has a favorable prognosis.

Tubular carcinoma. Tubular carcinoma is a very well-differentiated IDC and has been referred to in Chapter 10 because it must be differentiated from a benign process, most frequently a radial scar or complex sclerosing lesion. These tumors are often small and may be detected by mammography rather than by physical examination, although in some cases they present as a palpable mass.[83,90]

Features that point to a diagnosis of tubular carcinoma include invasion of the glandular elements in a haphazard pattern into the breast parenchyma beyond the confines of the lobular unit; open, rounded, uniform invasive tubules that may exhibit attenuation at one end and a prominent "bent teardrop" shape[89]; and gland-like structures that have lost their surrounding myoepithelial rim (i.e., they have only a single cell lining). The latter feature may be recognized more easily by using special stains to demonstrate basement membrane, most notably the periodic acid-Schiff (PAS) stain, but this cannot always be relied on.[86] The stain must be intense enough to demonstrate basement membrane, and histotechnologists should be instructed that this structure (rather than intraluminal mucin) is to be demonstrated. Associated areas of IDC, most commonly of cribriform and micropapillary patterns, are found within or adjacent to tubular carcinoma.[91] This finding may aid in differential diagnosis.

Tubular carcinoma, like radial scars, may be associated with nodular aggregates of elastic tissue and with fibrosis.[92] The cells lining the invasive glands characteristically are histologically bland and mitoses are rare. The tumors have an extremely favorable prognosis. Although lymph node metastases occur in over 10% of cases,[88] survival rates are very high.[84] However, to predict this favorable prognosis, most IDC (75% or greater) must exhibit classic tubular histology.

The mammographic features of pure tubular carcinoma are usually those of a spiculated mass of about 0.5 to 1.5 cm in diameter, sometimes with associated microcalcifications. The fibrotic reaction may extend beyond the mass.[85] These radiographic features overlap with those of less differentiated invasive ductal/lobular carcinomas. Occasionally, calcifications may be the only radiographic finding.[85] Classic calcifications of casting type may be present if DCIS is associated with the tubular carcinoma, either within the lesion or nearby. Screening mammography detects a significant proportion of tubular carcinomas that may remain clinically occult because of their relatively small size compared with more aggressive invasive breast cancers.[85]

When tubular carcinoma is associated with less differentiated IDC, the likelihood of metastatic cancer to the axillary nodes increases. Serial subgross and correlated radiographic method of examining mastectomy specimens indicated that tubular carcinoma may occur in as much as 7 to 8% of mastectomy specimens, of which 56% occurred in a multicentric association 5 cm or more from another in situ or invasive carcinoma.[87] Multifocal tubular carcinoma has also been reported.[82]

Mucinous carcinoma. Mucinous carcinoma, also referred to as *colloid* or *gelatinous carcinoma*, is a well-differentiated ductal cancer. The histologic appearance of this tumor is easily recognized and not often misdiagnosed. Mucinous carcinomas are composed of abundant extracellular mucin, in which small clusters of tumor cells appear to float. The tumor cells themselves generally show little pleomorphism, regular nuclear outlines, and small nucleoli with few mitoses. The rare benign mucocele-like lesion of the breast may provide a problem in differential diagnosis, particularly on fine needle aspiration.[98]

Mucinous carcinomas characteristically have a distinct, rounded outline or border. They do not show a prominent in situ component. The good prognosis and low incidence of patients with lymph node metastases are found only in cases of pure mucinous carcinoma.[97] When other types of IDC are found in association with mucinous carcinoma, the prognosis is worse. Even with pure mucinous carcinoma, tumor deaths may occur relatively late in the course of the disease.[94] Pure mucinous tumors may be more frequently found in older patients.[99] In most series of IDC, mucinous carcinomas (17 of 940) are less common than medullary carcinoma (41 of 940) but more common than invasive papillary carcinoma (4 of 940).[100]

The mammographic finding in mucinous carcinoma is usually an oval or irregular-shaped mass with circumscribed, lobulated, or obscured margins. The age range is generally postmenopausal; this special type of carcinoma may account for 7% of carcinomas in patients over 75.[101] The lesion size varies widely, depending on the method of detection, for example, by physical examination or by screening mammography. Because the presence of abundant mucin may make the mass similar in consistency on palpation to normal breast tissues, mucinous carcinomas may be quite large at the time of clinical presentation. Calcifications are not a typical feature but have been described.[96,101]

The ultrasound examination of mucinous carcinoma, based on limited numbers of patients, shows a solid demarcated lesion with fine internal echoes and a spectrum of excellent transmission of sound to slight shadowing.[93,95,101] A similar appearance would be expected both ultrasonographically and mammographically with the rare mucocele-like lesion of the breast in premenopausal women, which has been mentioned.[98]

Medullary carcinoma. Medullary carcinomas, in contrast to tubular carcinoma, usually present as palpable tumors. Despite their size and ominous histology, lymph node metastases are not as common as one might predict and survival is significantly better than that found in patients with IDC of no specific type.[108] The histopathologic features of medullary carcinoma are very large pleomorphic tumor cells and prominent nucleoli. Mitoses are not infrequent and tumor cells show virtually no glandular differentiation and a lack of cellular cohesion. The latter feature makes the distinction of medullary carcinoma from large cell lymphoma an important problem, and occasionally diagnosis by immunohistochemistry demonstrating epithelial markers (particularly low molecular weight keratins) may be necessary.

The cells of medullary carcinoma characteristically are arrayed in broad sheets with little evidence of associated intraductal carcinoma. The tumor margins are smooth and rounded without ragged infiltration into the surrounding normal tissue. A striking feature is the usually intense inflammatory infiltrate of mononuclear cells, frequently lymphocytes with some plasma cells, which surrounds the tumor cell sheets (Box 12-4).

Some tumors that do not exhibit all these classic features of medullary carcinomas have been recognized and categorized as *atypical* or *variant medullary carcinomas*. These tumors exhibit some but not all of the features of classic medul-

---

BOX 12-4 CLASSIC MEDULLARY CARCINOMA: PATHOLOGIC CRITERIA

1. Tumor well circumscribed
2. Syncytial architecture in >75% of tumor
3. Contains diffuse inflammatory infiltrate
4. Has atypical nuclei
5. Forms no glandular pattern

From Ridolfi RL, Rosen PP, Post AA, et al: Medullary carcinoma of the breast: a clinicopathologic study with 10 year follow-up, *Cancer* 40:1365, 1977.

Table 12-6 **Ten-year disease-free survival**

Histologic type	Survival rate
Typical medullary carcinoma	92%
Atypical medullary carcinoma	53%
Nonmedullary carcinoma	51%

From Rapin V, Contesso G, Mouriesse H, et al: Medullary breast carcinomas: a re-evaluation of 95 cases of breast cancer with inflammatory stroma, *Cancer* 61:2503, 1988.

lary carcinoma; for example, they may show minimal inflammatory infiltrate, tumor invasion, or glandular differentiation. They also have a prognosis that is closer to IDC of no special type than to classic medullary carcinoma [106,108] (Table 12-6). For this reason, the designation of atypical medullary carcinoma is probably important. Although medullary tumors tend to be larger than tubular cancers at the time of diagnosis, survival is improved if they are detected when less than 3 cm.

Typical medullary carcinoma of the breast as defined by strict criteria probably accounts for less than 2% of all IDC.[106] Less than one third of breast cancers with inflammatory stroma meet the strict criteria of typical medullary carcinoma.[106] Reported incidences of medullary carcinoma as 4% to 7% of invasive breast cancers probably include cases of atypical medullary carcinomas.[100,102,106,107]

Medullary carcinoma occurs in a wide age range (24 to 79 years) of women with a median age of 48 years.[105] It is diagnosed in young women and has been reported to account for 11% of breast cancers diagnosed in women less than age 35 years of age.[109] This fact, together with its well-circumscribed mammographic and ultrasonographic appearance, may help to explain the observation that medullary carcinoma may represent a larger percentage of the cancers in a mammographically false-negative group compared with a true positive group (5.5% versus 0.8%, respectively).[110]

Medullary carcinomas may also present as a clinically occult lesion which is mammographically detected. The lesion may be soft and may or may not contain areas of cystic degeneration.[101] Central necrosis is more often observed in the larger tumors.[108] Size range is generally 1.0 to 7.0 cm with a median diameter of 2.5 to 3.0 cm.[105,106]

Mammographically, medullary carcinomas are oval or round masses with well-circumscribed, lobulated, or slightly irregular margins. Calcifications are not a feature of this cancer type, although one case has been reported.[105,106] In at least one third of cases, the margins of the mass are partially obscured by either dense parenchyma or lymphocytic infiltrate.[105] A clear halo sign may be present in some cases and is therefore not a pathognomonic sign of a benign mass. No distinguishing imaging characteristics are noted either mammographically or ultrasonographically for medullary carcinoma.[104] The most common circumscribed breast carcinoma is IDC of no special type; medullary carcinomas make up only 30% to 40% of all circumscribed breast cancers.[106]

The ultrasonographic appearance of medullary carcinoma may mimic a benign lesion. The masses are usually well defined with inhomogeneous, hypoechoic texture. There is no attenuation of sound. Enhancement of through transmission of sound is usual.[105] Cystic spaces may be seen within the mass but are not pathognomonic and have been described as well in circumscribed ductal carcinomas, phyllodes tumors, and infrequently in fibroadenomas.[105] For medullary carcinoma to present clinically as a cystic mass is a rare occurrence.[103]

The prognosis for patients with the pure type of medullary carcinoma is considered good, with a 92% 10-year disease-free survival documented when strict histologic criteria are applied.[106]

Table 12-7 **Breast tumors with epithelial-myoepithelial features**

Tumor types	Biologic behavior
Pleomorphic adenoma	Benign
Adenomyoepithelioma	Benign—local recurrence possible
Adenoid cystic carcinoma	Malignant—generally favorable prognosis
Malignant adenomyoepithelioma (myoepithelial carcinoma)	Malignant—generally favorable prognosis
Metaplastic carcinoma	Malignant—poor prognosis

Papillary carcinoma. Invasive papillary carcinoma is rare.[111] The intracystic form of papillary carcinoma is discussed in Chapter 10. In situ papillary carcinoma has been discussed in this chapter under DCIS. Papillary invasive ductal carcinoma, as the name implies, may exhibit invasive growth of papillary epithelial structures with or without fibrovascular cores. Lymph node metastases are relatively uncommon and prognosis is good, similar to that found in mucinous carcinoma.[111] This tumor may occur in older and nonwhite patients with relatively high incidence.

Invasive cribriform carcinoma may be considered a variant of invasive papillary carcinoma, which resembles the cribriform pattern of DCIS. It is also associated with an excellent prognosis.[112]

Rare special types. Other distinct histologic varieties of IDC are recognized but are rare. Among these are tumors derived from both epithelial and myoepithelial cells (Table 12-7) and tumors characterized by abundant vacuolated cytoplasm.

Metaplastic carcinoma are tumors that are more likely to occur in older, postmenopausal women. These tumors exhibit a variety of histopathologic patterns and appear to be both epithelial and myoepithelial in origin, based on immunohistochemistry and electron microscopy.[126,129] A number of different tumor types are encompassed by the designation, *metaplastic carcinoma.* These include spindle cell carcinoma, carcinosarcoma, squamous cell carcinoma of ductal origin, matrix-producing carcinoma, and metaplastic carcinoma with osteoclastic giant cells.[126-130] Despite the differing histologic patterns, a single classification, that of metaplastic carcinoma, is favored.[120]

Prognosis for patients with metaplastic carcinomas is not good and is particularly poor for those with carcinosarcomas.[128] These tumors, particularly the spindle cell carcinomas, must be correctly classified and differentiated from either benign fibrous proliferations such as fibromatosis and fasciitis or the rare primary malignant fibrous histiocytoma of breast. Spindle cell carcinomas are malignant epithelial neoplasms, and nodal metastases occur. Immunohistochemistry for cytokeratins (high and low molecular weight), S-100 protein, and actin may be helpful in differential diagnosis. Also, the squamous cell carcinoma variant of metaplastic carcinoma must be differentiated from mucoepidermoid carcinoma, generally a low-grade neoplasm, and squamous cell metaplasia within ductal adenocarcinomas.[114]

Another group of tumors that are composed of both epithelial and myoepithelial cells are the *adenomyoepitheliomas.* These are even less common than the metaplastic carcinomas, and most reported cases are considered benign, despite local recurrences, and do not pursue an aggressive malignant course. Rare examples of lymph node metastases[124] and distant metastases resulting in the death of the patient have been reported.[117]

Pleomorphic adenomas (benign mixed tumors) and adenoid cystic carcinomas also have been reported as primary breast tumors. These neoplasms, found much more frequently as primary salivary gland and skin appendage tumors, also have a myoepithelial component. Both have characteristic histologic appearances. The benign mixed tumor typically has both glandular and stromal components, and the chondromyxoid stroma is characteristic.[118] The adenoid cystic carcinoma appears, according to most studies, to have an excellent prognosis.[116] Although it may be confused with invasive cribriform carcinoma, it demonstrates the distinctive hyalinized stroma that surrounds glands and is also present as masses of material located within the centers of cribriform spaces. Electron microscopic and immunochemical studies have demonstrated the myoepithelial origin of tumor cells in adenoid cystic carcinoma.[122]

Certain tumors are characterized by cells with abundant and frequently vacuolized cytoplasm. Secretory carcinoma of the breast is a rare tumor, which was first described in children and young women. Subsequently, tumors of similar histology have been described in older women as well.[125] Although the prognosis is very good in young patients, the tumors can metastasize, particularly in older women. The cells of secretory carcinoma are large with abundant cytoplasm containing secretory material. Similar material may also be present in an extracellular location. This material is neither lipid nor glycogen and in many cases can be shown to be either sulfated acid mucopolysaccharide or sialomucin.[125]

Other tumors of the breast characterized by abundant cytoplasm are the apocrine carcinoma, the lipid-rich carcinoma, and the glycogen-rich clear cell carcinoma. Both the latter two neoplasms are characterized by a predominant pattern of cells with abundant clear or vacuolated cytoplasm. Histochemistry shows distinct differences, with the cytoplasm of the lipid-rich carcinomas containing lipid as demonstrated by oil red O stains.[123] The clear cell carcinoma contains abundant cytoplasmic glycogen, demonstrated both by PAS stains and by electron microscopy.[115] This tumor and the lipid-rich carcinoma may be histologically aggressive tumors.

Ductal carcinomas characterized by a majority of cells showing apocrine differentiation have been recognized for some time.[119] Classic features of apocrine differentiation are abundant eosinophilic cytoplasm, somewhat pleomorphic large nuclei, and prominent luminal apocrine "snouts." These histologic features are distinctive, but most authors do not classify this tumor as a distinct subtype of IDC.[121] It has been suggested that immunohistochemical demonstration of the antigen GCDFP-15 in most tumor cells is a good marker of apocrine breast cancer.[113]

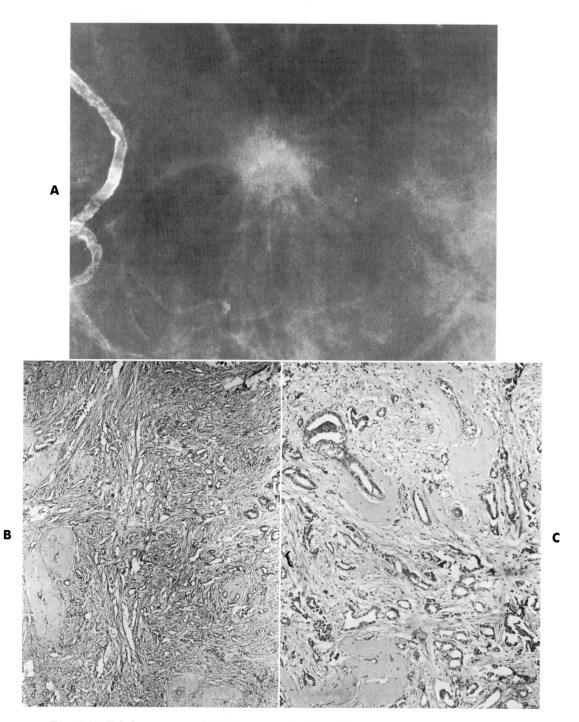

Fig. 12-37 Tubular carcinoma. **(A)** Classic example of a small (8 mm) spiculated mass associated with granular calcifications. **(B)** At low magnification the tubular carcinoma bears some resemblance to sclerosing adenosis. The infiltrating glands extend into the stroma in a ragged fashion, however, and lack the smooth borders and lobulocentric pattern of sclerosing adenosis. **(C)** At higher magnification the well-differentiated tubular structures can be appreciated. The amorphous material in the stroma represents elastosis, often prominent in tubular carcinomas.

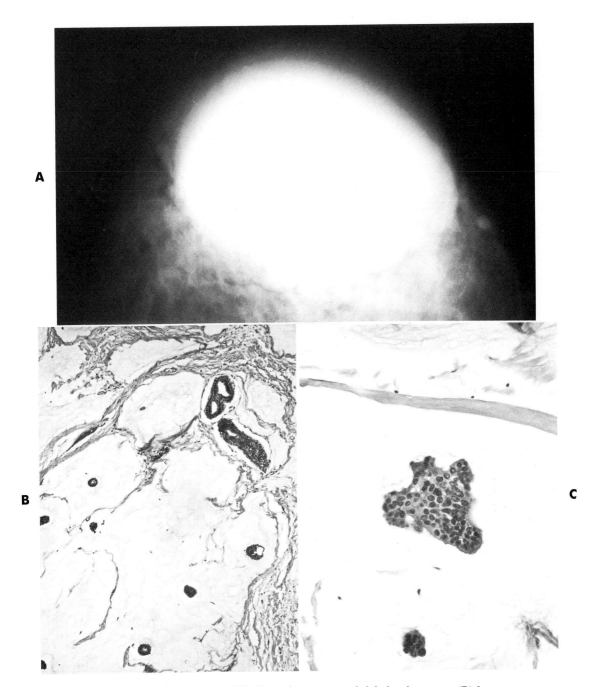

Fig. 12-38 Mucinous carcinoma **(A)** Classic large mass with lobulated margins. **(B)** Low magnification appearance of mucinous carcinoma characteristically is hypocellular. Much of the tumor is composed of large lakes of pale-straining mucin in which the small clusters of tumor cells appear to float. **(C)** At higher magnification these tumor cell clusters show small regular well-differentiated nuclei with little pleomorphism.

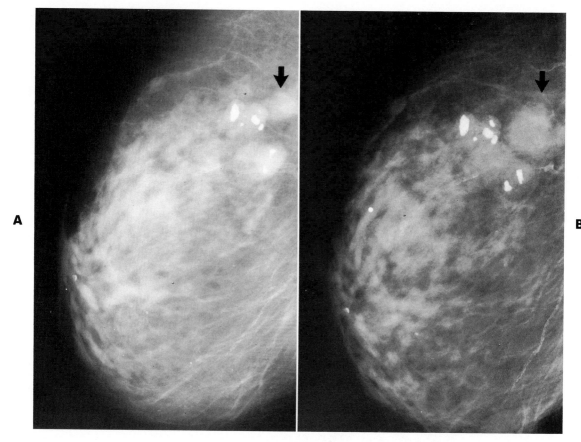

Fig. 12-39 Mucinous carcinoma: **(A)** mass *(arrows)* posterior to hyalinized fibroadenomas **(B)** increased in size over 2 years. (Case courtesy of Dr. Marie Lee, Seattle, Washington.)

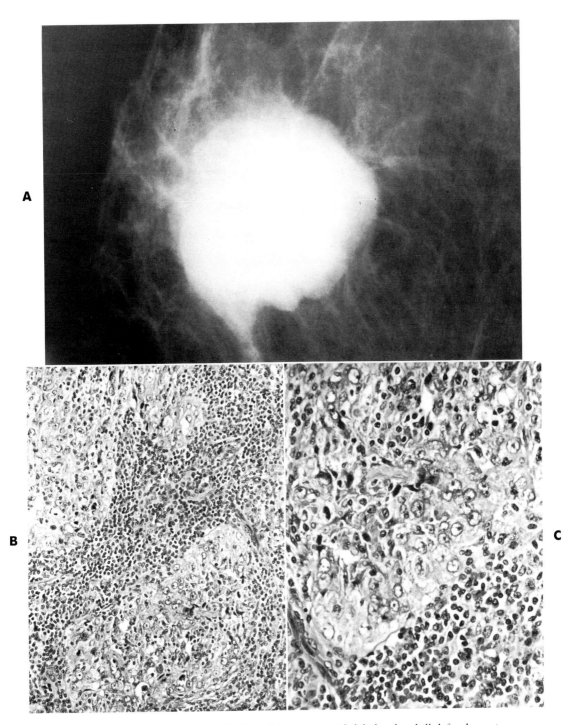

Fig. 12-40 Medullary carcinoma. **(A)** Round 4-cm mass with lobulated and ill-defined margins. **(B)** Loosely cohesive tumor cells are surrounded by a dense infiltrate of mature lymphocytes and plasma cells. **(C)** At high magnification the marked pleomorphism of the tumor cells can be seen. The cytoplasmic borders are indistinct. The nuclei are large and vesicular with prominent nucleoli. The infiltrate of small dark-staining lymphocytes can be seen to the right of the photomicrograph.

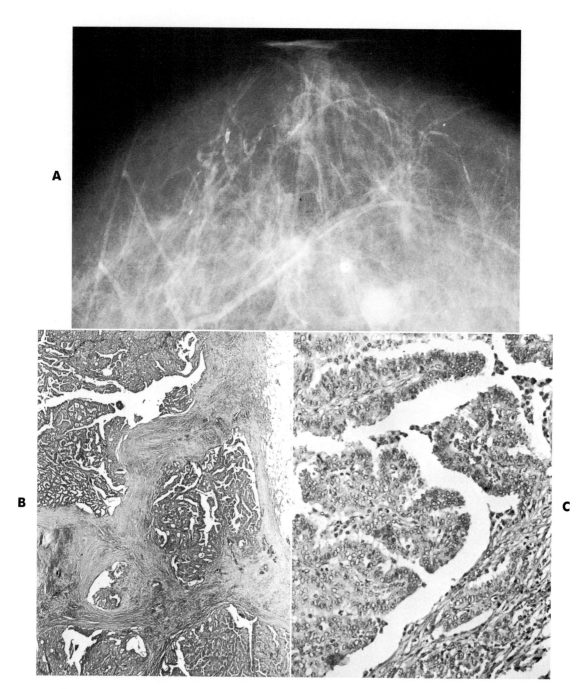

Fig. 12-41 Invasive papillary carcinoma. **(A)** Round mass with ill-defined margins had increased in size from the time of a prior mammogram in an elderly female. **(B)** At low magnification the papillary pattern of the invasive carcinoma can be readily identified. **(C)** At higher magnification the papillae can be seen to be composed of palisading epithelial cells arranged along fibrovascular stalks or forming solid epithelial fronds.

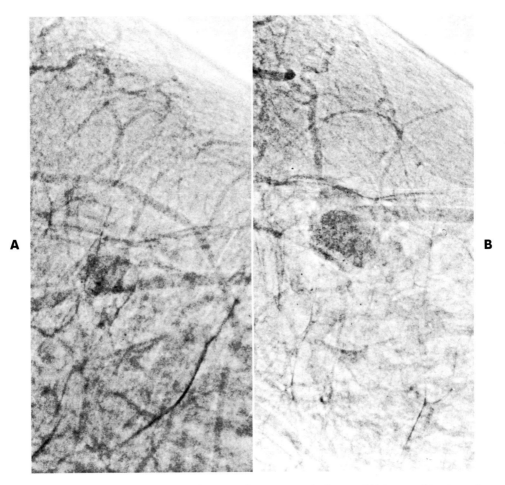

Fig. 12-42 Papillary carcinoma. Oval mass with punctate calcification **(A)** increased in size and developed more lobular margins over 1 year **(B).**

Fig. 12-43 Invasive cribriform carcinoma is considered a type of invasive papillary tumor. The cribriform cancer forms sheets of tumor cells with numerous well-defined lumens, resembling cribriform ductal carcinoma in situ.

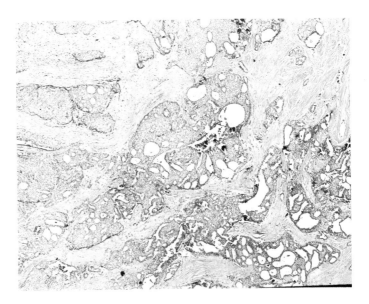

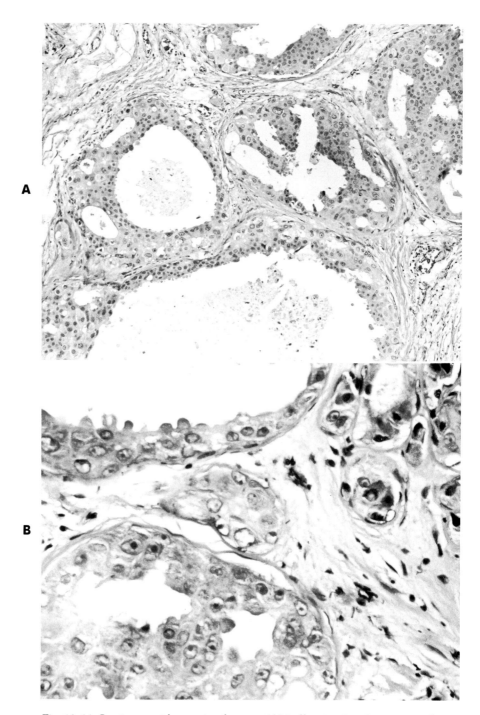

Fig. 12-44 Carcinoma with apocrine features. **(A)** Infiltrating ductal carcinoma showing prominent apocrine features. The tumor forms large masses with central lumens of varying sizes, as well as solid sheets. **(B)** At higher magnification the apocrine differentiation is more apparent. The tumor cells have large nuclei with prominent nucleoli. Cytoplasm is dense and eosinophilic and cytoplasmic luminal blebs (apical snouts) can be seen.

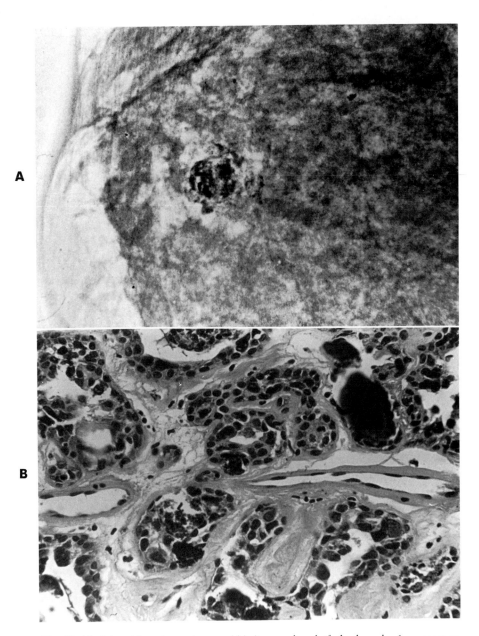

Fig. 12-45 Adenoid cystic carcinoma. **(A)** A coarsely calcified subareolar 1-cm mass on this xeromammogram proved to be an adenoid cystic carcinoma. **(B)** Histologically the tumor cells are arranged in sheets and tubules that are surrounded by amorphous hyaline material. These tumor cells are of myoepithelial origin. (Courtesy of Dr. Sandra Mc-Cann, Columbus, Georgia, and Dr. Robert Fechner, Charlottesville, Virginia.)

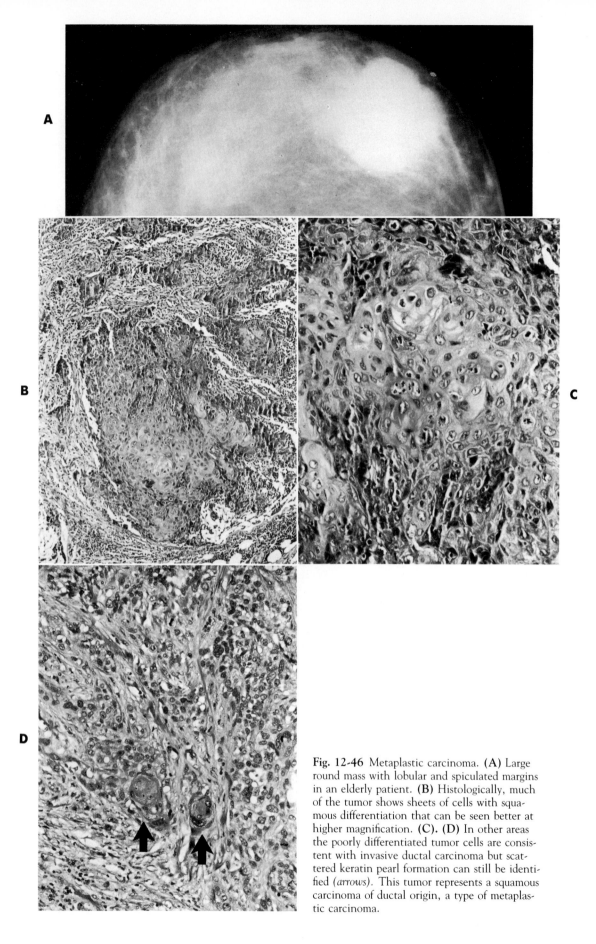

Fig. 12-46 Metaplastic carcinoma. **(A)** Large round mass with lobular and spiculated margins in an elderly patient. **(B)** Histologically, much of the tumor shows sheets of cells with squamous differentiation that can be seen better at higher magnification. **(C). (D)** In other areas the poorly differentiated tumor cells are consistent with invasive ductal carcinoma but scattered keratin pearl formation can still be identified (*arrows*). This tumor represents a squamous carcinoma of ductal origin, a type of metaplastic carcinoma.

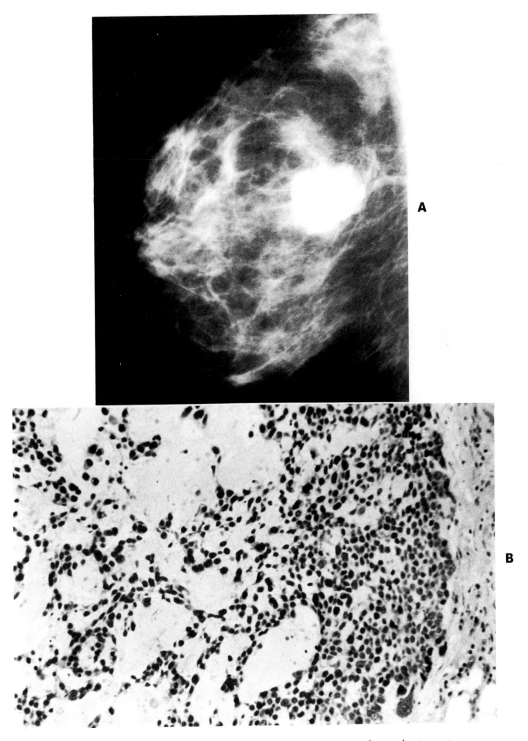

Fig. 12-47 Metaplastic carcinoma. **(A)** This carcinosarcoma, a type of metaplastic carcinoma, caused a 3-cm high-density mass with lobulated margins in a 37-year-old woman. **(B)** Histologically, the poorly differentiated tumor showed both cartilaginous and epithelial differentiation. (Courtesy of Dr. Ralph Smathers, Palo Alto, California.)

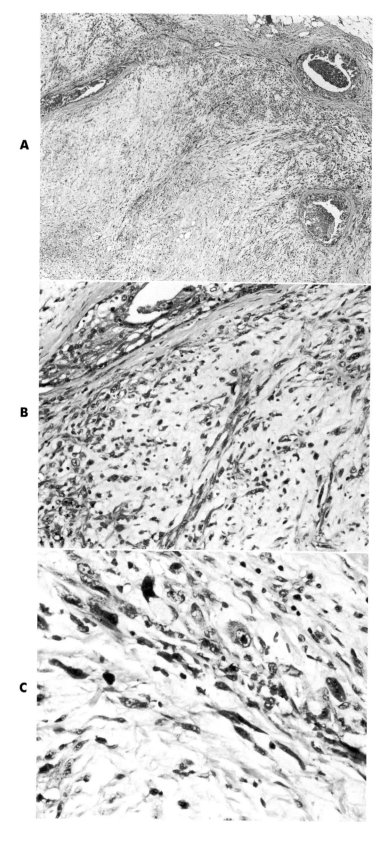

Fig. 12-48 Metaplastic carcinoma. **(A)** Another example of carcinosarcoma. At low magnification, ducts showing ductal carcinoma in situ (DCIS) can be seen at the periphery of the tumor. **(B)** At high magnification a portion of a duct involved by DCIS can be seen at the upper left. The invasive tumor shows chondroid differentiation. **(C)** The anaplastic tumor cells show considerable variation in morphology, with some polygonal in outline and others spindled in shape.

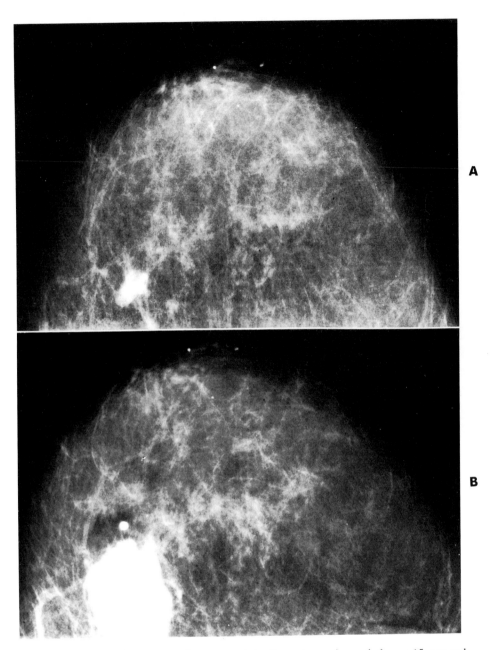

Fig. 12-49 Spindle cell carcinoma demonstrated significant interval growth from a 15-mm nodule **(A)** to a 3-cm lobulated mass **(B)** over a 1-year interval. (Courtesy of Gary Shapira, Richmond, Indiana.)

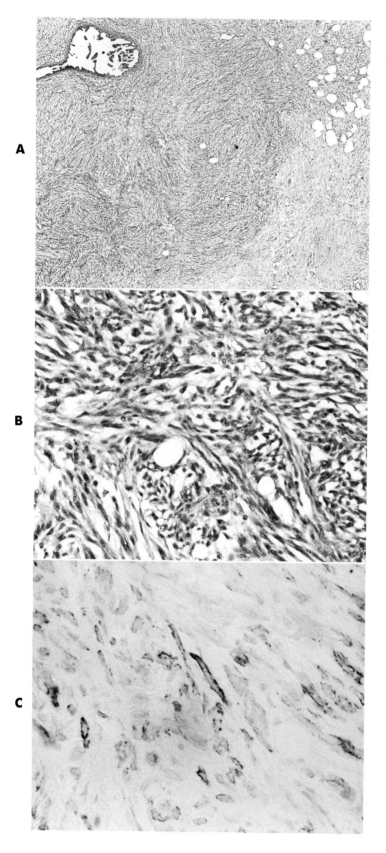

Fig. 12-50 Spindle cell carcinoma. **(A)** Spindle cell carcinoma, also a type of metaplastic carcinoma, is illustrated in these photomicrographs. A duct involved by ductal carcinoma in situ is seen at the upper left. The tumor infiltrates fatty tissue at right. **(B)** Individual tumor cells are predominantly elongated or spindled in appearance. **(C)** Immunochemical stains for low–molecular weight cytokeratins are positive in many of the tumor cells. (Courtesy of Dr. Gary Shapira, Richmond, Indiana.)

Invasive Lobular Carcinoma

Histopathology. Lobular carcinoma in both in situ and invasive forms is less common than ductal carcinoma. Invasive lobular carcinoma (ILC) accounts for approximately 10% of breast cancers.[131,135,136] Like its in situ form, the histology of this tumor is distinctive. The cells of ILC are small with round regular nuclei and inconspicuous nucleoli. Usually few mitoses are found. The cytoplasm is generally scant and may exhibit well-formed vacuoles that can be shown to contain mucin. Rather than forming well-defined glands or tubules, the tumor cells characteristically are arrayed in chains, the "Indian file" pattern; frequently, these chains of tumor cells ring around normal duct structures in a targetoid array.

Variations on the classic histologic pattern of ILC have been noted.[132,134,137] Although the cellular morphology of these lobular variant tumors is similar to classic ILC, the architectural patterns vary considerably from the Indian file growth pattern. Variant lobular carcinomas usually exhibit a solid, alveolar, or mixed pattern of growth. Like classic ILC, these carcinomas are frequently associated with LCIS and may be multicentric and bilateral. A recent study has suggested a slightly worse prognosis for variant lobular tumors, but the data were not statistically significant.[133] This same study demonstrated a better disease-free survival for stage I ILC than for stage I IDC, but the same results did not hold for stage II ILC. A high percentage of patients with classic ILC tend to be premenopausal.

It should be recognized that more than one type of mammary carcinoma—invasive or in situ—can exist within any biopsy or mastectomy specimen. When this is the case, our practice is to refer to each histologic pattern present as invasive mammary carcinoma (for example) with components of invasive lobular and tubular carcinoma. If desired or requested, the relative amounts of each tumor type can be specified in the surgical pathology report.

Signet ring cells characterized by a solitary mucin-containing cytoplasmic vacuole and compressed nucleus are seen not infrequently in ILC. Occasionally, these distinctive cells make up the major portion of a tumor, and the neoplasms have been designated as *signet ring cell carcinomas of the breast.* They appear to be more closely related to ILC than to IDC. In one study, all cases of signet ring carcinoma showed coexisting invasive or in situ lobular cancer.[139] They are histologically aggressive tumors, prone to metastasize and induce a striking desmoplasia in metastatic sites.

Certain tumors of the breast composed of uniform small cells with regular nuclei and marked cytoplasmic argyrophilia resembling classic carcinoid tumors of the intestine have been designated as *breast carcinoids.* Radiographically, they are not distinguishable from more conventional invasive carcinomas. Many clinicians consider them to be tumors of mammary epithelial rather than neuroendocrine origin. An excellent discussion of the topic is provided by Page and Anderson.[140]

Imaging. The mammographic appearance of ILC most often is either an asymmetric density with parenchymal distortion or a spiculated or ill-defined mass.[134a,136,138] It is not possible to differentiate ILC from IDC by the mammographic or gross morphologic features in most cases. Dystrophic calcifications may occur in both histologic types. The presence of distinct casting type calcifications suggest a ductal carcinoma component.

BOX 12-5 INVASIVE LOBULAR CARCINOMA: MAMMOGRAPHIC PATTERNS

Asymmetric density without definable margins
Architectural distortion
High-density mass with spiculated borders
No tumor discernible mammographically (breast may be dense or fatty)
Microcalcifications (uncommon)
Round, discrete mass (uncommon)

ILC may be difficult to diagnose by mammography, more so than other sub-types of breast cancer. The number of false-negative cases on mammography is nearly twice as high for ILC as for ductal carcinoma.[131,136] The tendency of ILC to infiltrate the parenchyma, glandular tissue, and fat in a diffuse and Indian file pattern may produce only a slight increase in parenchymal density, resulting in little appreciable mammographic abnormality. A subtle derangement of parenchymal architecture may be the only mammographic finding.[138] In a dense breast, ILC may present as a palpable mass or thickening and result in no mammographic finding. Physical examination is abnormal in a high percentage of cases (89%).[135,136] Even large cancers have been diagnosed in fatty breasts with no mammographic change.[135]

Breast ultrasound examination in most cases confirms a hypoechoic lesion with ill-defined margins.[134a] Microcalcifications may be present and prompt a biopsy but are usually associated with benign histology or associated ductal carcinoma histology (in situ or invasive or both). ILC only rarely causes a circumscribed mass.[136] By contrast ductal carcinoma, specific or nonspecific type, is a more common cause of a circumscribed mass on mammography.

In summation, ILC may produce very subtle or no mammographic findings because of its tendency to infiltrate the parenchyma and produce little or no increase in density or distortion even in a fatty breast. One should be suspicious of any abnormal physical finding regardless of the mammographic appearance.[135] Correlation of the physical examination with subtle and nonspecific mammographic findings is strongly encouraged.[141] Suspicious findings on physical examination should be pursued even in the presence of a normal mammogram. Undoubtedly, ILC is difficult to diagnose[136] (Box 12-5).

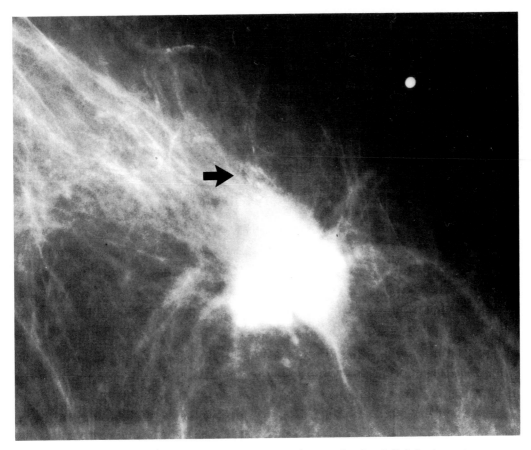

Fig. 12-51 Invasive lobular carcinoma. Irregular mass has spiculated and ill-defined margins and is associated with a small focus of heterogenous calcifications (*arrow*).

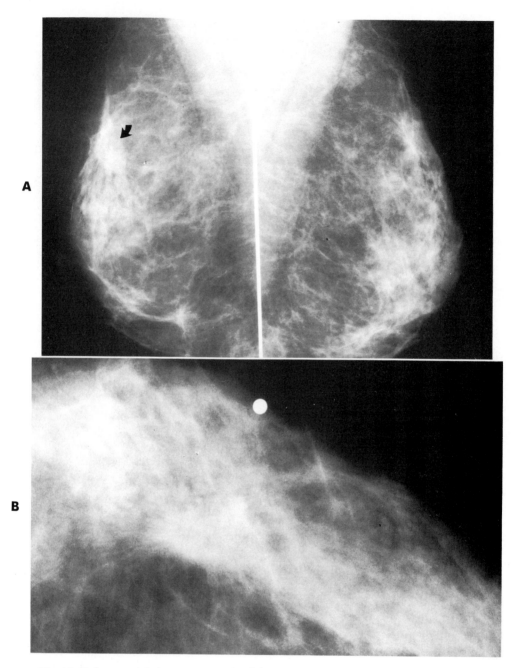

Fig. 12-52 Invasive lobular carcinoma. A subtle area of parenchymal distortion *(arrow)* in the upper outer quadrant of the right breast **(A)** was palpable in retrospect. A repeat craniocaudad view **(B)** demonstrates a focal density with spiculated margins corresponding to the palpable area of thickening marked by a bb on the skin.

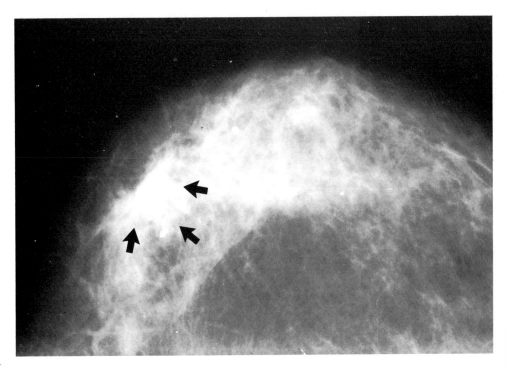

Fig. 12-53 Invasive lobular carcinoma. Area of parenchymal distortion and increased parenchymal density (*arrow*) correspond to firm palpable mass.

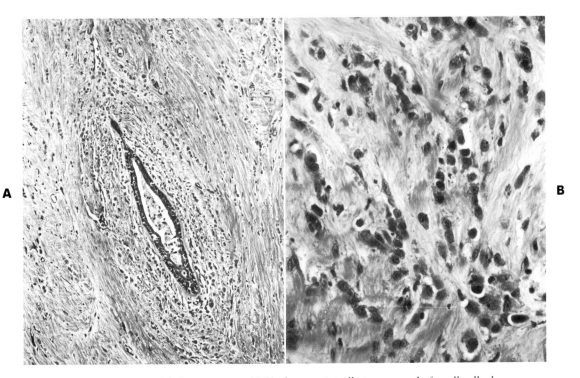

Fig. 12-54 Invasive lobular carcinoma (ILC) characteristically is composed of small cells that invade in cords or chains without evidence of tubular formation through a fibrous stroma. The targetoid pattern of infiltrating tumor cells ringing around an uninvolved duct is seen in **A.** The small tumor cells with hyperchromatic nuclei and scant cytoplasm are evident in **B.** This photomicrograph also illustrates the characteristic chains of cells or Indian file pattern of ILC.

CARCINOMAS WITH SPECIAL CLINICAL PRESENTATIONS

Paget's disease and inflammatory carcinoma represent two types of carcinoma with distinctive clinical presentations.

Paget's disease of the nipple

Paget's disease of the nipple presents with the specific clinical findings of a red ulcerated lesion of the nipple–areolar complex. The term *eczema of the nipple* is most often used to describe this clinical appearance. The ulceration and erythema are due to the presence of tumor cells within the epidermis of the nipple. The association of this rash with an underlying breast carcinoma was first described by Sir James Paget.[147] Despite the fact that a palpable breast mass may not be detected, carcinoma is invariably present in the breast. The lesion may be a pure DCIS, confined to the major lactiferous ducts, or it may be a clinically occult invasive carcinoma.[142]

The cells of Paget's disease are generally considered to be adenocarcinoma cells, which migrate into the epidermis of the nipple from cancer involving ducts in underlying breast tissue. Immunohistochemical and electron microscopic studies have shown that these cells show immunostaining patterns distinct from the surrounding epidermal keratinocytes and similar to those for mammary ductal epithelium and epithelium of apocrine and eccrine sweat glands.[143,146]

Recent molecular studies have suggested, however, that cells of mammary Paget's disease are polyclonal in origin, unlike cells from ductal adenocarcinoma, which are monoclonal.[148] This raises again the possibility that the cells of mammary Paget's disease may arise from precursor cells (possibly analogous to poral sweat gland cells) within the nipple, separate from the underlying breast cancer, a theory that has been suggested for the breast but more commonly accepted for extramammary Paget's disease.[145]

Although the nipple may frequently be involved by underlying breast cancer, the clinical presentation of Paget's disease is distinctly less common. By serial subgross and correlated radiographic technique, carcinoma involving the nipple was found in as many as 4.7% of 149 mastectomies but only 1 of 7 cases was recognized clinically.[144]

Most often the radiographic appearance demonstrates direct nipple involvement with nipple retraction or areolar edema associated with an underlying breast cancer, usually palpable. Less frequently the radiographic manifestation of Paget's disease of the nipple is that of casting type calcifications of ductal carcinoma extending into the ducts at the base of the nipple or into the nipple itself. A bright light may be required to examine the portion of the ducts that traverse the erectile tissue of the nipple in assessing extent of involvement mammographically. Masking of extraneous light is suggested to increase perception of nipple and subareolar mammographic changes.

Inflammatory carcinoma

Inflammatory carcinoma presents clinically as a swollen inflamed breast, resembling acute mastitis. The swelling and induration of the skin are the result of lymphedema secondary to tumor emboli in dermal lymphatics (dermal lymphatic carcinomatosis).[153] The extensive edema may make it difficult to detect the underlying invasive carcinoma by palpation. Diagnosis may be made by skin biopsy or by fine needle aspiration if the tumor can be palpated or mammographically localized.

Inflammatory carcinoma accounts for approximately 2.4% of cases of breast cancer in a large university clinic.[152] Inflammatory carcinoma has been reported in persons from age 12 to 75 years. The average age is the same for invasive breast cancer of no specific type.[160]

BOX 12-6 MAMMOGRAPHIC FINDINGS IN INFLAMMATORY CARCINOMA OF THE BREAST

Overall increased breast density
Increased skin thickness
Prominent subcutaneous lymphatics

BOX 12-7 DIFFERENTIAL DIAGNOSIS OF DIFFUSE SKIN THICKENING OF THE BREAST

Inflammatory breast cancer
Congestive heart failure[161]*
Superior vena cava obstruction*
Lymphatic obstruction due to lymphoma, Hodgkin's disease[154]
Breast abscess or mastitis[154]
S/P radiation therapy[151]
Myxedema*
Acromegaly[156]*
Surgery of chest wall or axilla[159]
Fat necrosis[154]

*May be bilateral.

The radiographic findings in patients with inflammatory breast cancer are most often a diffuse increased density within the breast parenchyma accompanied by skin thickening.[150] Frequently no focal mass nor area of calcifications is discernible within the breast. The appearance is nonspecific and can also be caused by diffuse mastitis. The mammographic finding of a diffuse increase in breast density may be subtle in some cases[152] (Box 12-6). There are several non-neoplastic causes of diffuse skin thickening of the breast (Box 12-7).

The physical examination of the patient with inflammatory carcinoma reveals a heavy, usually painful, indurated breast with warmth and erythema of the skin giving the clinical description of inflammatory carcinoma. A breast may be diffusely infiltrated with cancer and have skin edema due to dermal lymphatic cancer (peau d'orange), and yet not be associated with the classic erythema of inflammatory breast cancer.[158] Lymphatic obstruction in the axilla also causes skin edema without inflammation.[157] To qualify as inflammatory carcinoma of the breast, at least one third of the skin of the breast is found to be erythematous.[155]

The diagnosis of inflammatory breast cancer is most directly made by a skin biopsy that confirms tumor cells in the dermal lymphatics. Open biopsy or fine needle aspiration cytology may also confirm the diagnosis of cancer. However, the presence of cancer cells within dermal lymphatics is required to establish the clinical diagnosis of inflammatory breast cancer. The axillary lymph nodes are most often involved with metastatic carcinoma at the time of clinical presentation.

The prognosis of patients with inflammatory breast cancer is poor. Treatment is directed at reducing the tumor burden by chemotherapy or radiation therapy or both prior to mastectomy.

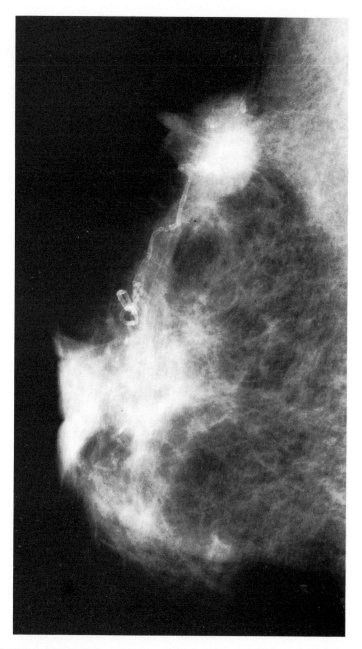

Fig. 12-55 Invasive ductal carcinoma and Paget's disease. Oblique projection shows large spiculated mass in upper outer quadrant with associated subareolar extent, areolar skin thickening, and nipple retraction. The findings illustrated are 9 months post-chemotherapy for inflammatory carcinoma with Paget's disease of the nipple.

Fig. 12-56 Paget's disease of the nipple. The large tumor cells with pale cytoplasm are distributed within the epidermis of the nipple, either singly close to the basemens membrane, or in clusters.

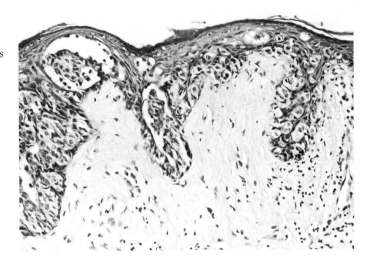

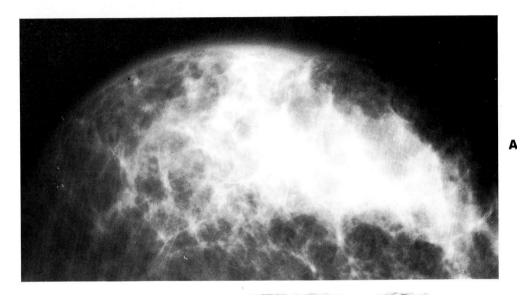

A

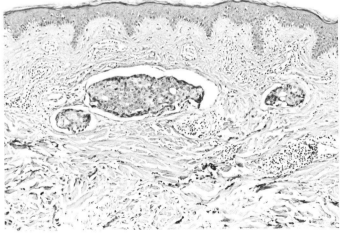

B

Fig. 12-57 Inflammatory breast cancer. **(A)** Classic skin thickening associated with diffuse increase in density of parenchyma. **(B)** The typical clinical appearance of inflammatory breast cancer is due to lymphedema of the skin secondary to numerous tumor emboli present in dermal lymphatic spaces, which are shown in this photomicrograph.

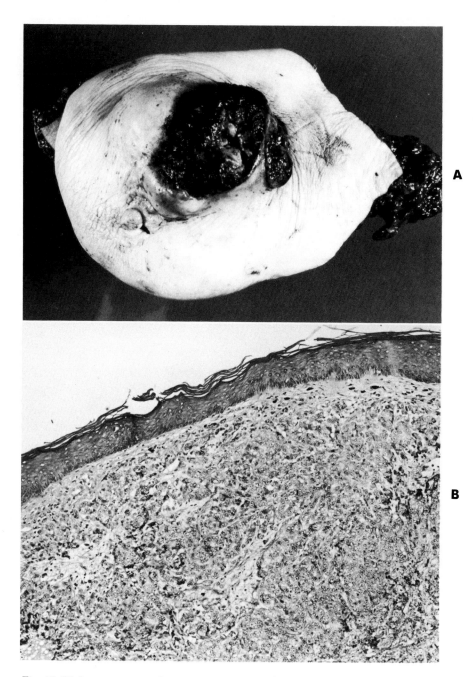

Fig. 12-58 In contrast to inflammatory carcinoma, this advanced breast cancer shows ulceration and invasion of skin by the underlying tumor **(A)**. The anaplastic tumor cells extend up to the epidermis in **B,** but lymphedema and tumor emboli are not present. (**A** is from Golden A, Powell DE, Jennings CD: *Pathology: Understanding human disease,* ed 2, Baltimore, 1985, Williams and Wilkins.)

REFERENCES

Introduction

1. Anderson DE: Familial versus sporadic breast cancer, *Cancer* 70:1740, 1992.
2. Donovan AJ: Bilateral breast cancer, *Surg Clin North Am* 70:1141, 1990.
3. Ephross SA, Morris PL, Hulka BS: Increases in breast cancer incidence and mortality rates between 1975 and 1986 in white and black Americans: a screening effect or an alarming trend? *Am J Epidemiol* 132:790, 1990.
4. Hall JM, Lee MK, Newman B: Linkage of early onset familial breast cancer to chromosome 17q 21, *Science* 250:1684, 1990.
5. Glass A, Hoover RN: Changing incidence of breast cancer, *J Natl Cancer Inst* 80:1076, 1988.
6. Harris JR, Lippman M, Veronesi U, et al: Breast cancer, *N Engl J Med* 327:319, 1992.
7. Lynch HT, Watson P, Conway TA, et al: Natural history and age at onset of hereditary breast cancer, *Cancer* 69:1404, 1992.
8. Miller BA, Feuer EJ, Hankey BF: The increasing incidence of breast cancer since 1982: relevance of early detection, *Cancer Causes Control* 2:67, 1991.
9. Skolnick MH, Cannon-Albright LA: Genetic predisposition to breast cancer, *Cancer* 70:1747, 1992.
10. Wellings SR: A hypothesis of the origin of human breast cancer from the terminal ductal lobular unit, *Pathol Res Pract* 166:515, 1980.
11. Wellings SR, Jensen HM: On the origin and progression of ductal carcinoma in the human breast, *J Natl Cancer Inst* 50:1111, 1973.

In situ carcinoma
Ductal carcinoma in situ

12. Ashikari R, Hajdu SI, Robbins GF: Intraductal carcinoma of the breast (1960-1969), *Cancer* 28:1182, 1971.
13. Azzopardi JG: *Problems in breast pathology* vol 11, London, 1979, In *Major problems in pathology series*, WB Saunders.
14. Betsill WL, Rosen PP, Lieberman PH: Intraductal carcinoma: long-term follow-up after treatment by biopsy alone, *JAMA* 239:1863, 1978.
15. D'agincourt L: Early detection of DCIS broadens therapy options, *Diagn Imaging* pg. 80, September 1992.
16. Dershaw DD, Abramson A, Kinne DW: Ductal carcinoma in situ: mammographic findings and clinical implications, *Radiology* 170:411, 1989.
17. Franceschi D, Crowe J, Zollinger R, et al: Breast biopsy for calcifications in nonpalpable breast lesions, *Arch Surg* 125:170, 1990.
18. Harris JR, Lippman ME, Veronesi U, et al: Medical progress: breast cancer (second of three parts), *N Engl J Med* 327(6):390, 1992.
19. Hall FM: Mammography in the diagnosis of in situ breast carcinoma, *Radiology* 168:279, 1988.
20. Holland R, Hendriks JHCL, Verbeek ALM, et al: Clinical practice: extent, distribution and mammographic/histological correlations of breast ductal carcinoma in situ, *Lancet* 335:519, 1990.
21. Homer MJ, Safaii H, Smith TJ, et al: The relationship of mammographic microcalcifications to histologic malignancy: radiologic-pathologic correlation, *AJR Am J Roentgenol* 153:1187, 1989.
22. Ikeda DM, Andersson I: Ductal carcinoma in situ: atypical mammographic appearances, *Radiology* 172:661, 1989.
23. Ikeda DM, Andersson I: Ductal carcinoma in situ: atypical mammographic appearance (Letter), *Radiology* 175:285, 1990.
24. Lagios MD, Margolin FR, Westdahl RR, et al: Mammographically detected duct carcinoma in situ: frequency of local recurrence following tylectomy and prognostic effect of nuclear grade on local recurrence, *Cancer* 63:618, 1989.
25. Lilleng R, Hagman BM, Nesland JM: C-erb B-2 protein and neuroendocrine expression in intraductal carcinomas of the breast, *Mod Pathol* 5:41, 1992.
26. Meyer JE, Eberlein TJ, Stomper PC, et al: Biopsy of occult breast lesions, analysis of 1261 abnormalities, *JAMA* 263:2341, 1990.
27. Meyer JS: Cell kinetics of histologic variants of in situ breast carcinoma, *Breast Cancer Res Treat* 7:171, 1986.
28. Mitnick JS, Roses DF, Harris MN, et al: Circumscribed intraductal carcinoma of the breast, *Radiology* 170:423, 1989.
29. Mitnick JS, Roses DF, Harris MN, et al: Circumscribed intraductal carcinoma of the breast, *Radiology* 172:579, 1989 (letter).
29a. Page DL, Anderson TJ: Diagnostic histopathology of the breast, London, Churchill Livingstone, p. 172.
30. Page DL, Dupont WD, Rogers LW, et al: Intraductal carcinoma of the breast: follow-up after biopsy only, *Cancer* 49:751, 1982.
31. Rosen PP: Axillary lymph node metastases in patients with occult noninvasive breast carcinoma, *Cancer* 46:1298, 1980.

32. Schuh ME, Nemoto T, Penetrante RB, et al: Intraductal carcinoma: analysis of presentation, pathologic findings, and outcome of disease, *Arch Surg* 121:1303, 1986.
33. Schnitt SJ, Silen W, Sadowsky NL, et al: Current concepts: ductal carcinoma in situ (intraductal carcinoma) of the breast, *N Engl J Med* 318:898, 1988.
34. Schwartz GF, Patchefsky AS, Finklestein SD, et al: Nonpalpable in situ ductal carcinoma of the breast: predictors of multicentricity and microinvasion and implications for treatment, *Arch Surg* 124:29, 1989.
35. Shaw de Paredes E, Langer TG: Subtle signs of carcinoma, *Appl Radiol* p 15, September 1992.
36. Sickles EA: Mammographic features of "early" breast cancer, *AJR Am J Roentgenol* 143:461, 1984.
37. Silverstein MJ, Rosser RJ, Gierson ED, et al: Axillary lymph node dissection for intraductal breast carcinoma: is it indicated? *Cancer* 59:1819, 1987.
38. Stomper PC, Connolly JL: Ductal carcinoma in situ of the breast: correlation between mammographic calcification and tumor subtype, *AJR Am J Roentgenol* 159:483, 1992.
39. Stomper PC, Connolly JL, Meyer JE, et al: Clinically occult ductal carcinoma in situ detected with mammography: analysis of 100 cases with radiologic-pathologic correlation, *Radiology* 172:235, 1989.
40. Wilson JF, Destouet JM, Winchester DP, et al: 1991 RSNA Special Focus Session: current controversies in the management of ductal carcinoma in situ of the breast, *Radiology* 185:77, 1992.
41. Wong JH, Kopald KH, Morton DL: The impact of microinvasion on axillary metastases and survival in patients with intraductal breast cancer, *Arch Surg* 125:1298, 1990.

Lobular carcinoma in situ

42. Beute BJ, Kalisher L, Hutter RVP: Lobular carcinoma in situ of the breast: clinical, pathologic and mammographic features, *AJR Am J Roentgenol* 157:257, 1991.
43. Foote FW Jr, Stewart FW: Lobular carcinoma in situ: a rare form of mammary cancer, *Am J Pathol* 17:491, 1941.
44. Haagensen CD, Lane N, Bodian C: Coexisting lobular neoplasia and carcinoma of the breast, *Cancer* 51:1468, 1983.
45. Haagensen CD, Lane N, Lattes R, Bodian C: Lobular neoplasia (so-called lobular carcinoma *in situ*) of the breast, *Cancer* 42:737, 1978.
46. Hutter RVP, Synder RE, Lucas JC, et al: Clinical and pathologic correlation with mammographic findings in lobular carcinoma in situ, *Cancer* 23:826, 1969.
47. McDivitt RW, Hutter RVP, Foote FW Jr, Stewart FW: In situ lobular carcinoma: a prospective follow-up study indicating cumulative patient risks, *JAMA* 201:82, 1967.
48. Page DL, Kidd JE, Dupont WD, et al: Lobular neoplasia of the breast: higher risk for subsequent invasive cancer predicted by more extensive disease, *Hum Pathol* 22:1232, 1991.
49. Pope TL, Fechner RE, Wilhelm MC, et al: Lobular carcinoma in situ of the breast: mammographic features, *Radiology* 168:63, 1988.
50. Rosen PP, Lieberman PH, Braum DW, et al: Lobular carcinoma *in-situ* of the breast, *Am J Surg Pathol* 2:225, 1978.
51. Snyder RE: Mammography and lobular carcinoma in situ, *Surg Obstet Gynecol* 122:255, 1966.
52. Sonnenfeld MR, Frenna TH, Weidener V, Meyer JE: Lobular carcinoma in situ: mammographic-pathologic correlation of results of needle-directed biopsy, *Radiology* 181:363, 1991.

Invasive carcinoma
Invasive ductal carcinoma

53. Baak JPA: Mitosis counting in tumors, *Hum Pathol* 21:683, 1990.
54. Baak JPA, Von Dop H, Jurver PHJ, et al: The value of morphometry to classic prognosticators in breast cancer, *Cancer* 56:374, 1985.
55. Bloom HJ, Richardson WW: Histological grading and prognosis in breast cancer, *Br J Cancer* 11:359, 1957.
56. Boyages J, Recht A, Connolly J, et al: Factors associated with local recurrence as a first site of failure following the conservative treatment of early breast cancer, *Recent Results Cancer Res* 115:92, 1989.
57. Donegan WL: Evaluation of a palpable breast mass, *N Engl J Med* 327:937, 1992.
58. Donegan WL: Prognostic factors: stage and receptor status in breast cancer, *Cancer* 70:1755, 1992.
59. Elston CW: *Grading of invasive carcinoma of the breast.* In Page DL, Anderson TJ, editors: *Diagnostic histopathology of the breast,* London, Churchill Livingstone, p 303.
60. Elston CW, Gresham GA, Rao GS, et al: The Cancer Research Campaign (King's/Cambridge) trial for early breast cancer: clinico-pathological aspects, *Br J Cancer* 45:655, 1982.
61. Fisher ER, Redmond C, Fisher B: Histologic grading of breast cancer, *Pathol Ann* 15:239, 1980.
62. Gallager HS, Martin JE: Early phases in the development of breast cancer, *Cancer* 24:1170, 1969.
63. Gallagher HS, Martin JE: An orientation to the concept of minimal breast cancer, *Cancer* 28:1505, 1971.
64. Hartman WH: Minimal breast cancer: an update, *Cancer* 53:681, 1984.

65. Hilsenbeck SG, Allred DC: Improved methods of estimating mitotic activity in solid tumors, *Hum Pathol* 23:601, 1992.
66. Jackson VP, Dines KA, Bassett LW, et al: Diagnostic importance of the radiographic density of noncalcified breast masses: analysis of 91 lesions, *AJR Am J Roentgenol* 157:25, 1991.
67. Kopans DB, Swann CA, White G, et al: Asymmetric breast tissue, *Radiology* 171:639, 1989,
68. Lagios MD, Westdahl PR, Rose MR: The concept and implications of multicentricity in breast carcinoma, *Pathol Ann* 16(2):83, 1981.
69. Le Doussal V, Tubiana-Hulin M, Friedman S, et al: Prognostic value of histologic grade nuclear components of Scarff-Bloom-Richardson (SBR): an improved score modification based on a multivariant analysis of 1262 invasive ductal carcinomas, *Cancer* 64:1914, 1989.
70. McGuire WL, Clark GM: Prognostic factors and treatment decisions in axillary node-negative breast cancer, *N Engl J Med* 326:1756, 1992.
71. Newstead GM, Baute PB, Toth HK: Invasive lobular and ductal carcinoma: mammographic findings and stage at diagnosis, *Radiology* 184:623, 1992.
72. Page DL, Anderson TJ: Diagnostic histopathology of the breast, London, Churchill Livingstone, pp 278-279.
73. Page DL: Prognosis and breast cancer, *Am J Surg Pathol* 15:334, 1991.
74. Parl FF, DuPont WD: A retrospective cohort study of histologic risk factors in breast cancer patients, *Cancer* 50:2410, 1982.
75. Sickles EA: Mammographic features of 300 consecutive nonpalpable breast cancers, *AJR Am J Roentgenol* 146:661, 1986.
76. Simpson JF, Duff PL, Page DL: Expression of mitoses per thousand cells and cell density in breast carcinomas: a proposal, *Hum Pathol* 23:608, 1992.
77. Stekvist B, Westman-Nalser S, Vegelius J, et al: Analysis of reproducibility of subjective grading systems for breast carcinoma, *J Clin Pathol* 32:979, 1979.
78. Stomper PC, Connolly JL: Mammographic features predicting an extensive intraductal component in early-stage infiltrating ductal carcinoma. *AJR Am J Roentgenol* 158:269, 1992.
79. Stomper PC, Davis SP, Weidner N, et al: Clinically occult, noncalcified breast cancer: serial radiologic-pathologic correlation in 27 cases, *Radiology* 169:621, 1988.
80. Swann CA, Kopans DB, Koerner FC, et al: The halo sign and malignant breast lesions, *AJR Am J Roentgenol* 149:1145, 1987.
81. vanDiest PJ, Baak JPA, Matze-Cok P, et al: Reproducibility of mitosis counting in 2469 breast cancer specimens: results from the multicenter morphometric mammary carcinoma project, *Hum Pathol* 23:603, 1992.

Tubular carcinoma

82. Carstens PHB: Tubular carcinoma of the breast: a study of frequency, *Am J Clin Pathol* 70:204, 1978.
83. Carstens PHB, Huvas AG, Foote PW, Ashikari R: Tubular carcinoma of the breast, *Am J Clin Pathol* 58:231, 1972.
84. Cooper HS, Patchefsky AS, Krall RA: Tubular carcinoma of the breast, *Cancer* 42:2334, 1978.
85. Feig SA, Shaber GS, Patchefsky AS, et al: Tubular carcinoma of the breast: mammographic appearance and pathological correlation, *Radiology* 129:311, 1978.
86. Flotte TJ, Bell DA, Greco MA: Tubular carcinoma and sclerosing adenosis: the use of basal lamina as a differential feature, *Am J Surg Pathol* 4:75, 1980.
87. Lagios MD, Rose MR, Margolin FR: Tubular carcinoma of the breast: association with multicentricity, bilaterality, and family history of mammary carcinoma, *Am J Clin Pathol* 73:25, 1980.
88. Oberman HA, Fidler WJ: Tubular carcinoma of the breast, *Am J Surg Pathol* 13:387, 1979.
89. Page DL, Anderson TJ: *Diagnostic histopathology of the breast*, London, Churchill Livingstone, p 210.
90. Patchefsky AS, Shaber GS, Schwartz GJ, et al: The pathology of breast cancer detected by mass population screening, *Cancer* 40:1659, 1977.
91. Taylor HB, Norris HJ: Well-differentiated carcinoma of the breast, *Cancer* 25:687, 1970.
92. Tremblay G: Elastosis in tubular carcinoma of the breast, *Arch Pathol* 98:302, 1974.

Mucinous carcinoma

93. Bassett LW, Gold RH, Kimme-Smith C: *Hand held and automated breast ultrasound*, Thorofare, NJ, Slack, p. 120.
94. Clayton F: Pure mucinous carcinoma of the breast, *Hum Pathol* 17:34, 1986.
95. Cole-Beuglet C, Soriano RZ, Kurtz AB, et al: Ultrasound analysis of 104 primary breast carcinomas classified according to histopathologic type, *Radiology* 147:191, 1983.
96. Koehl RL, Snyder RE, Hutter RVP, et al: The incidence and significance of calcifications within operative breast specimens, *Am J Clin Pathol* 53:3, 1970.
97. Rasmussen BB, Rose C, Christensen I: Prognostic factors in primary mucinous breast carcinoma, *Am J Clin Pathol* 87:155, 1987.
98. Rosen PP: Mucocele-like tumors of the breast, *Am J Surg Pathol* 10:464, 1986.

99. Rosen PP, Lesser ML, Kinne DW: Breast carcinoma at the extremes of age: a comparison of patients younger than 35 years and older than 75 years, *J Surg Oncol* 28:90, 1985.
100. Schneider JA: Invasive papillary breast carcinoma: Mammographic and sonographic appearance, *Radiology* 171:377, 1989.
101. Troupin RH: Mammographic-pathologic correlation. In Feig SA, editor: *ARRS categorical course syllabus: breast imaging,* 1988, p 79.

Medullary cancer

102. Bloom HJG, Richardson WW, Fields JR: Host resistance and survival in carcinoma of breast: a study of 104 cases of medullary carcinoma in a series of 1,411 cases of breast cancer followed for 20 years, *Br Med J* 3:181, 1970.
103. Howell LP, Kline TS: Medullary carcinoma of the breast: an unusual cytologic finding in cyst fluid aspirates, *Cancer* 65:277, 1990.
104. Kopans DB: Medullary carcinoma of the breast, *Radiology* 171:876, 1989 (Letter).
105. Meyer JE, Amin E, Lindfors KK, et al: Medullary carcinoma of the breast: mammographic and US appearance, *Radiology* 170:79, 1989.
106. Rapin V, Contesso G, Mouriesse H, et al: Medullary breast carcinomas: a re-evaluation of 95 cases of breast cancer with inflammatory stroma, *Cancer* 61:2503, 1988.
107. Richardson WW: Medullary carcinoma of the breast: a distinctive tumor type with a relatively good prognosis following radical mastectomy, *Br J Cancer* 10:415, 1956.
108. Ridolfi RL, Rosen PP, Post A, et al: Medullary carcinoma of the breast: a clinicopathologic study with 10 year follow-up, *Cancer* 40:1365, 1977.
109. Rosen PP, Lesser ML, Kinne DW, et al: Breast carcinoma in women 35 years of age or younger, *Ann Surg* 199:133, 1984.
110. Wallis MG, Walsh MT, Lee JR: A review of false negative mammography in a symptomatic population, *Clin Radiol* 44:13, 1991.

Papillary carcinoma

111. Fisher ER, Palekar AS, Redmond C, et al: Pathologic findings from the national surgical adjuvant breast project (Protocol No. 4). VI: Invasive papillary cancer, *Am J Clin Pathol* 73:313, 1980.
112. Page DL, Dixon JM, Anderson TJ, et al: Invasive cribiform carcinoma of the breast, *Histopathology* 7:525, 1983.

Rare special types

113. Eusebi V, Millis RR, Castani MG, et al: Apocrine carcinoma of the breast: a morphologic and immunochemical study, *Am J Pathol* 123:532, 1986.
114. Fisher ER, Gregorio RM, Palekar AS, Paulson JD: Mucoepidermoid and squamous cell carcinomas of breast with reference to squamous metaplasia and giant cell tumors, *Am J Surg Pathol* 7:15, 1983.
115. Hull MT, Warfel KA: Glycogen-rich clear cell carcinomas of the breast: a clinicopathologic and ultrastructural study, *Am J Surg Pathol* 10:553, 1986.
116. Leeming R, Jenkins M, Mendehlson G: Adenoid cystic carcinoma of the breast, *Arch Surg* 127:233, 1992.
117. Loose JH, Patchefsky AS, Hollander IJ, et al: Adenomyoepithelioma of the breast: a spectrum of biologic behavior, *Am J Surg Pathol* 16:868, 1992.
118. Moran CA, Suster S, Carter D: Benign mixed tumors (pleomorphic adenomas) of the breast, *Am J Surg Pathol* 14:913, 1990.
119. Mossler JA, Barton TK, Brinkhous AD, et al: Apocrine differentiation in human mammary carcinoma, *Cancer* 46:2463, 1980.
120. Oberman HA: Metaplastic carcinoma of the breast: a clinicopathologic study of 29 patients, *Am J Surg Pathol* 11:918, 1987.
121. Page DL, Anderson TJ: *Diagnostic histopathology of the breast,* London, 1987, Churchill Livingston, p 294.
122. Peters GN, Wolff M: Adenoid cystic carcinoma of the breast, *Cancer* 52:680, 1982.
123. Ramos CV, Taylor HB: Lipid-rich carcinoma of the breast: a clinicopathologic analysis of 13 examples, *Cancer* 33:812, 1974.
124. Tavassoli FA: Myoepithelial lesions of the breast: myoepitheliosis, adenomyoepithelioma and myoepithelial carcinoma, *Am J Surg Pathol* 15:554, 1991.
125. Tavassoli FA, Norris HJ: Secretory carcinoma of the breast, *Cancer* 45:2404, 1980.
126. Wargotz ES, Deos PH, Norris HJ: Metaplastic carcinomas of the breast II. Spindle cell carcinoma, *Hum Pathol* 20:732, 1989.
127. Wargotz ES, Norris HJ: Metaplastic carcinomas of the breast I. Matrix producing carcinoma, *Hum Pathol* 20:628, 1989.
128. Wargotz ES, Norris HJ: Metaplastic carcinomas of the breast III. Carcinosarcoma, *Cancer* 64:1490, 1989.
129. Wargotz ES, Norris HJ: Metaplastic carcinoma of the breast IV. Squamous cell carcinomas of ductal origin, *Cancer* 65:272, 1990.
130. Wargotz ES, Norris HJ: Metaplastic carcinoma of the breast V. Metaplastic carcinoma with osteoclastic giant cells, *Hum Pathol* 21:1142, 1990.

Invasive lobular carcinoma

131. Adler OB, Engel A: Invasive lobular carcinoma: mammographic pattern, *ROFO* 152(4):460, 1990.
131a. Bussolati G, Papotti M, Sapino A, et al: Endocrine markers in argyrophilic carcinomas of the breast, *Am J Surg Pathol*, 11:248, 1987.
132. Dixon JM, Anderson TJ, Page DL, et al: Infiltrating lobular carcinoma of the breast, *Histopathology* 6:149, 1982.
133. DiCostanzo D, Rosen PP, Gareen I, et al: Prognosis in infiltrating lobular carcinoma: an analysis of "classical" and variant tumors, *Am J Surg Pathol* 14:12, 1990.
134. Fechner R: Histologic variants of invasive lobular carcinoma of the breast, *Hum Pathol* 6:373, 1975.
134a. Helvie MA, Paramagul C, Oberman HA, Adler DD: Invasive lobular carcinoma: imaging features and clinical detection, *Invest Radiol*, 28:202, 1993.
135. Hilleren DJ, Anderson IT, Lindholm K, et al: Invasive lobular carcinoma: mammographic findings in a 10-year experience, *Radiology* 178:149, 1991.
136. LeGal M, Ollivier L, Asselain B, et al: Mammographic features of 455 invasive lobular carcinomas, *Radiology* 185:705, 1992.
137. Martinez V, Azzopardi JG: Invasive lobular carcinoma of the breast: incidence and variants, *Histopathology* 3:467, 1979.
138. Mendelson EB, Harris KM, Doshi N, et al: Infiltrating lobular carcinoma: mammographic patterns with pathologic correlation, *AJR Am J Roentgenol* 153:265, 1989.
139. Merino MJ, LiVolsi VA: Signet ring carcinoma of the female breast: a clinicopathologic analysis of 24 cases, *Cancer* 48:1830, 1981.
140. Page DL, Anderson TJ: *Diagnostic histopathology of the breast*, Churchill Livingstone, London, 1987, p 261.
141. Sickles EA. The subtle and atypical mammographic features of invasive lobular carcinoma, *Radiology* 178:25, 1991.

Carcinomas with special clinical presentations
Paget's disease of the nipple

142. Ashikari R, Park K, Huvos AG, et al: Paget's disease of the breast, *Cancer* 26:680, 1970.
143. Chaudary MA, Millis RR, Lane B, et al: Paget's disease of the nipple: a ten year review including clinical, pathological and immunohistochemical findings, *Breast Cancer Res Treat* 8:139, 1986.
144. Lagios MD, Gates EA, Westdahl PR, et al: A guide to the frequency of nipple involvement in breast cancer: a study of 149 consecutive mastectomies using a serial subgross and correlated radiographic technique, *Am J Surg* 138:135, 1979.
145. Nadji M, Morales AR, Girlanner RE, et al: Paget's disease of the skin: a unifying concept of histogenesis, *Cancer* 50:2203, 1982.
146. Ordonez NG, Awalt H, Mackay B: Mammary and extramammary Paget's disease: an immunocytochemical and ultrastructural study, *Cancer* 59:1173, 1987.
147. Paget J: On disease of the mammary areola preceding cancer of the mammary gland, *St Barth Hosp Rep* 10:87, 1874.
148. Remotti H, Watson L, Barsky S: Mammary Paget's disease: evidence for a multicentric polyclonal-epithelial "field" neoplasm lacking true epithelial invasion, *Mod Pathol* 5:17A, 1992 (abstract).
149. Toker C: Some observations on Paget's disease of the nipple, *Cancer* 14:653, 1961.

Inflammatory carcinoma

150. Berger SM: Inflammatory carcinoma of the breast. *AJR Am J Roentgenol* 88:1109, 1962.
151. Bloomer WD, Berenberg AL, Weissman BN: Mammography of the definitively irradiated breast, *Radiology* 118:425, 1976.
152. Droulias CA, Sewell CW, McSweeney MB, et al: Inflammatory carcinoma of the breast: a correlation of clinical, radiologic, and pathological findings, *Ann Surg* 184:217, 1976.
153. Ellis DL, Teitelbaum SL: Inflammatory carcinoma of the breast: a pathologic definition, *Cancer* 33:1045, 1974.
154. Gold RH, Montgomery CK, Minagai H, et al: The significance of mammary skin thickening in disorders other than primary carcinoma: a roentgenologic-pathologic correlation, *AJR Am J Roentgenol* 112:613, 1971.
155. Haagensen CD: *Diseases of the breast*, ed 2, Philadelphia, 1971, WB Saunders.
156. Hall DA, Kalisher L: The breast as mirror of systemic diseases, *Rev Interam Radiol* 2(4):211, 1977.
157. Kushner LN: Hodgkin's disease simulating inflammatory breast carcinoma on mammography, *Radiology* 92:350, 1969.
158. Lucas FV, Perez-Mesa C: Inflammatory carcinoma of the breast, *Cancer* 41:1595, 1978.
159. Morrish HF: The significance and limitations of skin thickening as a diagnostic sign in mammography, *AJR Am J Roentgenol* 96:1041, 1966.
160. Nichini FM, Goldman L, Lapayowker MS, et al: Inflammatory carcinoma of the breast in a 12-year-old girl, *Arch Surg* 105:505, 1972.
161. Stoltz JL, Friedman AK, Arger PH: Breast cancer simulation: mammography in congestive heart failure mimics acute mastitis and advanced carcinoma, *JAMA* 229:682, 1974.

CHAPTER 13

Stromal, Vascular, Hematolymphoid, and Metastatic Breast Lesions

Carol B. Stelling
Deborah E. Powell

Stromal lesions
    Sarcomas
        Fibrosarcoma and malignant fibrous histiocytoma
        Liposarcoma
        Leiomyosarcoma
    Fibromatoses and benign stromal tumors
        Fibromatosis or extraabdominal desmoid
        Diabetic mastopathy
        Focal fibrosis
        Granular cell tumor
        Other benign stromal tumors
Vascular lesions
    Benign vascular lesions
        Mondor's disease
        Angiosarcoma
        Hemangiopericytoma
Hematolymphoid breast lesions
    Lymphoma and Hodgkin's disease
    Pseudolymphoma
    Hematologic malignancies
Metastatic disease

STROMAL LESIONS

Sarcomas

Sarcomas of the breast are rare and may arise from any of the stromal elements. Fibrosarcoma and liposarcoma are reported more frequently among the various histologic types. Angiosarcomas are described in the section on vascular lesions. Malignant fibrous histiocytoma, leiomyosarcoma, chondrosarcoma, and osteogenic sarcoma also occur as primary lesions within the breast but are extremely rare.[12,14,16,19] Other rare histologic types of sarcoma have been described (Box 13-1).[18] The prognosis associated with each type of sarcoma is related to the cell of origin as well as to the histologic grade of the tumor.[2]

Sarcomas represent less than 1% of all malignant tumors of the breast.[9,16] Primary sarcomas are seen most commonly as a painless palpable mass, 2 to 13 cm in diameter, occurring in persons of various ages.[16] However, symptoms of pain, tenderness, nipple retraction, and skin thickening have also been described.[8,16] Clinical lymphadenopathy may be present but is most often due to reactive hyperplasia.[8] Metastatic spread is invariably hematogenous and usually pulmonary, and it occurs generally within 5 years of diagnosis.[16]

BOX 13-1 STROMAL SARCOMAS OF THE BREAST

Fibrosarcoma
Malignant fibrous histiocytoma
Liposarcoma
Leiomyosarcoma
Osteogenic sarcoma
Chondrosarcoma
Neurogenic sarcoma
Alveolar soft part sarcoma
Rhabdomyosarcoma
Others

Prior radiation therapy to the breast is a known risk factor for development of sarcoma, but most lesions arise de novo.[16]

Sarcomas of the breast must be distinguished from the malignant phyllodes tumor discussed in Chapter 9 and the more common metaplastic or spindle cell carcinomas discussed in Chapter 12. The phyllodes tumor has the characteristic leaf-like growth pattern, which frequently can be recognized grossly. It also has a recognizable benign epithelial component, although this may be less prominent in the malignant phyllodes tumors.

Spindle cell carcinomas may be particularly difficult to distinguish from true sarcomas of the breast. The distinction is important and is not simply a matter of pathologic accuracy. Spindle cell carcinomas are epithelial tumors that metastasize to regional lymph nodes; node sampling must be part of the treatment procedure for these patients. In contrast, true breast sarcomas rarely if ever metastasize to regional lymph nodes[7]; hence, treatment should be directed toward removing all of the breast tumor with adequate margins and assessing the patient for distant metastatic spread and possible adjunctive chemotherapy. Although in persons with spindle cell (and metaplastic) carcinomas, epithelial differentiation can often be recognized with extensive sampling of the tumor, sometimes immunohistochemistry is required for correct diagnosis. True sarcomas are vimentin positive but stain negative for low molecular weight cytokeratins.[14] As mentioned in Chapter 12, spindle cell carcinomas are cytokeratin positive in at least some areas, although they also frequently stain positively for vimentin.

Although many sarcomas of the breast show evidence of histologic differentiation as smooth muscle, fat, or fibroblasts, often the predominant pattern is a proliferation of spindle cells. Berg and associates[3] suggested that these tumors be classified simply as stromal sarcomas. Their series of 25 patients had a somewhat more favorable prognosis than a group of 40 patients with malignant phyllodes tumors. They suggested that attempts to further classify stromal tumors as to cell of origin might be unimportant (except in the case of angiosarcomas) and that the important distinction was to differentiate them from phyllodes tumors. This notion has not been widely accepted, however, and usually investigators attempt to define the cell of origin of breast sarcomas using electron microscopy and, more recently, immunohistochemistry, if necessary. This approach is based on the strong impression that cell of origin in addition to tumor grade is an important predictor of recurrence and prognosis.[2,15] In addition to histologic grade, tumor contour and mitotic counts are of importance in predicting aggressive behavior for breast sarcomas in general.[2]

In the following sections, the specific histologic subtypes of fibrosarcoma and malignant fibrous histiocytoma, liposarcoma, and leiomyosarcoma are discussed.

Fibrosarcoma and malignant fibrous histiocytoma. Pure fibrosarcoma (FS) of the breast occurs in less than 1% of a symptomatic population.[9] Histopathologically, the FS is composed of spindle cells frequently arranged in interwoven bundles or fascicles in a recognizable pattern referred to as *herringbone*. A related tumor, the malignant fibrous histiocytoma (MFH), also is composed of spindle cells capable of collagen synthesis. The cell of origin is considered to be a primitive mesenchymal cell, which can differentiate into other forms as well as fibroblasts; therefore, the MFH can also show histiocytic differentiation including multinuclear giant cells.

The classic pattern of MFH is the storiform or swirled pattern of spindle cells, which stream out in a radial fashion from around small vessels. MFH also is more histologically varied than FS, frequently showing admixed giant cells and mononuclear inflammatory cells.

A recent study by Jones and associates[11] has grouped these two malignant tumors of fibroblastic origin, FS and MFH, into one category. In this study of 32 tumors, the herringbone or FS pattern was identified in 14, and the storiform or MFH pattern was found in 17. Neither pattern was found in one case. The authors found that the herringbone pattern was more predictive of good prognosis than the storiform or MFH pattern. However, the two more important features predicting favorable prognosis for these tumors were mitotic rate and degree of cytologic atypia. Low-grade FS/MFH tumors, although capable of local recurrence, resulted in no deaths for the 16 patients in this group. The recurrence rate was found to be related both to tumor size and to infiltrating rather than circumscribed margins. Low-grade tumors had an average mitotic activity of 2 mitoses per 10 high-power fields (hpf; range 0 to 5). Sixty-nine percent of tumors showed mild cytologic atypia, and the rest had moderate atypia. In contrast, 69% of the 16 high-grade tumors had marked cytologic atypia. The average mitotic count for these high-grade tumors was 12 per 10 hpf (range 4 to 30). The authors found a useful predictor of tumor aggressiveness to be the score of mitotic rate times cytologic atypia. This score was 6 or less for low-grade tumors and 12 or more for high-grade tumors. Thirty-one percent of patients with high-grade tumors died of their disease, and 25% developed distant metastases.

As seen on mammograms, fibrosarcomas are dense, with some portion of the margin indistinct.[8] No spiculation has been described. The radiographic size corresponds to the palpable size.[4] On ultrasonography, fibrosarcomas are either solid or complex masses. If hemorrhage or necrosis is present, hypoechoic or cystic spaces may be detected within the mass lesion.

Liposarcoma. Liposarcoma, another rare breast tumor, appears to be more aggressive biologically than other sarcomas such as FS/MFH and leiomyosarcoma. In a large series reported by Austin and Dupree[1] recurrence or metastases occurred in 20% and two patients (10%) died of their tumors. All recurrences occurred within 1 year of the original diagnosis. Pleomorphic liposarcoma and myxoid liposarcoma are the histologic patterns associated with recurrence or metastasis.[1,5,10,13] Well-differentiated liposarcomas apparently do not metastasize or do so only rarely.

Like other primary breast sarcomas, liposarcomas do not metastasize to axillary lymph nodes, and metastasis is hematogenous, predominantly to bones and lung. Several cases of fatal liposarcoma have been reported in patients who were pregnant or lactating.[1,10,13] It has been suggested that the increased vascularity of the breast associated with these physiologic states may facilitate tumor metastasis.[13] In addition to arising as primary sarcomas of mammary parenchyma, liposarcomas may occur as the predominant pattern of stromal overgrowth in a malignant phyllodes tumor.[1,17] Liposarcomas must be distinguished from benign proliferations such as fat necrosis (discussed in Chap. 14) and from signet ring cell carcinoma (mentioned in Chap. 12).

The imaging features of liposarcoma have not been described. A large mass containing some lipomatous elements would be expected. A history of a breast mass enlarging over months to years is reported.[1] Grossly, either pushing or infiltrative margins are described.[1]

Leiomyosarcoma. Smooth muscle tumors of the breast are rare. Benign leiomyomas have been reported, most frequently arising in the nipple. Malignant smooth muscle tumors are even less common. Some of the cases of leiomyosarcoma of the breast have been confirmed by electron microscopy.[6] In other cases, the diagnosis has been made purely by appearance on light microscopy. Immunohistochemical studies are not reported. Characteristically, smooth muscle tumors are composed of interwoven bundles of spindle cells with tapering eosinophilic cytoplasm and blunt-ended nuclei that lack either a storiform or a herringbone pattern. Even malignant smooth muscle tumors have relatively low mitotic activity. A patient with proven hepatic metastases, which appeared 15 years after the original surgery, had 3 mitoses per 10 hpf.[6]

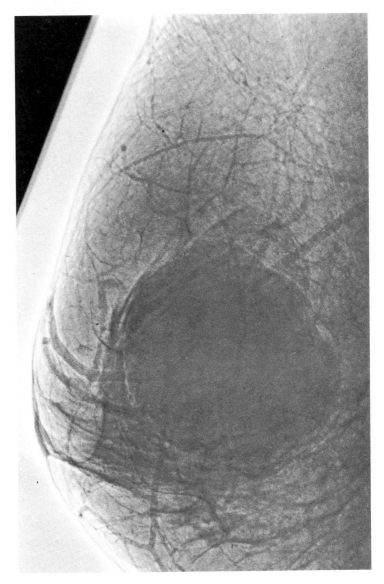

Fig. 13-1 Fibrosarcoma with liposarcoma component imaged by xeromammography as large circumscribed mass with lobulated margins. (Courtesy of Dr. Phil Evans, Dallas, Texas.)

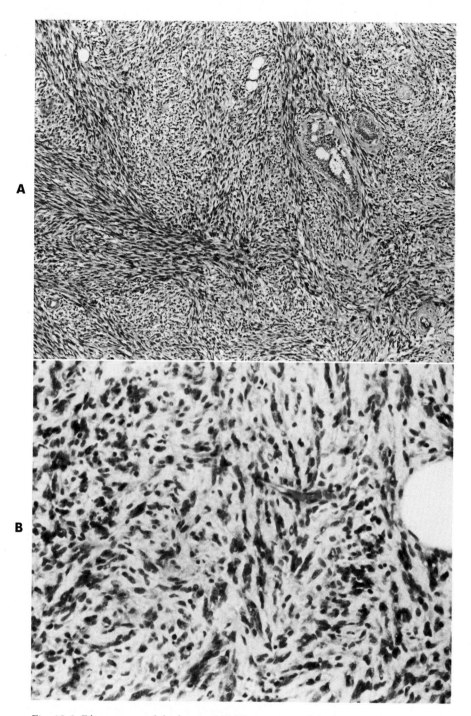

Fig. 13-2 Fibrosarcoma of the breast. **(A)** Fibrosarcoma of the breast is characterized by intersecting bundles of spindle cells that infiltrate the stroma and surround normal ducts. **(B)** At higher magnification, the spindled cytoplasm and some degree of nuclear pleomorphism can be seen.

Fig. 13-3 Malignant fibrous histiocytoma of breast. Low-power photomicrographs show the spindle cell neoplasm infiltrating mammary adipose tissue **(A)** and around preserved breast lobules **(B).** Higher magnification **(C)** shows the marked cellular pleomorphism of the tumor and multinucleated giant cells *(arrows)*.

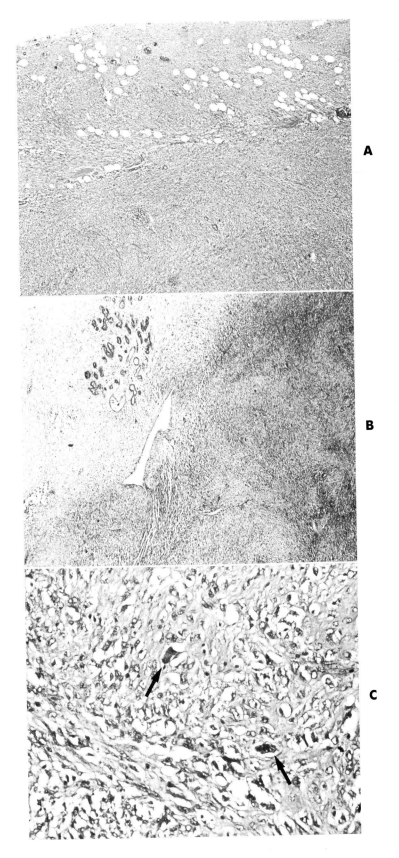

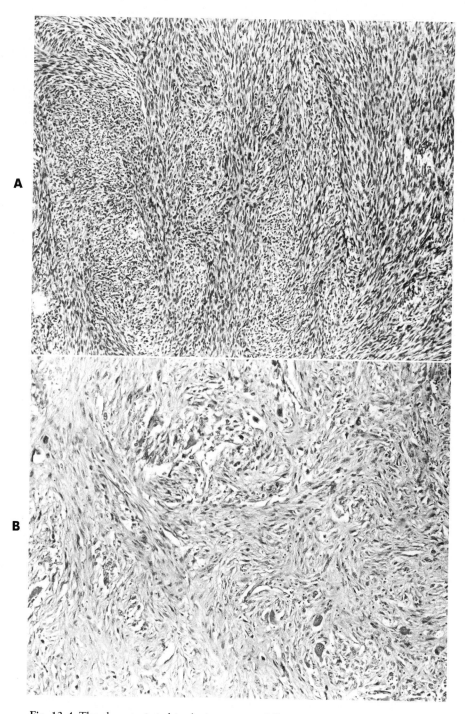

Fig. 13-4 The characteristic histologic patterns of fibrosarcoma (FS) and malignant fibrous histiocytoma (MFH) are compared in these two photomicrographs. FS, illustrated in **A,** shows a uniform population of spindle cells arranged in a classical herringbone pattern of interlacing bundles. MFH, illustrated in **B,** has a varied histologic appearance of multinucleated giant cells and spindle cells that show a swirling or storiform pattern.

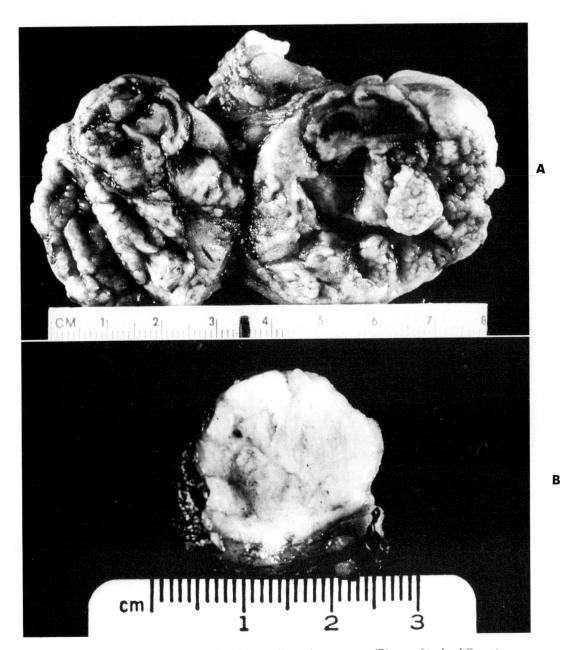

Fig. 13-5 Phyllodes tumor (**A**) and malignant fibrous histiocytoma (**B**) can often be differentiated by their gross as well as microscopic pattern. The lobulated, irregular fronds or convolutions of the phyllodes tumor can be seen here, while the malignant fibrous histiocytoma presents a more solid appearance.

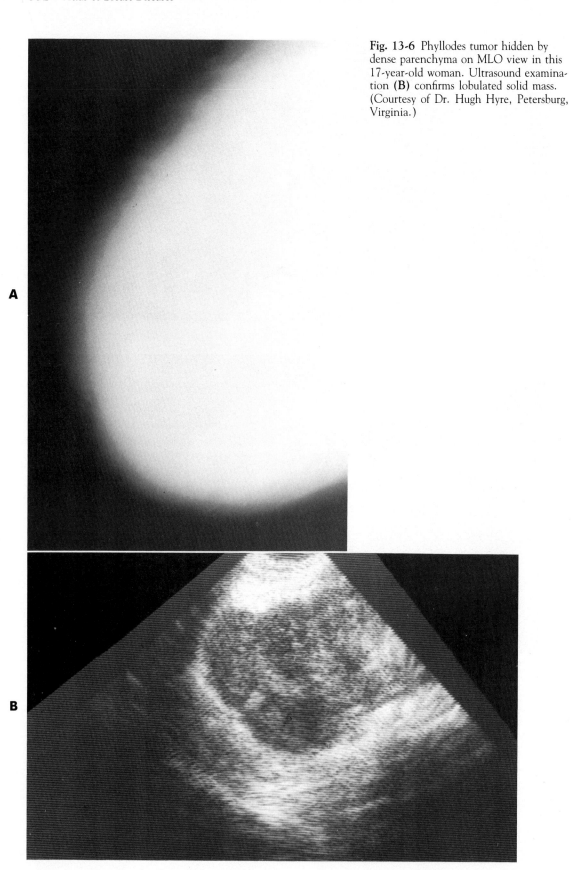

Fig. 13-6 Phyllodes tumor hidden by dense parenchyma on MLO view in this 17-year-old woman. Ultrasound examination **(B)** confirms lobulated solid mass. (Courtesy of Dr. Hugh Hyre, Petersburg, Virginia.)

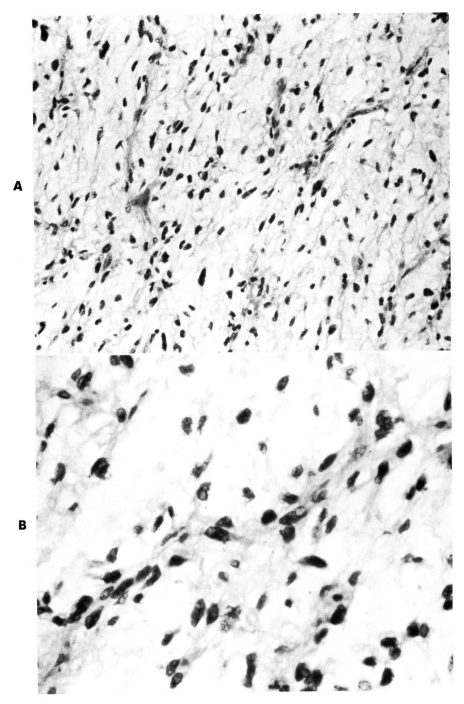

Fig. 13-7 Liposarcoma of the breast. (**A**) Low-power photomicrograph of the tumor shows a loose myxoid–appearing neoplasm composed of spindle cells. Prominent small branching vessels can be seen and are characteristic of this tumor. (**B**) At high magnification, tumor cells with vacuoles within the cytoplasm and overlying the nucleus can be seen, which are characteristic of lipoblasts.

Fibromatoses and benign stromal tumors

A number of distinct disorders that have fibrosis as a prominent feature occur in the breast (Box 13-2). Most of these conditions can clinically mimic breast cancer. Some conditions such as fibromatosis (also known as *extraabdominal desmoid*) may be locally aggressive, whereas others remain locally well circumscribed. Recognition of these uncommon conditions may help prevent unnecessarily radical surgery in selected patients. In addition, a few benign stromal tumors including granular cell tumor, neurilemoma, leiomyoma, and benign spindle cell tumor are discussed in this section.

Fibromatosis or extraabdominal desmoid. The breast is one of the more uncommon locations for extraabdominal desmoid (EAD). This disorder is characterized by a fibroblastic proliferation without inflammation or neoplasia. A desmoid is characteristically associated with the fascia or aponeurosis of muscle. Therefore, in the breast these lesions may be positioned close to the pectoral muscle. Some authors require the presence of ducts or lobules to affirm that the process arises within the mammary parenchyma rather than in the skin or chest wall.[39]

In the breast, the desmoid produces a spiculated mass without calcifications. Not only does the mammographic appearance mimic invasive breast cancer but the clinical examination of a firm nontender mass is suspicious for cancer.[28]

The histopathology of EAD is that of a proliferative and infiltrative lesion of bland fibroblastic cells, usually remarkably devoid of either marked cytologic atypia or increased mitotic activity. Although cases of EAD have not been reported to metastasize, they have been shown to recur locally, occasionally many times. The best predictor of local recurrence is the presence of the lesion in the margins of excision.

The pathologic differential diagnosis of EAD includes well-differentiated fibrosarcoma, reactive fibrosis (such as keloid and nodular fasciitis), and fibrous histiocytoma.[22,39]

EAD may occur in a person of any age and is more common in women than in men. A traumatic cause of EAD has been proposed such as external trauma or prior surgical procedure.[22] Hormonal manipulation (antiestrogen therapy) has been prescribed with some success.[32]

Diabetic mastopathy. Diabetic mastopathy (fibrous disease of the breast in type I diabetes) is a distinct clinicopathologic entity recognized in women with long-standing insulin-dependent diabetes mellitus. First described in 1984 by Soler and Khardori,[34] this uncommon entity has also been described in the radiographic and pathologic literatures.[30,37]

BOX 13-2 FIBROMATOSES AND BENIGN STROMAL TUMORS

Fibromatoses
Fibromatosis (extraabdominal desmoid)
Diabetic mastopathy
Focal fibrosis

Benign stromal tumors
Granular cell tumor (myoblastoma)
Neurilemoma (schwannoma)
Neurofibroma
Leiomyoma
Benign spindle cell breast tumor

Diabetic mastopathy consists of focal, dense keloid-like areas of fibrosis, which show lymphocytic lobulitis and ductitis and also lymphocytic vasculitis (predominately B-cell). Many patients have peculiar epithelioid cells, *epithelioid fibroblasts*, embedded in dense fibrous stroma.[37]

The clinical presentation of diabetic mastopathy is that of one or more palpable breast masses in a woman with insulin-dependent diabetes mellitus. The mammographic findings are not specific. Dense parenchyma is described, and in some cases an area of dense asymmetric tissue is reported.[26,30] Ultrasonographic examination shows marked acoustical shadowing as a consistent feature.[30] Fine needle aspiration is difficult to perform because the fibrotic tissue makes movement of the needle characteristically difficult. Most often the cellular material aspirated is insufficient for analysis.[30]

Unnecessary biopsy may be averted if the clinical setting meets the criteria put forth by Logan. If the lesion is solitary, care must be taken not to misdiagnose a malignancy.

The incidence of diabetic fibrous mastopathy varies according to the target population. In a busy clinical breast practice, an incidence of 1 in 1700 women has been reported.[30] In an endocrinology practice specializing in diabetes, diabetic mastopathy was described in 13% of insulin-dependent diabetic women less than age 40 years.[34]

The cause of diabetic mastopathy is unknown but an autoimmune phenomenon is suggested. Most patients with this condition also have nephropathy, retinopathy, or neuropathy.[37]

Focal fibrosis. Focal fibrosis is a poorly recognized lesion consisting of abundant fibrous stroma with a few scattered ductal and lobular elements. No cysts or inflammatory cells are present. Some authors suggest that this condition may be a variant of involution rather than a pathologic entity.[20] No increased risk for breast cancer has been reported.

Focal fibrosis, discussed briefly in Chapter 11, is usually ignored or not recognized by the pathologist. It is histologically difficult to differentiate from the parenchymal replacement by dense collagen, which is often seen as a component of fibrocystic change. If focal fibrosis is suspected radiographically, consultation between radiologist and pathologist is advisable, with review of both mammograms and histologic slides.

The reported mammographic findings in focal fibrosis consist of an oval or round mass with a circumscribed or indistinct margin.[27] The density appears isodense to an equivalent volume of breast parenchyma. When the margins are indistinct, this solid mass, palpable or clinically occult, may be considered suspicious for malignancy. As the numbers of screening mammograms increase, more of these areas of focal fibrosis may be evaluated, providing more information concerning the natural history of this breast lesion.

Granular cell tumor. Granular cell tumor of the breast (myoblastoma) is a lesion that is clinically benign but may mimic carcinoma of the breast on both physical examination and mammography.[21,23] About 6% of granular cell tumors occur in the breast.[38] The lesion is more common in blacks and can be seen in males or females, usually in middle age.[33]

The granular cell tumor is characteristically a nonencapsulated, poorly circumscribed lesion composed of clusters of distinctive cells arrayed between dense bundles of collagen and infiltrating into fat. The cells have indistinct cytoplasmic borders, small nuclei lacking prominent nucleoli, and abundant granular cytoplasm. The granules are membrane-bound vacuoles containing cellular debris, and they have a distinct appearance by electron microscopy. Some are surrounded by recognizable basal laminae.[25] The cells have been shown to be positive for S-100 protein by immunochemical staining techniques.[35] They do not contain glycogen.

The mammographic features of myoblastoma are those of a mass with an ill-defined, indistinct margin or a few spiculations extending into surrounding tissue. Calcifications are not a reported feature. Appearance on ultrasonography would be expected to be that of a solid mass with shadowing. The usual working diagnosis is a mass suspicious for cancer.

Frozen-section diagnosis of granular cell tumor is to be discouraged because it may be confused with rare forms of breast cancer such as the histiocytoid variant.[33] Malignant forms of granular cell tumors are very uncommon.[25]

The histogenesis of granular cell tumor is still uncertain.[25] Originally, the cells were thought to be muscular in origin; hence, the name *granular cell myoblastoma*. More recently, based on electron microscopic and immunochemical studies, their origin has been considered to be more probably from nerve sheath. Most pathologists now consider the granular cell tumor to be of neural derivation, although a few believe that the tumor may represent altered histiocytes or may derive from primitive mesenchymal cells.[25]

Other benign stromal tumors. A variety of benign stromal tumors may occur in the breast. Some, such as the lipomas, have been discussed previously in Chapter 9. Some others are mentioned here. Hemangiomas are discussed later in this chapter.

Neurofibroma/neurilemoma. Neurofibromas may occur singly or as one of many in von Recklinghausen's disease (neurofibromatosis); neurilemomas are most often single and rarely a component of this syndrome. Neurofibromatosis is a phacomatosis that affects 1 of 3000 persons in the population. The condition is recognized by the association of café-au-lait spots, multiple neurofibromas, and, rarely, multiple neurilemomas. Neurofibromas may involve a neural plexus or a peripheral nerve sheath. Neurilemomas are encapsulated nerve sheath tumors characterized by two histologic patterns known as Antoni A and Antoni B.

In the breast, peripheral neurofibromas are apparent clinically. They are imaged most often as elevated skin lesions producing soft tissue nodules with a margin sharply delineated by air. When subcutaneous in location, neurofibromas produce less distinct soft tissue nodules imaged in the subcutaneous fatty tissues. A solitary neurofibroma or neurilemoma is more likely to cause diagnostic confusion in a clinical breast practice than multiple lesions do.[29] A neurilemoma may be hard on palpation and may cause skin retraction.[33]

Leiomyoma. Benign smooth muscle tumors arise most frequently in the uterus and the gastrointestinal tract. When they occur in other sites, they are commonly associated with vascular walls.

In the breast, however, benign smooth muscle tumors have been reported in the nipple, where they appear to arise from smooth muscle at the base of the nipple or areola.[31]

Benign spindle cell breast tumor. Spindle cell tumor, described by Toker and colleagues[36] in 1981, is composed of groups of spindle cells, which by electron microscopy have been shown to be a varied population of primitive mesenchymal cells, myofibroblasts, fibroblasts, and smooth muscle cells. Some fat cells are seen but appear to be trapped within the spindle cell proliferation. The authors point out the similarity of this tumor to spindle cell lipomas, a distinctive lesion most commonly located in the posterior neck and shoulder region of males.[24] It is interesting that of the four cases of benign spindle cell breast tumor reported by Toker and colleagues,[36] three were in men. Regardless of whether it is related to spindle cell lipoma, benign spindle cell breast tumor appears to be a benign lesion, cured by local excision.[36]

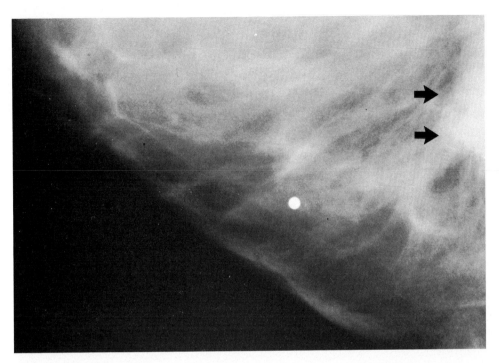

Fig. 13-8 Extraabdominal desmoid tumor imaged as palpable mass with ill-defined margins (*arrows*) deep in right inferior breast in this magnified MLO view. (Courtesy of Dr. Marie Lee, Seattle, Washington.)

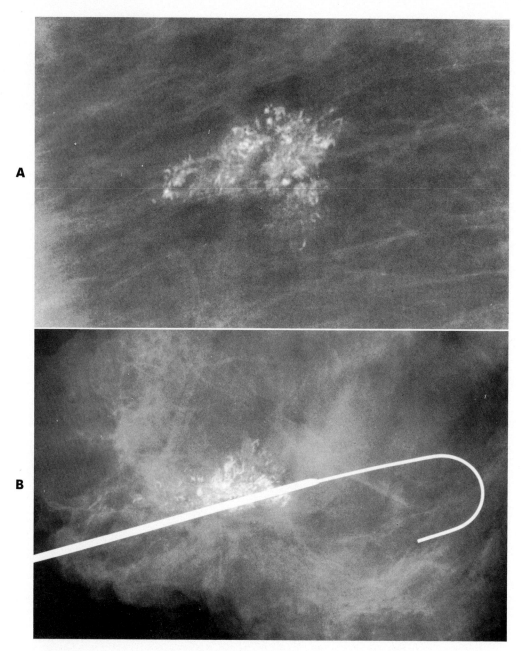

Fig. 13-9 Focal fibrosis. Bizarre branching calcifications (**A**) were suspicious for comedocarcinoma. (**B**) Wire-directed excisional biopsy was performed. Pathologic diagnosis was focal fibrosis with calcifications.

Fig. 13-10 Stromal fibrosis with calcifications. This low-magnification photomicrograph shows dense, sparsely cellular stroma composed of collagen. Small clustered obliterated ducts or lobules can be seen immediately adjacent to the darkly staining irregular calcifications.

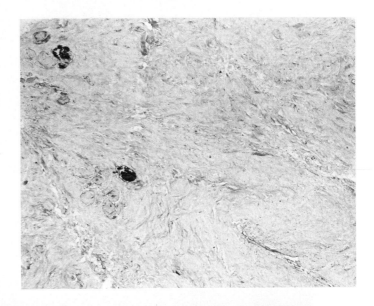

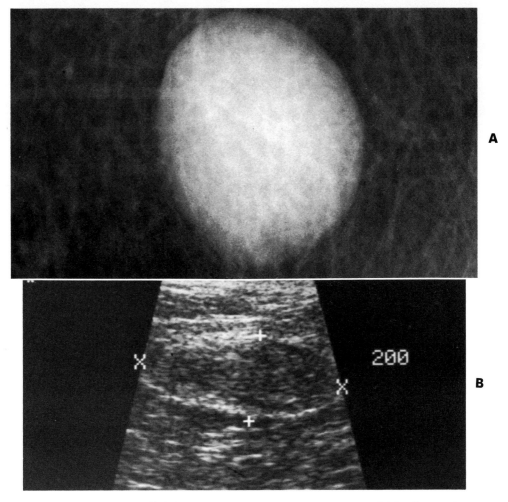

Fig. 13-11 Round mass with slightly indistinct posterior margin **(A)** was solid by ultrasound examination **(B).** Pathologic diagnosis was fibrous tissue with atrophic ducts. (Courtesy of Dr. Richard Bird, Charlotte, North Carolina.)

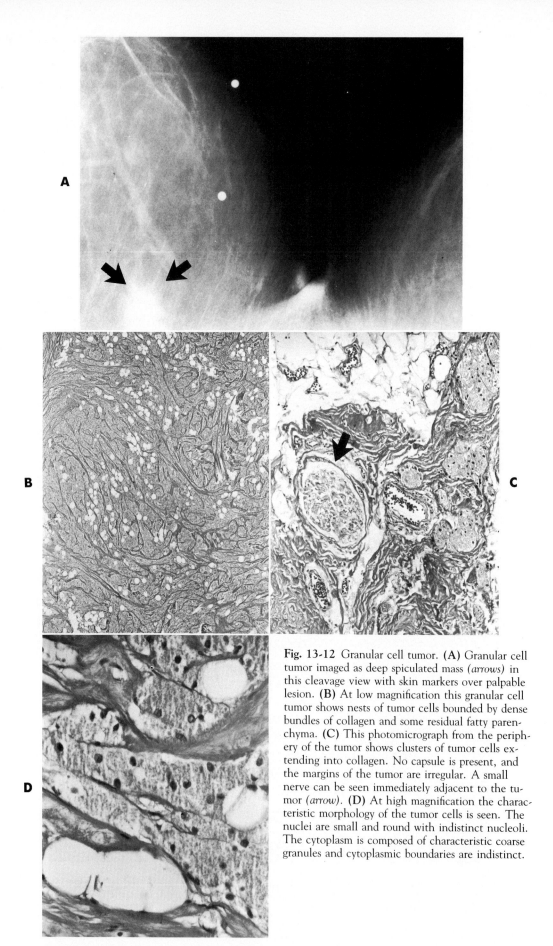

Fig. 13-12 Granular cell tumor. **(A)** Granular cell tumor imaged as deep spiculated mass *(arrows)* in this cleavage view with skin markers over palpable lesion. **(B)** At low magnification this granular cell tumor shows nests of tumor cells bounded by dense bundles of collagen and some residual fatty parenchyma. **(C)** This photomicrograph from the periphery of the tumor shows clusters of tumor cells extending into collagen. No capsule is present, and the margins of the tumor are irregular. A small nerve can be seen immediately adjacent to the tumor *(arrow)*. **(D)** At high magnification the characteristic morphology of the tumor cells is seen. The nuclei are small and round with indistinct nucleoli. The cytoplasm is composed of characteristic coarse granules and cytoplasmic boundaries are indistinct.

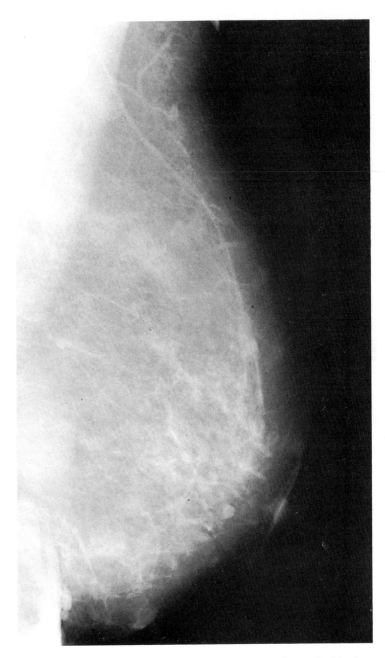

Fig. 13-13 Multiple peripheral neurofibromas in a woman with von Recklinghausen's disease imaged as circumscribed cutaneous and subcutaneous masses. (Courtesy of Dr. Marie Lee, Seattle, Washington.)

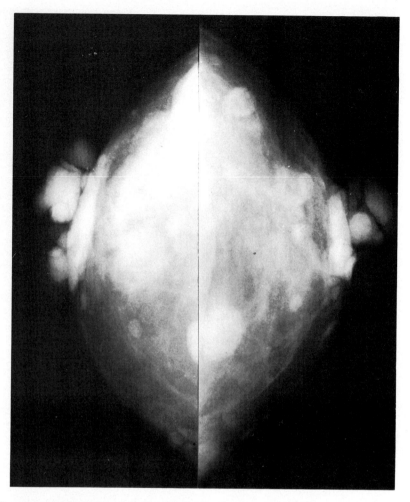

Fig. 13-14 Multiple bilateral elevated skin lesions are caused by cutaneous neurofibromas in this woman with von Recklinghausen's disease.

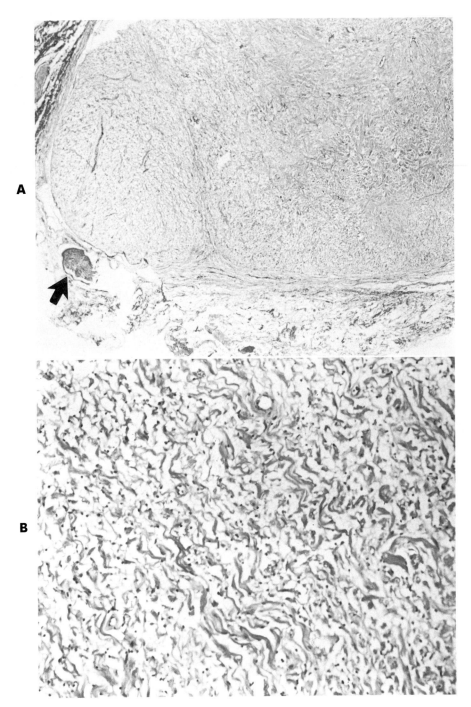

Fig. 13-15 Neurofibroma. (**A**) Low-magnification photomicrograph of a neurofibroma shows a well-demarcated tumor composed of wavy spindle cells, collagen bundles, and small blood vessels. A small nerve trunk is seen adjacent to the tumor (*arrow*). (**B**) High-magnification photomicrograph shows a tumor composed of wavy spindle cells and collagen with a myxoid stroma and a few infiltrating mononuclear cells.

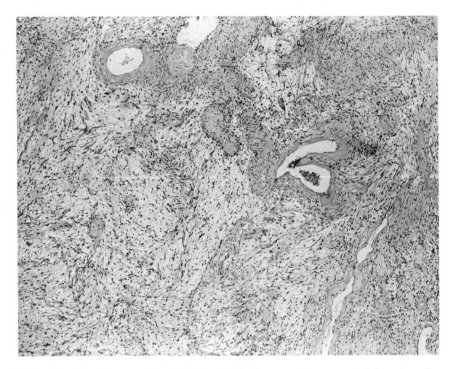

Fig. 13-16 Neurilemoma. The histology of neurilemomas is more varied than that of neurofibromas. Two patterns, termed Antoni A and Antoni B, can be recognized and are illustrated in this photomicrograph. Antoni A areas consist of compact bundles of spindle cells, often with palisaded nuclei. Antoni B areas are looser and more myxoid and can be seen in the lower left portion of this photomicrograph.

VASCULAR LESIONS

Vascular lesions of the breast demonstrate a wide diversity of biologic potential. First, various benign tumors with no aggressive potential are discussed (Box 13-3). Venous thrombosis in the breast, more popularly known as *Mondor's disease*, is presented because of its clinical and mammographic findings. Finally, the aggressive lesions of angiosarcoma and hemangiopericytoma are presented.

Benign vascular lesions

Benign vascular tumors of the breast are known to occur as both microscopic and grossly visible lesions. Although it rarely occurs, a number of these lesions may be detected mammographically.[41] Microscopic lesions, usually termed *perilobular hemangiomas*, may involve either mammary stroma or intralobular connective tissue.[47] The larger lesions, termed *hemangiomas*, range in size from 0.3 to 2.5 cm. Most are less than 2.0 cm. Both lesions are formed by small capillary-sized vessels, frequently containing erythrocytes. Tumor borders are usually rounded and well circumscribed, but occasionally irregular borders extending into fat are described.[43] Features described as atypical within hemangiomas are focal endothelial hyperplasia, endothelial nuclear hyperchromasia, anastomosing vascular channels, and invasive margins.[41] When adequately excised, none of these benign lesions has metastasized or caused the death of a patient. In a recent study of atypical hemangiomas, it is suggested that the diagnosis of hemangioma or atypical hemangioma be considered for any vascular mammary lesions less than 2 cm.[41] Caution is urged not to overinterpret these lesions as low-grade angiosarcomas.

Other benign vascular lesions of the breast are composed of larger vascular channels, usually containing smooth muscle within the vessel walls. These lesions, termed *angiomatoses* and *venous hemangiomas*, are very rare in the breast and resemble similarly titled lesions found in soft tissues in other parts of the body.[46] Angiomatoses are large, diffusely infiltrating lesions composed of a mixture of vascular and lymphatic channels.[44] Some lesions may be congenital. Because of their size and diffuse growth pattern, complete excision may be difficult without mastectomy and the lesions may recur. Patients with venous hemangiomas usually present with palpable, well-circumscribed masses (1.0 to 5.0 cm) formed by thick-walled venous channels containing varying amounts of smooth muscle and fibrous tissue within their walls.[46]

Finally, vascular lesions of mammary parenchyma should not be confused with vascular lesions arising within skin or subcutaneous tissues of the breast.[45] A variety of vascular lesions can occur in these sites, including capillary and cavernous hemangiomas, juvenile hemangiomas, venous hemangiomas, papillary endothelial hyperplasia, and angiolipomas. Angiolipomas can also occur within breast parenchyma.[40] Clinically, these parenchymal lesions are often considered to be carcinomas or lipomas. Histologically, they are easily recognized when removed from subcutaneous tissues. However, because these lesions

---

BOX 13-3 BENIGN VASCULAR LESIONS OF THE BREAST

Perilobular hemangioma
Hemangioma
Lymphangioma
Cavernous hemangioma
Venous hemangioma
Angiomatoses
Angiolipoma

are rarely found in the breast, the pathologist must be careful not to overdiagnose them as well-differentiated angiosarcomas invading adipose tissue, particularly because the capsule of the lipoma is usually not apparent. Lack of endothelial atypia is helpful in diagnosis, as is consultation with the surgeon and the mammographer.

Another lesion that must be differentiated from angiosarcoma of the breast is pseudoangiomatous hyperplasia of mammary stroma (PHMS).[48] This relatively recently described lesion may be found (but not always recognized) in a fairly high (23%) percentage of breast biopsies.[42] Usually, however, PHMS is an inconspicuous component of the biopsy. Rarely, it may present as a large mass or density within the breast. Histologically, a proliferation of dense fibrous stroma containing slit-like spaces lined by elongated cells is found. These have been shown by immunochemical and electron microscopic studies to be fibroblasts rather than endothelial cells.[42] PHMS may involve both interlobular and intralobular stroma.

Mondor's disease. Thrombosis of a superficial vein of the breast or anterior chest wall is called Mondor's disease. This entity pathologically is a phlebitis-periphlebitis, which is seen more often in women than in men. The thoracoepigastric veins are most often affected over the lateral breast.[49] Bilateral involvement is uncommon.

The diagnosis of Mondor's disease is made by clinical examination and is not difficult if the examiner is aware of the entity. The classic finding on physical examination, similar to any thrombophlebitis, is a linear rope or cord-like thickening palpable in the subcutaneous tissues over 2 or more cm. Skin retraction along the line of the palpable cord is common and can be exaggerated by stretching the skin. Pain, warmth, or erythema may be present if the event is acute. The condition is self-limiting over several weeks.

The cause of Mondor's disease is often unknown. In some patients, a history of antecedent trauma, dehydration, or inflammatory condition may be elicited. The trauma may be iatrogenic in nature, such as a recent breast biopsy.[52] Mondor's disease secondary to using the breast as a site for intravenous drug abuse has been reported.[50]

Mammography may be requested in an appropriate age group to clarify uncertain physical findings. One study recommends mammography to assess possible associated malignancy.[49] In this report, 12% of 63 patients with Mondor's disease collected in cancer centers over a period of 10 years were associated with malignancy.[49] This high rate of associated cancers may reflect the bias of the population studied.

The mammographic finding of Mondor's disease is a dilated vein or subcutaneous thickening that parallels the palpable cord.[51,53] No permanent mammographic residua have been described.

Angiosarcoma. Angiosarcomas occur in deep soft tissues of the head and extremities. Angiosarcomas arising in parenchyma of the breast constitute about 9% of angiosarcomas.[57] Breast origin is to be differentiated in presentation from cutaneous angiosarcoma. Both types have poor prognoses. The Stewart-Treves syndrome is the occurrence of lymphangiosarcoma in the lymphademetous arm of a woman following mastectomy and usually radiation therapy.[61,64] Cutaneous angiosarcoma of the breast also has been described following lumpectomy and radiation therapy.[60]

Angiosarcoma of the breast is rare in breast malignancy, occurring once in every 2000 to 3500 breast cancers.[63] The neoplasm has been reported in women from 20 to 70 years of age but the mean age (35 to 42 yr) is younger than for women with breast carcinomas.[33,57] The presenting symptom is a palpable spongy mass. No clinically occult cases of angiosarcoma have been reported.[57] In some women (17% to 30%), overlying bluish, violaceous, or black discoloration of the skin is noted.[33,57] The mean size of the sarcoma is about 3.5 cm in various series. The tumor may be multifocal. Rapid growth and hematologic metastases are common.[58,59] Bilateral breast involvement occurs, and it may not be clear whether the contralateral lesion is a metastasis or a second primary tumor.[54,62]

Angiosarcomas of the breast have been considered to be the most common vascular neoplasms of the breast and the most lethal of breast sarcomas. Histologically, these lesions exhibit considerable variation in growth pattern. Although well-differentiated tumors show invasive readily identifiable vascular spaces lined by endothelial cells with enlarged nuclei and occasional mitoses, high-grade tumors may consist mainly of anaplastic spindle cell masses with areas of hemorrhage, necrosis, and atypical mitosis.

Two recent studies have suggested that tumor grade of angiosarcomas is highly predictive of biologic behavior.[58,59] High-grade tumors have poor survival rates, whereas well-differentiated tumors may recur locally but metastasize less frequently. Tumor size does not appear to be related to survival, nor does duration of tumor prior to biopsy. Histologic criteria for diagnosis of angiosarcoma include size greater than 2 cm, invasive growth pattern with lobular or parenchymal destruction, anastomosing vascular channels, endothelial hyperchromasia and nuclear enlargement, papillary endothelial tufting, mitotic activity, and sarcomatous foci with necrosis and hemorrhage.[55] One caveat to be noted is that these tumors are histologically varied and must be well sampled. High-grade tumors may contain multiple areas of well-differentiated neoplasm, which may be more common at the periphery of the tumor.[59] Therefore, the entire tumor must be removed and generously sampled to establish the correct histologic grade.

Angiosarcomas, like other breast sarcomas, rarely metastasize to axillary lymph nodes. The route of metastases is hematogenous, with lung, liver, bones, and skin as preferred sites.[58,59] Metastases to the opposite breast are not uncommon.

The imaging features of angiosarcomas are nonspecific. Most women have a solitary mass with indistinct margins. Multiple nodules have been reported. In about one third of women, no mammographic abnormality is present; this may be the expected situation in younger women with dense breast parenchyma. Calcifications are an uncommon feature and, if present, are pleomorphic, not branching forms. Skin thickening has been described but would be more typical for cutaneous origin. The sonographic features are also variable. In general, the mass is a solid, multilobulated, not well-circumscribed, inhomogeneous mass with areas of hyperechogenicity and hypoechogenicity. Shadowing has not been described. Variability through transmission of sound has been reported.[56,57]

Hemangiopericytoma. Hemangiopericytoma is an uncommon soft tissue neoplasm that is most often benign in biologic behavior. Aggressive behavior with local recurrence or distant metastases is associated with cellular atypia, a high mitotic rate, and necrosis.[65] The breast is an extremely unusual site for hemangiopericytoma. Only 3 of 80 vascular neoplasms of the breast from the AFIP files in 1981 were hemangiopericytomas.[66]

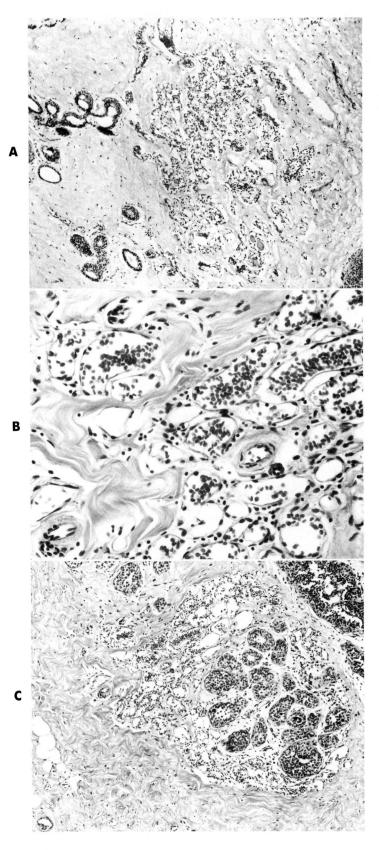

Fig. 13-17 Perilobular hemangioma. At low magnification this perilobular hemangioma can be seen adjacent to an atrophic lobule with dilated small ductules **(A)**. At high magnification the small capillary-like vascular spaces with thin walls lined by endothelial cells and filled with red blood cells can be seen **(B)**. Another example of perilobular hemangioma surrounds a lobule showing atypical lobular hyperplasia **(C)**.

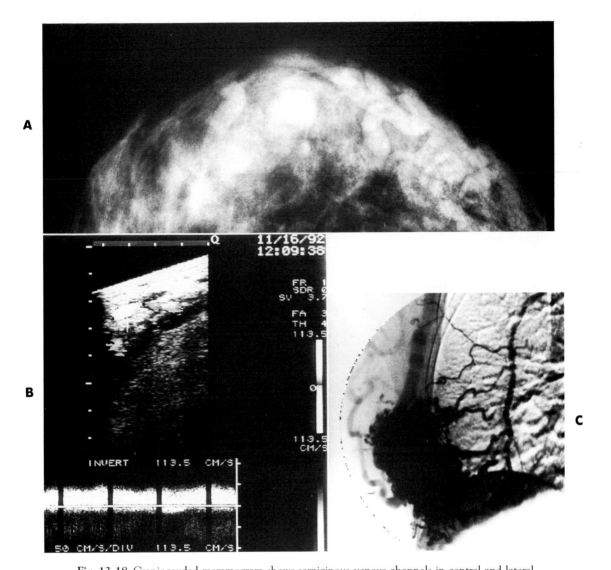

Fig. 13-18 Craniocaudad mammogram shows serpiginous venous channels in central and lateral right breast **(A).** Venous flow demonstrated over dilated vascular channel by Doppler ultrasound **(B).** Internal mammary arteriogram shows arteriovenous malformation of central right breast **(C).** (Courtesy of Dr. Keith Lawrence, Tupelo, Mississippi.)

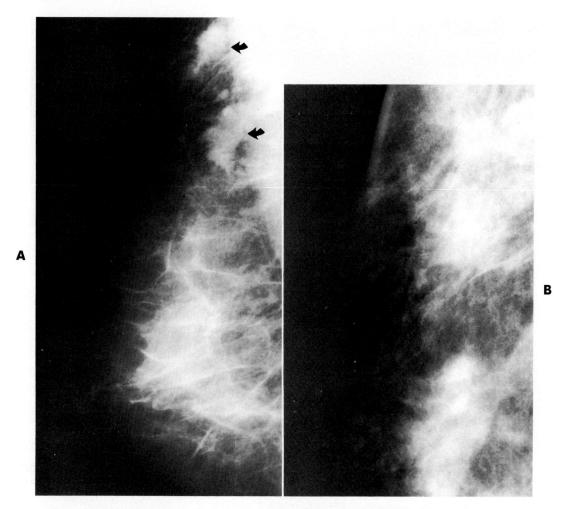

Fig. 13-19 Two lymphangiomas (*arrows*) in axillary tail of right breast imaged as dense irregular masses (**A**). Magnification view (**B**) shows ill-defined margins. (Courtesy of Dr. Ralph Smathers, Palo Alto, California.)

Fig. 13-20 (A) Palpable mass (marked by skin bb) in left breast axillary tail shows phleboliths on this chest wall mammogram. Probable cavernous hemangioma. **(B)** Cavernous hemangioma in the subcutaneous tissue of the breast. The overlying epidermis and dermis are elevated by the lesion which is composed of vascular spaces of varying size which are distended and filled by red blood cells.

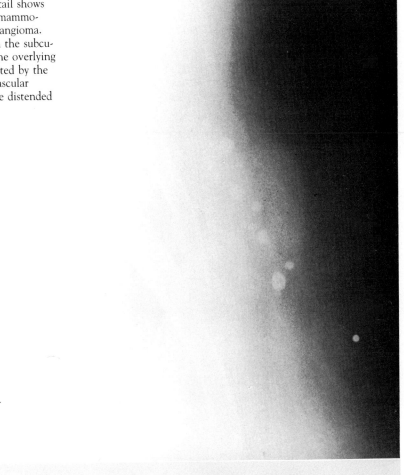

A

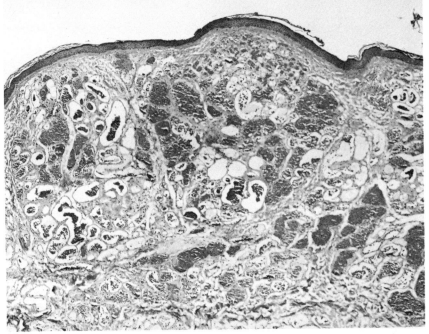

B

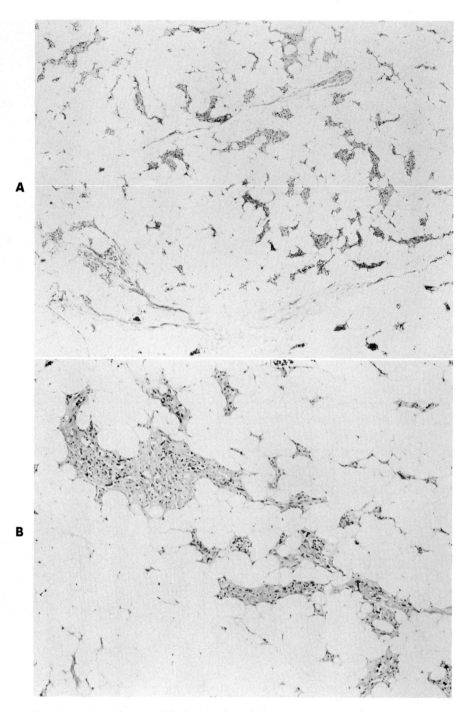

Fig. 13-21 Angiolipoma of the breast. Angiolipoma can occur in subcutaneous tissue or in the mammary parenchyma, as in this case. They are composed of mature adipose tissue and collections of small vascular structures **(A).** Often a capsule is not apparent in histologic sections. The lesion should not be misdiagnosed as angiosarcoma. At higher magnification the lack of cellular atypia in the vessels can be seen and is helpful in establishing the correct diagnosis **(B).**

Fig. 13-22 Atypical hemangioma of the breast. At low magnification this vascular lesion shows somewhat irregular margins **(A).** At higher magnification, anastomosing vascular channels of varying size can be seen **(B).** The lesion is also characterized by enlargement and hyperchromasia of endothelial cells, seen in this photomicrograph, and occasional mitoses *(arrow)* **(C).** This small lesion measured 1.5 cm.

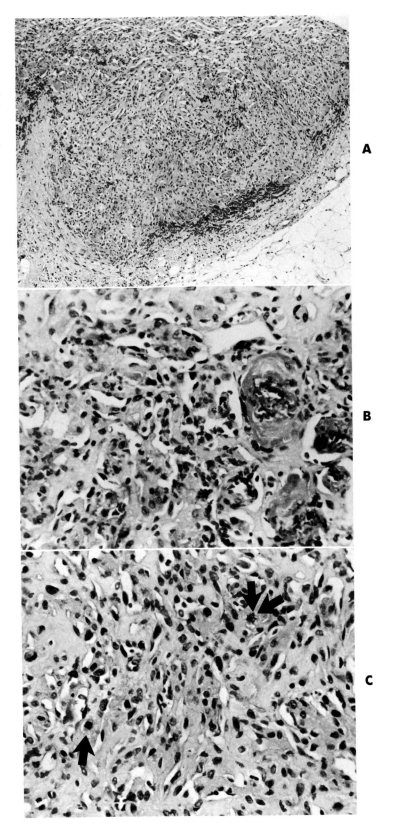

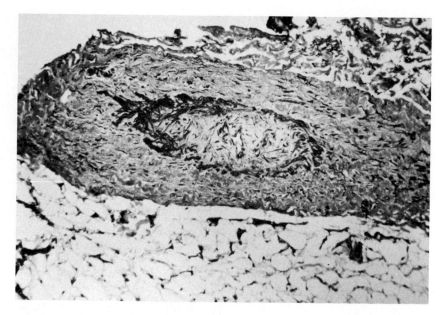

Fig. 13-23 Mondor's disease. Mondor's disease represents venous thrombosis in the breast or anterior chest wall. In this case venous occlusion by old organized thrombus is found in the axillary tail of the breast. The vessel is surrounded by collagen and, more peripherally, by adipose tissue.

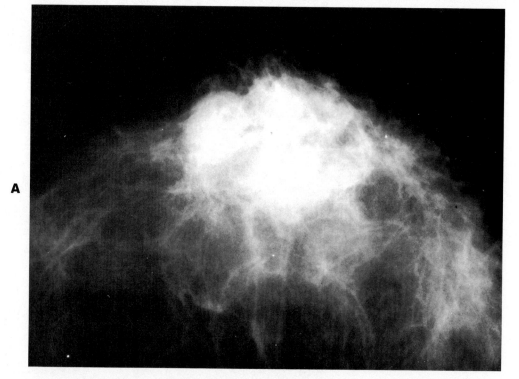

Fig. 13-24 Angiosarcoma of the breast. **(A)** Angiosarcoma produces a dense lobulated mass with irregular margins centrally in this craniocaudad view.

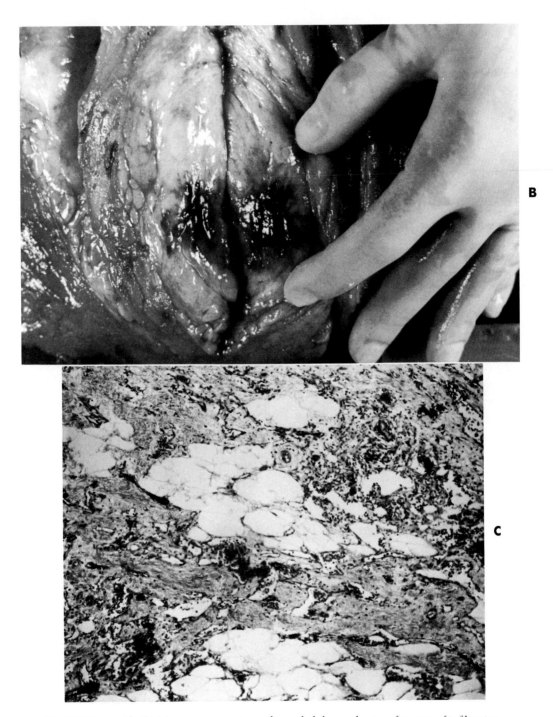

Fig. 13-24, cont'd (B) Mastectomy specimen shows dark hemorrhagic soft tumor of infiltrating angiosarcoma in breast parenchyma. (C) In this photomicrograph, neoplastic vascular channels of varying size containing red blood cells infiltrate through fibrofatty mammary parenchyma.

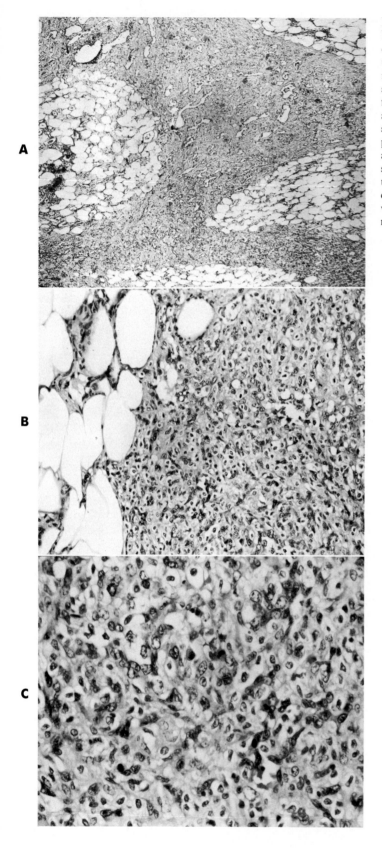

Fig. 13-25 Angiosarcoma of the breast. The histology of angiosarcoma can be varied even within the same tumor. This low-magnification photomicrograph shows tumor exhibiting well-formed vascular structures in some areas and other foci of more solid sheets of spindle cells **(A)**. Higher power of one of these more solid areas shows small rudimentary vessels and single tumor cells infiltrating fat **(B)**. Individual tumor cells show marked pleomorphism, vesicular nuclei with nucleoli, and mitotic figures **(C)**.

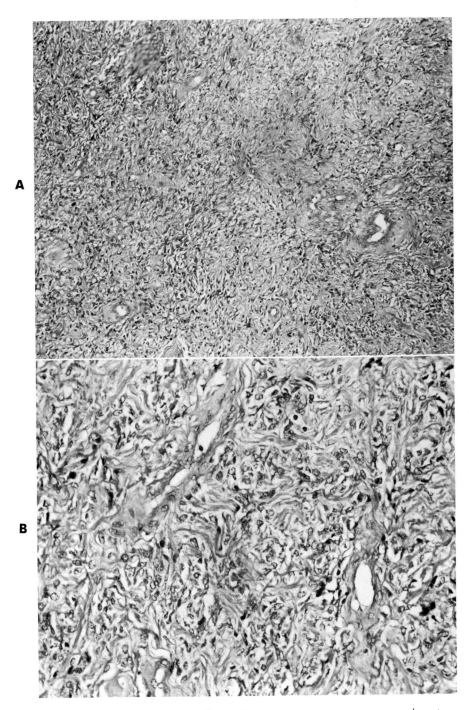

Fig. 13-26 Hemangiopericytoma. Hemangiopericytoma is an uncommon neoplasm in the breast. The tumor at low magnification shows prominent, often branching vessels **(A).** At higher magnification, the proliferating tumor cells surround and compress small blood vessels, which often can be difficult to recognize **(B).**

HEMATOLYMPHOID BREAST LESIONS

The hematolymphoid breast lesions include three groups of Hodgkin's and non-Hodgkin's lymphoma, pseudolymphoma, and hematologic malignancies including chloroma and plasmacytoma. In many patients, a history of preexisting or simultaneous extramammary disease facilitates appropriate clinical diagnosis of a palpable breast mass or lymphadenopathy. However, in rare cases the breast may be the presenting manifestation and the only site of involvement of a hematolymphoid disorder.

Lymphoma and Hodgkin's disease

Non-Hodgkin's lymphoma and Hodgkin's disease arising primarily in the breast are rare, accounting for about 0.1% to 0.5% of primary breast malignancies.[69,80] Of the two conditions, non-Hodgkin's lymphoma is more common as gauged by reports in the literature. Only rare cases of primary Hodgkin's disease of the breast have been reported.[78]

For the breast to be considered the primary site of lymphoma, certain criteria have been proposed.[80] No concurrent or past evidence of extramammary disease should be present. Ipsilateral lymph node involvement is acceptable, provided that it is simultaneous in onset to the breast lesion. There must be close association histopathologically between the breast and nodal involvement. Primary breast lymphoma defined in this manner has been shown to have a prognosis similar to that of localized lymphoma at other sites.[79] Because little data are available on Hodgkin's disease primary to the breast, the following discussion will concern primary non-Hodgkin's lymphoma of the breast.

The reported age range for persons with non-Hodgkin's lymphoma is broad: 21 to 86 years with a median of 57 years in one large study.[67] As many as one third of patients are in their sixth decade,[69] and the mean age is the same as that for patients with adenocarcinoma of the breast.[67] Women are affected more frequently than men.[67,69,77] The lesion is more often in the right breast,[77,80] and the upper outer quadrant is a common location.[69] Bilaterality is reported, either synchronously or metachronously.[69,80]

The typical presenting symptom of non-Hodgkin's lymphoma is a painless breast mass; however, accompanying tenderness, discomfort, pain, or redness has been reported.[72] Less frequently, diffuse breast swelling is the chief complaint. Skin ulceration or fixation is rare. There are usually no systemic B-cell symptoms with primary breast lymphoma,[79] although they have been noted rarely.[78] The size of the breast mass is reported to vary from 1.5 cm to 12 cm.[79] Size is not a distinguishing feature since 30% may be 2 cm or less in diameter.[67] There are no characteristic clinical findings.

Similarly, there are no characteristic imaging findings in non-Hodgkin's lymphoma patients. The mammographic findings cover a spectrum from masses with indistinct borders or areas of increased parenchymal density considered suspicious for malignancy to a well-circumscribed round or oval mass or multiple smooth nodules consistent with a benign condition.[76,77] Slightly lobular margins have also been described.[77] No microcalcifications or parenchymal distortion is seen,[77] and lymphoma cells infiltrate between or into mammary ducts without destroying structure.[67,80]

Ultrasonographic findings are also variable.[72] The only clue to diagnosis of non-Hodgkin's lymphoma may be enlarged axillary nodes, usually oval and smoothly marginated.[74,76] Because advanced breast cancer may be accompanied by ipsilateral lymphadenopathy, this sign is not specific for lymphoma. Breast edema due to lymphatic obstruction by enlarged axillary nodes may simulate inflammatory breast carcinoma mammographically.[75] Bilateral axillary lymph node enlargement should increase the level of suspicion for lymphoma.[77]

Histologically, the most common pattern for primary lymphoma of the breast is a diffuse large cell or mixed lymphoma.[67,73] Other types of lymphoma including follicular lymphomas of both mixed and small cleaved cell types have occurred.[67] Small lymphocytic lymphomas and Hodgkin's disease are rare.[67,78] Although most non-Hodgkin's lymphomas of the breast that have been immunophenotyped have been shown to be of B-cell derivation,[73] at least one case of T-cell lymphoblastic lymphoma has been described.[70] The suggestion has been made that lymphomas of the breast may present in two distinct clinical patterns.[70] One presentation, uncommon in North American patients but more common in those from Africa and Italy, occurs in pregnant or lactating women as a Burkitt's type lymphoma, which is bilateral at presentation and rapidly progressive.

A second and more common presentation of primary lymphoma is that of a unilateral breast mass in an older patient, which may mimic carcinoma and which may be caused by a variety of different histologic types, most frequently large cell or mixed cell lymphomas.

Hugh and associates[70] have suggested that some primary breast lymphomas may represent MALT lymphomas (malignant lymphomas of mucosal-associated lymphoid tissues). These lymphomas were suggested to arise in a setting of lymphoid hyperplasia; this may be true for breast as well as other organ sites.[71] The breast is a hormone-dependent MALT site, and it is noteworthy that two of the lymphomas reported by Hugh and associates[70] were estrogen receptor-positive. No other report exists of estrogen receptor-positive breast lymphomas. However, estrogen receptor positivity on lymphoid cells—benign as well as malignant—has been reported.[68]

Pseudolymphoma

Pseudolymphoma of the breast is a recognized but uncommon nonmalignant lymphoid infiltrate of the breast. It is poorly studied, and its incidence is as low as 5 in 8654 breast surgical specimens.[83]

The clinical presentation of pseudolymphoma is that of a mass in a young or middle-aged woman (26 to 57 years of age). A dull aching sensation has been described. The right and left breasts are equally involved.[83] In some women, a prior history of trauma to the area can be elicited.

The histopathologic criteria include a polymorphic lymphoid infiltrate composed of a mixture of mature lymphocytes, histiocytes, plasma cells, and occasionally eosinophils.[81,83] Germinal centers are frequently seen, and occasionally fat necrosis is present. The imaging features have been reported in one case to be that of a round 2.5 cm mass with lobulated margins and a halo effect along 50% of the circumference.[81] Although only one case has been reported, this description is probably characteristic since the gross morphology of the lesions is described as round to ovoid and homogeneously tan. A capsule is not present. The typical preoperative diagnosis is a fibroadenoma or occasionally fibrocystic disease.[83]

Pseudolymphoma is generally a term that is increasingly suspect. Some of these lymphoid processes at other sites have been shown to have clonal immunoglobulin gene rearrangements and are considered to be part of a spectrum of B-cell neoplasia and preneoplasia, which may eventually develop into overt malignant lymphoma.[82,84] In particular, many MALT type lymphomas of the stomach and lung have been included in this group in the past. Follow-up in the study on pseudolymphoma of the breast by Lin and associates[83] was 2 to 8 years. However, this time interval may not be sufficient to exclude a low-grade lymphoma in all cases, particularly since patients diagnosed with pseudolymphoma may develop a malignant lymphoma after a number of years.

Hematologic malignancies

As in other parts of the body, the breast may be infiltrated by tumor cells of a malignant hematologic process. Occasionally, this process may present as a mass and appear before the leukemia or bone marrow malignancy has manifested itself. Involvement of the breast by malignant myeloid cells forming a solid mass (chloroma or granulocytic sarcoma) occurs occasionally before the myeloid leukemia is diagnosed. The same may occur with plasma cells producing a plasmocytoma either as an isolated finding or as part of plasma cell myeloma. In the latter instance, bony abnormalities and serum or urine protein electrophoreses demonstrating monoclonal gammopathy may be helpful. History of a known hematologic disorder (leukemia or myeloma) will assist in proper diagnosis of these uncommon breast masses. Any hematolymphoid infiltrate is possible in the breast; one case of myeloid metaplasia has been reported.[85] Breast involvement by cells of acute lymphocytic leukemia has also been described.[87] The malignant cellular infiltrate may produce either diffuse infiltration or discrete masses, unilateral or bilateral. Bilateral axillary adenopathy is more common than breast involvement.

Granulocytic sarcoma is a destructive tumor of immature cells in the granulocytic series. The term *granulocytic sarcoma* has been proposed since such tumors may not have a characteristic green color as the term *chloroma* implies. Such soft tissue tumor involvement may precede evidence of leukemia in the peripheral blood or bone marrow.[86] Although granulocytic sarcoma may be seen with either acute or chronic myeloid leukemia, it is more often associated with the acute form. The age range is wide (15 to 75 years).[86]

The histologic differential diagnosis of a granulocytic sarcoma includes large cell lymphoma and infiltrating lobular carcinoma.[86] The latter is included because of the tendency for the infiltrating tumor cells to form an "Indian file." A characteristic histopathologic finding in granulocytic sarcoma is the presence of scattered eosinophilic myelocytes.[88] However, special stains such as the Leder stain for esterase (an enzyme found in granulocytic cells), immunohistochemical stains, or electron microscopy frequently may be required for accurate diagnosis.

The imaging features of granulocytic sarcoma and plasmacytoma are nonspecific. Ill-defined masses or vague areas of increased density within the tissue parenchyma are reported.[77] Calcifications and secondary changes of skin or nipple retraction are not described. The masses range from 1.5 to 4.5 cm in diameter.[77] Involvement of lymph nodes by the hematolymphoid process may produce either unilateral or bilateral axillary adenopathy.

Fig. 13-27 Lymphoma of the breast. Primary lymphoma arising in the breast causes a 1.5 cm dense mass with ill-defined margins **(A)**. (Courtesy of Dr. Abe Pollack, Brooklyn, New York.) **(B)** Large cell lymphomas are the most common primary lymphomas occurring in the breast. This low-magnification photomicrograph shows preserved mammary ducts at the left of the picture. The malignant cell infiltrate is seen at center and to the right. **(C)** At high magnification the tumor cells exhibit considerable nuclear pleomorphism. Individual cells exhibit nucleoli and scant cytoplasm. Lack of cytoplasm and of cell cohesion help to differentiate this neoplasm from poorly differentiated carcinoma. In some cases, however, immunohistochemistry may be required for correct diagnosis.

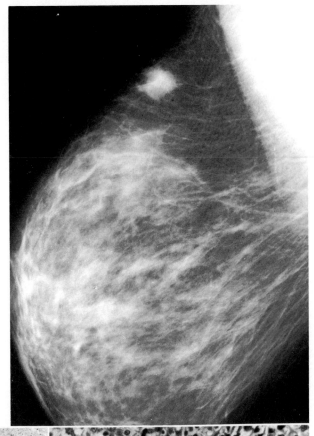

A

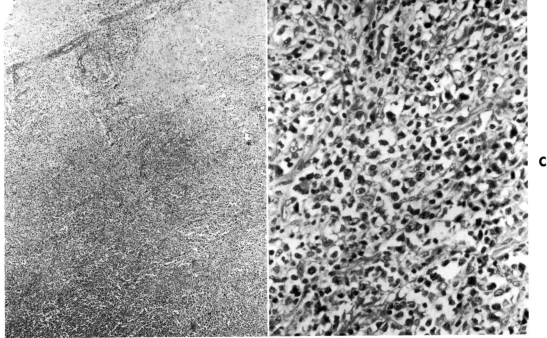

B

C

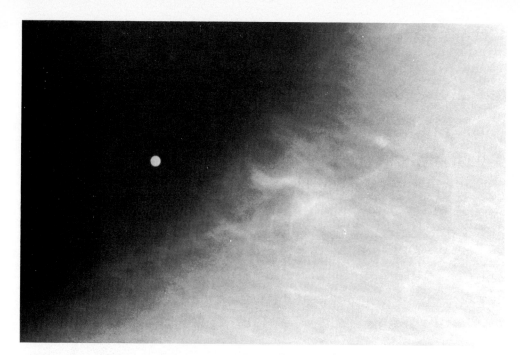

Fig. 13-28 Lymphoma involving deep dermis and subcutaneous fat in tail of right breast of a 59-year-old woman who had had a previous diagnosis of mixed small and large cell lymphoma of parotid gland. The mammogram shows an area of asymmetric density with poorly defined margins. The lymphoma infiltrated the fat without producing a lesion on gross inspection. (Courtesy of Dr. Marie Lee, Seattle, WA).

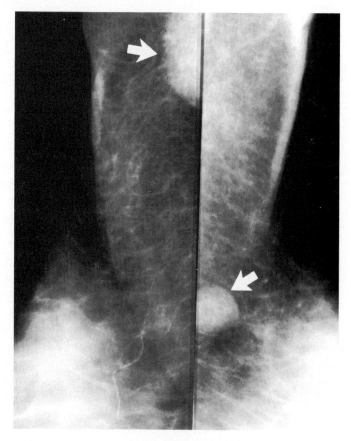

Fig. 13-29 Bilateral axillary lymphadenopathy *(arrows)* was caused by systemic lymphoma in this woman as imaged by upper portion of bilateral MLO views.

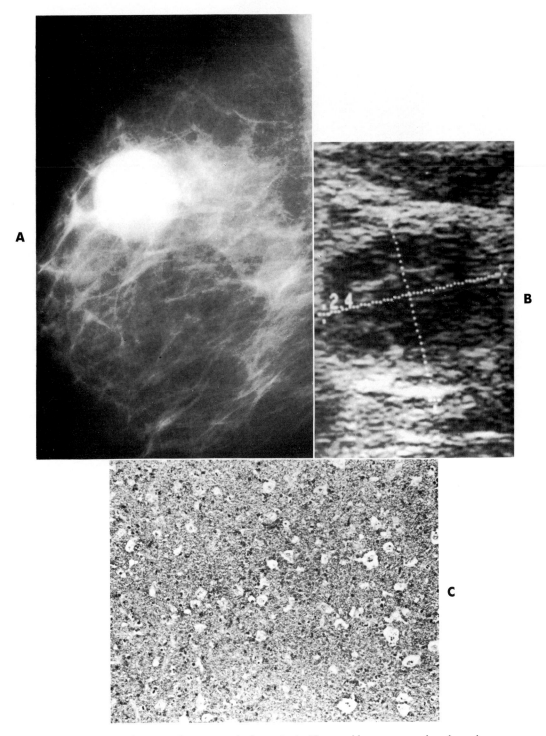

Fig. 13-30 Round mass with circumscribed margin in 37-year-old woman was thought to be a cyst because of rapid enlargement over 2 weeks (**A**). However, ultrasound examination showed a 2.4-cm solid mass (**B**). The pathologic diagnosis was Burkitt's lymphoma (**C**). At low magnification this undifferentiated lymphoma shows a "starry sky" pattern of large macrophages in the cleared areas, which are phagocytizing debris from necrotic cells in this rapidly proliferating neoplasm. The darker areas represent the closely packed malignant cells. (Courtesy of Dr. Phil Evans, Dallas Texas.)

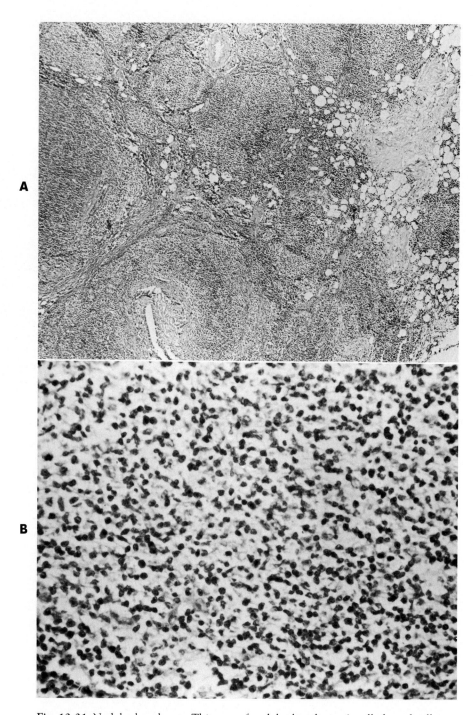

Fig. 13-31 Nodular lymphoma. This case of nodular lymphoma (small-cleaved cell type) represents a somewhat unusual histologic pattern for lymphoma presenting as a breast mass. The nodular pattern can be appreciated in the low-magnification photomicrograph **(A)**. The lymphoma surrounds a normal duct, seen at the bottom of the picture. The small tumor cells seen in **B** have dense, regular nuclei and indistinct nucleoli.

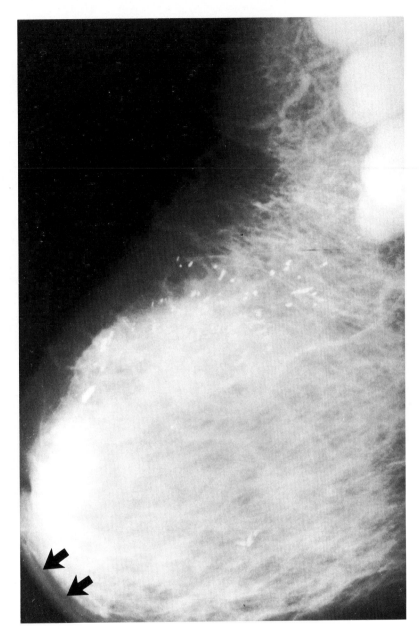

Fig. 13-32 Leukemic infiltrate mimics inflammatory breast carcinoma with diffuse breast edema, skin thickening *(arrows)*, and enlarged axillary lymph nodes. Note benign secretory duct calcifications. (Courtesy of Dr. Phil Evans, Dallas, Texas.)

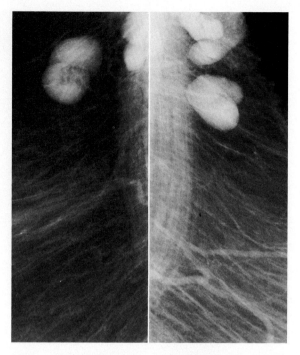

Fig. 13-33 Bilateral symmetric axillary adenopathy is secondary to chronic lymphocytic leukemia.

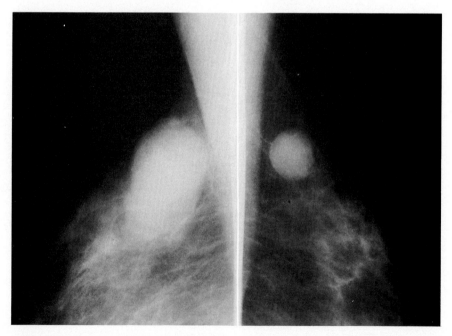

Fig. 13-34 Bilateral intramammary lymph node enlargement secondary to myelocytic leukemia.

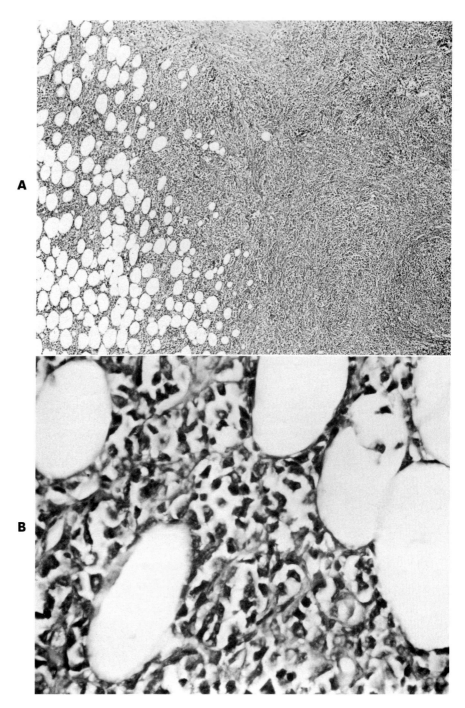

Fig. 13-35 Granulocytic sarcoma. Granulocytic sarcoma is an infiltrate of immature myeloid cells which may occur with or preceding a diagnosis of myeloid leukemia. In this example tumor cell infiltrate diffusely the fibrofatty parenchyema of the breast **(A)**. At high magnification, cellular pleomorphism with immature myeloid cells with eosinophilic cytoplasm (eosinophilic myelocytes) are seen. Characteristically the tumor cells do not form cohesive sheets **(B)**.

METASTATIC DISEASE

Blood-borne metastatic disease to the breast from an extramammary primary solid tumor is uncommon.[94] For purposes of our discussion, lymphoma, leukemia, myeloma, and other hematolymphoid disorders are not included in this group but have been discussed in the preceding section of this chapter. The incidence of metastatic disease to the breast varies depending on whether the report is a clinical or an autopsy series.[95] The extramammary malignancies that most often metastasize to the breast are melanoma and lung cancer, particularly small cell type.[89,94] Other primary sites are carcinoma of the ovary, thyroid, stomach, and pancreas, head and neck squamous cell carcinomas, and soft tissue sarcomas such as rhabdomyosarcoma.[89,94,95,97] Metastatic carcinoid also occurs and may be misdiagnosed as primary breast cancer, particularly on frozen section.[93]

Most reports indicate that these metastatic lesions are nontender. However, pain and discomfort are described in some series.[91,95] Mass lesions up to 4.5 cm in diameter are present, either as single or multiple lesions. An upper outer quadrant location is common. The mammographic features are most often those of a mass with circumscribed or sometimes indistinct margins. Diffuse skin thickening and asymmetry of density are reported but are less common than masses.[95]

Desmoplastic response is not a feature of blood-borne metastases, and spiculation of the mass is not seen. Therefore, the size of the mass as seen by mammography and physical examination is comparable.[89] Microcalcifications are not a feature except in rare cases of psammoma bodies in metastatic ovarian papillary cystadenocarcinoma, of which as few as three cases have been reported.[94,96] Therefore, the mammographic features mimic those of simple cysts or noncalcified fibroadenomas.[92] Age of patient is not helpful, since both fibroadenomas and metastatic disease to the breast may occur in the young age group. The fact that the metastatic lesion in the breast may be the first evidence of a primary malignancy may further obscure the diagnosis. In addition to cyst and fibroadenoma, the mammographic differential diagnosis includes circumscribed ductal carcinoma, medullary carcinoma, mucinous carcinoma, and papillary carcinoma.[89] Metastases to the breast are also reported in male patients, most often from prostate cancer.[97]

The ultrasonography of blood-borne metastases is that of a round or oval mass with medium- to low-level internal echoes.[90] The wall may be regular (50%) or irregular (50%). Characteristically, no acoustic shadowing is seen. If multiple metastases occur, the ultrasound pattern of all lesions are similar. Breast ultrasonography may be used to monitor response to chemotherapy.[90]

Clues to the diagnosis of blood-borne metastases to the breast are listed in Box 13-4. Generally the diagnosis is most evident when the patient has a history of an extramammary malignancy and known soft tissue metastases. When a solitary metastasis to the breast is the presenting finding, special histochemical stains and ultrastructural studies may be necessary to reach the correct diagnosis of metastatic disease.

BOX 13-4 CLINICAL CLUES SUGGESTING METASTASES TO THE BREAST

History of extramammary malignancy
Known soft tissue metastases
Rapid growth of mass or masses
Location of mass in subcutaneous fat
Associated axillary adenopathy
Lack of desmoplasia and microcalcifications

Modified from Paulus DD, Libshitz HI: Metastases to the breast, *Radiol Clin North Am* 20:561, 1982.

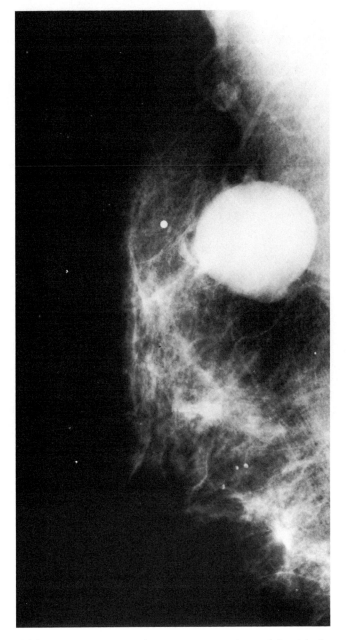

Fig. 13-36 Melanoma metastatic to the upper outer quadrant of the right breast produces a round, dense, palpable mass with circumscribed margins.

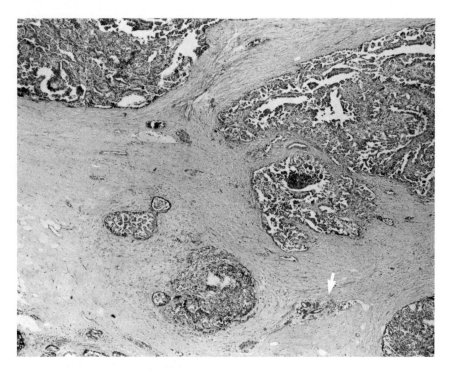

Fig. 13-37 Metastatic ovarian carcinoma. This metastatic papillary adenocarcinoma from the ovary to the breast shows multiple tumor masses of varying size and a prominent papillary growth pattern. A small, preserved, normal lobule can be identified *(arrow)*. This tumor may be misdiagnosed as primary papillary carcinoma of the breast. The lack of an in situ component is helpful in making the correct diagnosis.

REFERENCES
Stromal lesions
Sarcomas

1. Austin RM, Dupree WB: Liposarcoma of the breast: a clinico-pathologic study of 20 cases, *Hum Pathol* 17:906, 1986.
2. Barnes L, Pietruszka M: Sarcomas of the breast: a clinico-pathologic analysis of ten cases, *Cancer* 40:1577, 1977.
3. Berg JW, DeCrosse JJ, Fracchia AA, et al: Stromal sarcomas of the breast: a unified approach to connective tissue sarcomas other than cystosarcoma phyllodes, *Cancer* 15:418, 1962.
4. Berger SM, Gershon-Cohen J: Mammography of breast sarcoma, *AJR Am J Roentgenol* 87:76, 1962.
5. Breckenridge RL: Liposarcoma of the breast: report of a case, *Am J Clin Pathol* 24:954, 1954.
6. Chen KTK, Kuo TT, Hoffman KD: Leiomyosarcoma of the breast: a case of long survival and late hepatic metastasis, *Cancer* 47:1883, 1981.
7. Christensen L, Schidt T, Blichers-Taft M, et al: Sarcomas of the breast: a clinico-pathological study of 67 patients with long term follow-up, *Eur J Surg Oncol* 14:241, 1988.
8. Elson BC, Ikeda DM, Anderson I, et al: Fibrosarcoma of the breast: mammographic findings in five cases, *AJR Am J Roentgenol* 158:993, 1992.
9. Epstein EE: Fibrosarcoma of the breast: a case report, *S Afr Med J* 57:288, 1980.
10. Ii K, Hizawa K, Okagaki K, et al: Liposarcoma of the breast: fine structural and histochemical study of a case, *Tokushima J Exp Med* 27:45, 1980.
11. Jones MW, Norris HJ, Wargotz ES, et al: Fibrosarcoma malignant fibrous histiocytoma of the breast: a clinico-pathologic study of 32 cases, *Am J Surg Pathol* 16:667, 1992.
12. Ladefoged C, Nielsen BB: Primary chondrosarcoma of the breast: a case report and review of the literature, *Breast Dis* 10:26, 1984.
13. Livendahl RA: Liposarcoma of the mammary gland. *Surg Gynecol Obstet* 50:81, 1930.
14. Mufarrji AA, Feiner HD: Breast sarcoma with giant cells and osteoid: a case report and review of the literature, *Am J Surg Pathol* 11:225, 1987.
15. Norris HJ, Taylor HB: Sarcomas and related mesenchymal tumors of the breast, *Cancer* 22:22, 1968.

16. Pollard SG, Marks PV, Temple LN, et al: Breast sarcoma: a clinicopathologic review of 25 cases, *Cancer* 66:941, 1990.
17. Qizilbash AH: Cystosarcoma phyllodes with liposarcomatous stroma, *Am J Clin Pathol* 65:321, 1976.
18. Reynolds J, Mies C, Daly JM: *Mesenchymal infiltrating tumors.* In Bland KI, Copeland EM III, editors: *The breast, comprehensive management of benign and malignant disease*, Philadelphia, 1991, WB Saunders.
19. Watt AC, Haggar AM, Krasicky GA: Extraosseous osteogenic sarcoma of the breast: mammographic and pathologic findings, *Radiology* 150:34, 1984.

Fibromatoses and Benign Stromal Lesions

20. Azzopardi JG, Ahmed A, Millis RR: *Problems in breast pathology.* In *Major problems in pathology*, vol II, London, 1979, WB Saunders, pp. 89-90.
21. Bassett LW, Cove HC: Myoblastoma of the breast, *AJR Am J Roentgenol* 132:122, 1979.
22. Casillas J, Sais GJ, Greve JL, et al: Imaging of intra and extraabdominal desmoid tumors, *RadioGraphics* 11:959, 1991.
23. D'Orsi CJ: Zebras of the breast, *Contemp Diag Radiol* 10:1, 1987.
24. Enzinger TM, Weiss SW: *Soft tissue tumors.* St. Louis, 1983, CV Mosby pp. 211-214.
25. Enzinger TM, Weiss SW: *Soft tissue tumors.* St. Louis, 1983, CV Mosby, pp. 745-756.
26. Garstin WIH, Kaufman Z, Michell MJ, et al: Fibrous mastopathy in insulin dependent diabetes, *Clin Radiol* 44:89, 1991.
27. Hermann G, Schwartz IS: Focal fibrous disease of the breast: mammographic detection of an unappreciated condition, *AJR Am J Roentgenol* 140:1245, 1983.
28. Kalisher L, Long JA, Peyster RG: Extra-abdominal desmoid of the axillary tail mimicking breast carcinoma, *AJR Am J Roentgenol* 126:903, 1976.
29. Krishnan MMS, Krishnan R: An unusual breast lump: neurilemmoma, *Aust N Z J Surg* 52:612, 1982.
30. Logan WW, Hoffman NY: Diabetic fibrous breast disease, *Radiology* 172:667, 1989.
31. Nascimento AG, Karas M, Rosen PP, et al: Leiomyoma of the nipple, *Am J Surg Pathol* 3:151, 1979.
32. Reitämo JJ, Hayry P, Nykyri E, et al: The desmoid tumor. I. Incidence, sex-, age- and anatomical distribution in the Finnish population, *Am J Clin Pathol* 77:665, 1982.
33. Sloane JP: *Biopsy pathology of the breast*, New York, 1985, John Wiley & Sons.
34. Soler NG, Khardori R: Fibrous disease of the breast, thyroiditis, and cheiroarthropathy in type I diabetes mellitus, *Lancet* 1:193, 1984.
35. Stefansson K, Wollman RL: S-100 protein in granular cell tumors (granular cell myoblastoma), *Cancer* 49:1834, 1982.
36. Toker C, Tang CK, Whitely JF, et al: Benign spindle cell breast tumor, *Cancer* 48:1615, 1981.
37. Tomaszewski JE, Brooks JS, Hicks D, et al: Diabetic mastopathy: a distinctive clinico-pathologic entity, *Hum Pathol* 23:780, 1992.
38. Umansky C, Bullock WK: Granular cell myoblastoma of the breast, *Ann Surg* 168:810, 1968.
39. Wargotz ES, Norris HJ, Austin RM, et al: Fibromatosis of the breast: a clinical and pathological study of 28 cases, *Am J Surg Pathol* 11:38, 1987.

Vascular lesions

40. Brown RW, Bhathal PS, Scott PR: Multiple bilateral angiolipomas of the breast: a case report, *Aust N Z J Surg* 52:614, 1982.
41. Hoda SA, Cranor ML, Rosen PP: Hemangiomas of the breast with atypical histological features: further analysis of histological subtypes confirming their benign character, *Am J Surg Pathol* 16:553, 1992.
42. Ibrahim RE, Sciotto CG, Weidner N: Pseudoangiomatous hyperplasia of mammary stroma: some observations regarding its clinicopathologic spectrum, *Cancer* 63:1154, 1989.
43. Jozefczyk MA, Rosen PP: Vascular tumors of the breast: II. Perilobular hemangiomas and hemangiomas, *Am J Surg Pathol* 9:491, 1985.
44. Rosen PP: Vascular tumors of the breast: III. Angiomatosis, *Am J Surg Pathol* 9:652, 1985.
45. Rosen PP: Vascular tumors of the breast: V. Nonparenchymal hemangiomas of mammary subcutaneous tissues, *Am J Surg Pathol* 9:723, 1985.
46. Rosen PP, Jazefczyk MA, Boram LH: Vascular tumors of the breast: IV. The venous hemangioma, *Am J Surg Pathol* 9:659, 1985.
47. Rosen PP, Ridolfi RL: The perilobular hemangioma: a benign microscopic vascular lesion of the breast, *Am J Clin Pathol* 68:21, 1977.
48. Vuitch MF, Rosen PP, Erlandson RA: Pseudoangiomatous hyperplasia of mammary stroma, *Hum Pathol* 17:185, 1986.

Mondor's Disease

49. Catania S, Zurrida S, Veronesi P, et al: Mondor's disease and breast cancer, *Cancer* 69:2267, 1992.
50. Cooper RA: Mondor's disease secondary to intravenous drug abuse, *Arch Surg* 125:807, 1990.

51. Hoeffken W, Lanyi M: *Mondor syndrome.* In *Mammography: technique, diagnosis, differential diagnosis, results,* Philadelphia, 1977, WB Saunders, pp. 144-146.
52. Skipworth GB, Morris JB, Goldstein N: Bilateral Mondor's disease, *Arch Dermatol* 95:95, 1967.
53. Tabar L, Dean PB: Mondor's disease: clinical mammographic and pathologic features, *Breast, Dis* 7:18, 1981.

Angiosarcoma

54. Chen KTK, Kirkegaard DD, Bocian JJ: Angiosarcoma of the breast, *Cancer* 46:368, 1980.
55. Donnell RM, Rosen PP, Lieberman PH, et al: Angiosarcoma and other vascular tumors of the breast: pathologic analysis as a guide to prognosis, *Am J Surg Pathol* 5:629, 1981.
56. Grant EG, Holt RW, Chun B, et al: Angiosarcoma of the breast: sonographic, xeromammographic, and pathologic appearance, *AJR Am J Roentgenol* 141:691, 1983.
57. Lieberman L, Dershaw DD, Kaufman RJ, et al: Angiosarcoma of the breast, *Radiology* 183:649, 1992.
58. Merino MJ, Berman M, Carter D: Angiosarcoma of the breast, *Am J Surg Pathol* 7:53, 1983.
59. Rosen PP, Kimmel M, Ernsberger D: Mammary angiosarcoma: the prognostic significance of tumor differentiation, *Cancer* 62:2145, 1988.
60. Rubin E, Maddox WA, Mazur MT: Cutaneous angiosarcoma of the breast 7 years after lumpectomy and radiation therapy, *Radiology* 174:258, 1990.
61. Sordillo PP, Chapman R, Hajdu SI, et al: Lymphangiosarcoma, *Cancer* 48:1674, 1981.
62. Steingaszner LC, Enzinger FM, Taylor HB: Hemangiosarcoma of the breast, *Cancer* 18:352, 1965.
63. Stewart FW: *Tumors of the breast,* In *Atlas of tumor pathology.* Fascicle 34, Section 9, Washington, DC, Armed Forces Institute of Pathology, 1950.
64. Stewart FW, Treves N: Lymphangiosarcoma in post mastectomy lymphedema: a report of six cases in elephantiasis chirurgica, *Cancer* 1:64, 1948.

Hemangiopericytoma

65. Enzinger FM, Smith BH: Hemangiopericytoma analysis of 106 cases, *Hum Pathol* 7:61, 1976.
66. Tavassoli FA, Weiss S: Hemangiopericytoma of the breast, *Am J Surg Pathol* 5:745, 1981.

Hematolymphoid breast lesions
Lymphoma and Hodgkin's Disease

67. Brustein S, Filippa DA, Kimmel M, et al: Malignant lymphoma of the breast: a study of 53 patients, *Ann Surg* 205:144, 1987.
68. Danel L, Souweine G, Monier JC, et al: Specific estrogen binding sites in human lymphoid cells and thymic cells, *J Steroid Biochem* 18:559, 1983.
69. Giardini R, Piccolo C, Rilke F: Primary non-Hodgkin's lymphomas of the female breast, *Cancer* 69:725, 1992.
70. Hugh JC, Jackson FI, Hanson J, et al: Primary breast lymphoma: an immunohistologic study of 20 new cases, *Cancer* 66:2602, 1990.
71. Isaacson PG, Spencer J: Malignant lymphoma of mucosa-associated lymphoid tissue. *Histopathology* 11:445, 1987.
72. Jackson FI, Zulfikarali HL: Breast lymphoma: radiologic imaging and clinical appearances, *Can Assoc Radiol J* 42:48, 1991.
73. Jeon HJ, Akagi T, Hoshida Y, et al: Primary non-Hodgkin's malignant lymphoma of the breast: an immunohistochemical study of seven patients and literature review of 152 patients with breast lymphoma in Japan, *Cancer* 70:2451, 1992.
74. Kalisher L: Xeroradiography of axillary lymph node disease, *Radiology* 114:67, 1975.
75. Kushner LN: Hodgkin's disease simulating inflammatory breast carcinoma on mammography: a case report, *Radiology* 92:350, 1969.
76. Meyer JE, Kopans DB, Long JC: Mammographic appearance of malignant lymphoma of the breast, *Radiology* 135:623, 1980.
77. Paulus DD: Lymphoma of the breast, *Radiol Clin North Am* 28:833, 1990.
78. Schouten JT, Weese JL, Carbone PD: Lymphoma of the breast, *Ann Surg* 194:749, 1981.
79. Smith MR, Brustein S, Straus DJ: Localized non-Hodgkin's lymphoma of the breast, *Cancer* 59:351, 1987.
80. Wiseman C, Liao KT: Primary lymphoma of the breast, *Cancer* 29:1705, 1972.

Pseudolymphoma

81. Fisher ER, Palekar AS, Paulson JD, et al: Pseudolymphoma of the breast, *Cancer* 44:258, 1979.
82. Knowles DM, Athan E, Ubriaco A, et al: Extranodal noncutaneous lymphoid hyperplasias represent a continuous spectrum of B-cell neoplasia: demonstration by molecular genetics analysis, *Blood* 73:1635, 1989.
83. Lin JJ, Farha GJ, Taylor RJ: Pseudolymphoma of the breast. I. A study of 8,654 consecutive tylectomies and mastectomies, *Cancer* 45:973, 1980.
84. Myhre MJ, Isaacson PG: Primary B-cell gastric lymphoma: a reassessment of its histogenesis, *J Pathol* 152:1, 1987.

Hematologic Malignancies

85. Brooks JJ, Krugman DT, Damjanov I: Myeloid metaplasia presenting as a breast mass, *Am J Surg Pathol* 4:281, 1980.
86. Gartenhaus WS, Mir R, Pliskin A, et al: Granulocytic sarcoma of breast: aleukemic bilateral metachronous presentation and literature review, *Med Pediatr Oncol* 13:22, 1985.
87. Kennedy BJ, Bornstein R, Brunning RD, et al: Breast involvement in acute leukemia, *Cancer* 25:693, 1970.
88. Pascoe HR: Tumors composed of immature granulocytes occurring in the breast in chronic granulocytic leukemia, *Cancer* 25:697, 1970.

Metastatic disease

89. Bohman LG, Bassett LW, Gold RH, et al: Breast metastases from extramammary malignancies, *Radiology* 144:309, 1982.
90. Derchi LE, Rizzato G, Giuseppetti GM, et al: Metastatic tumors in the breast: sonographic findings, *J Ultrasound Med* 4:69, 1985.
91. Hadju SI, Urban JA: Cancers metastatic to the breast, *Cancer* 29:1691, 1972.
92. Jochimsen PR, Brown RC: Metastatic melanoma in the breast masquerading as fibroadenoma, *JAMA* 236:2779, 1976.
93. Kashlan RB, Powell RW, Nolting SF: Carcinoid and other tumors metastatic to the breast, *J Surg Oncol* 20:25, 1982.
94. Paulus DD, Libshitz HI: Metastases to the breast, *Radiol Clin North Am* 20:561, 1982.
95. McCrea ES, Johnston C, Haney PJ: Metastases to the breast, *AJR Am J Roentgenol* 141:685, 1983.
96. Moncada R, Cooper RA, Garces M, et al: Calcified metastases from malignant ovarian neoplasm, *Radiology* 113:31, 1974.
97. Toombs BD, Kalisher L: Metastatic disease to the breast: clinical, pathologic, and radiographic features, *AJR Am J Roentgenol* 129:673, 1977.

CHAPTER 14

Inflammatory, Granulomatous, and Male Breast Disorders

Carol B. Stelling
Deborah E. Powell

Inflammatory conditions of the breast
 Mastitis
 Breast abscess
 Duct ectasia
 Squamous metaplasia of lactiferous ducts
 Unusual infections
 Granulomatous mastitis
 Traumatic fat necrosis
Systemic inflammatory conditions
 Sarcoidosis of the breast
 Wegener's granulomatosis
 Amyloid
Disorders of the male breast
 Gynecomastia
  Physiologic versus pathologic gynecomastia
 Cancer of the male breast
 Other male breast disorders
  Inflammatory conditions of the male breast
  Benign breast lesions in the male

In this chapter some of the more common inflammatory diseases of the breast are discussed in addition to some systemic diseases that may involve mammary tissue as well as other organs. A discussion of some of the common benign and malignant conditions involving the male breast is included in this chapter.

INFLAMMATORY CONDITIONS OF THE BREAST
Mastitis

Acute mastitis is usually observed in women of childbearing years. For the most part, it is a clinical entity in the lactating breast and there is no need for breast imaging studies. An appropriate trial of an antistaphylococcal antibiotic usually results in a clinical cure. If mammograms are requested, the image demonstrates a diffuse increase in density of the parenchyma. Subacute or chronic infection may occur if the antibiotic chosen is inappropriate or if the patient stops the medication prematurely. The presence of an abscess may be suspected if a focal mass is palpable or if persistent fevers occur. Mammography in the subacute stage may show a localized ill-defined mass, most often subareolar in location. Biopsy of the lesion is seldom carried out.

Breast abscess

A localized collection of pus in the breast constitutes an abscess. Unless the abscess can drain through the ductal system, an incision and drainage procedure may be required. Patients with breast abscess are acutely ill with pain and fever.

Mammography is not recommended until the acute symptoms of breast abscess have subsided, usually with appropriate antibiotic therapy. Women with a breast abscess cannot tolerate the compression required for proper mammography. If imaging is needed to determine whether the infection is a diffuse mastitis or a localized abscess, breast ultrasound examination is the procedure of choice. Diffuse microabscesses are not amenable to drainage, and aggressive medical therapy is recommended. Mammography may be performed after the abscess has cleared to rule out a more suspicious process. Mammographic appearance of abscess is usually an oval or round mass with ill-defined or fuzzy margins. This appearance is indistinguishable from breast cancer. Microcalcifications are not a feature of breast abscess.

Duct ectasia

Duct ectasia is characterized by widened and dilated duct spaces, which may show an irregular luminal diameter and may or may not be associated with periductal fibrosis.[1,2] These ectatic ducts are part of the major duct system of the breast and differ from the cysts of fibrocystic change in that they do not originate in the lobule. They are commonly found close to the nipple, or areola. A large number of names have been given to the condition of duct ectasia (see Box 14-1).

The mammographic finding in patients with duct ectasia is a grouping of prominent ducts in the retroareolar area, usually bilaterally symmetric. Less frequently, duct ectasia may be the cause of an asymmetric retroareolar tubular structure. Its ultrasonographic appearance is a branching fluid-filled structure in the subareolar region. If cellular debris is present, a "target" lesion may be seen on transverse ultrasound scans.[3] The mammographic width of the visualized duct includes the periductal fibrosis and is not representative of the true lumen size.

In some patients with duct ectasia, benign calcifications are demonstrated mammographically. Calcification of intraluminal secretions produce long linear calcifications that are oriented toward the nipple and are most often bilateral and symmetric.[6] These secretory duct calcifications are sufficiently characteristic in their appearance that they do not cause diagnostic confusion with the more variable casting type calcifications of comedocarcinoma.

In some women duct ectasia is associated with periductal inflammation, often with a prominent infiltration of plasma cells, known as *plasma cell mastitis*. Resulting calcifications of plasma cell mastitis resemble hollow beads and are circumductal or periductal in location.[4] In more florid cases, a granulomatous response with numerous macrophages and giant cells may be seen. This is adjacent

---

BOX 14-1 SYNONYMS FOR DUCT ECTASIA

Varicocele tumor
Plasma cell mastitis
Comedomastitis
Mastitis obliterans (obliterative mastitis)
Periductal mastitis
Mammary duct ectasia
Secretory disease of the breast

From Rees BI, Gravelle IH, Hughes LE: Nipple retraction in duct ectasia, *Br J Surg* 64:577, 1977.

to the large dilated ducts, and because of the association, can be distinguished from other granulomatous diseases in the breast. The chronic inflammation may progress to scarring, which frequently surrounds the ducts. The associated destruction of periductal elastic tissue contributes to the dilatation. The ducts are lined by a flattened epithelium, and hyperplasia and apocrine change are rarely present.

Squamous metaplasia of lactiferous ducts

Squamous metaplasia of lactiferous ducts is commonly referred to in the literature as *subareolar abscess*. Patients with this condition frequently present clinically with episodes of chronic, recurring abscesses in the subareolar area, which frequently develop draining fistulous tracts.[9] These abscesses typically occur in younger women and fail to respond to antibiotic therapy, often requiring surgical treatment. The lesion is thought to develop in the lactiferous ducts beneath the nipple[8] or in the ducts of the glands of Montgomery, which empty onto the areola.[7] The mechanism is felt to be replacement of the duct epithelium by metaplastic squamous epithelium, which produces keratin and leads to plugging and obstruction of the ducts by keratinaceous debris. This may lead to secondary infection of inspissated secretions with abscess formation and ultimately to rupture and draining fistula formation. The glands of Montgomery are particularly susceptible to this process because they are smaller and more tortuous than the major lactiferous ducts and have decreased elastic tissue within their walls. This leads to an increased propensity for decreased drainage with the resulting sequence of inflammatory metaplasia and abscess formation.

No specific imaging features indicate squamous metaplasia. The clinical entity can be suggested in the presence of a history of recurring subareolar abscess or periareolar fistula. Mammographic findings of a subareolar inflammatory process may be present.

Unusual infections

The breast may also be a site of unusual breast infections including tuberculosis, fungus, and parasites (Box 14-2). With an increase in autoimmune disorders such as AIDS and the influx of refugees from underdeveloped countries, unusual infection should be considered in an appropriate clinical setting.

Tuberculosis and fungal diseases produce a nonspecific, ill-defined parenchymal mass. Axillary lymphadenopathy may or may not be present. The mammographic findings are nonspecific. Caution must be exercised in these affected

---

BOX 14-2 UNUSUAL BREAST INFECTIONS

Tuberculosis
  Mycobacterium tuberculosis
  Mycobacterium avium-intracellulare

Fungi
  Actinomycosis
  Blastomycosis (Seymour, 1982)
  Histoplasmosis

Syphilis

Parasites
  Cysticercosis
  Guinea worm (Stelling, 1982)
  Hydatid disease (Mirza, 1979)
  Loa loa

women. Coexisting cancer may be present.[22] A cavitary breast mass with gas/fluid interface has been described in one patient with disseminated systemic blastomycosis.[20] Histochemical techniques may be useful in identifying organisms, and special staining for fungi and acid-fast bacilli in particular should be used for identifying granulomas, even when classic patterns of caseation necrosis are not present.

With the increasing incidence of atypical mycobacterial infections, Fite stains may be more useful than conventional stains for *Mycobacterium tuberculosis hominis*. The use of DNA probes and molecular diagnostic techniques can greatly facilitate early diagnosis.

Granulomatous mastitis

Granulomatous mastitis is an uncommon recently recognized condition, which is characterized pathologically by extensive involvement of breast lobules by noncaseating epithelioid granulomas, some with giant cells and with microabscess formation. Granulomatous mastitis was first described in 1972 by Kessler and Wolloch in five women.[16] Since that time additional reports and literature reviews have been made. As of 1990, about 30 cases have been reported.[15] The diagnosis is one of exclusion of other causes of granulomatous processes, such as typhoid, fungal infections, filaria, and tuberculosis.[10,15,19]

Granulomatous mastitis occurs predominantly in women of reproductive age (17–42 years), with a mean age of about 32 years.[15] A common factor of reported cases is that all women are parous.[15] No consistent association with lactation or use of oral contraceptives has been found.[14] A possible autoimmune etiology has not been confirmed. Association with duct ectasia is not a feature of granulomatous mastitis, which distinguishes it from plasma cell mastitis with duct ectasia, which may exhibit granuloma formation.[14] Granulomatous mastitis frequently involves lobules, a feature that has suggested the name "granulomatous lobular mastitis."[14] This feature also differentiates this lesion from plasma cell mastitis (Table 14-1).

Most women with granulomatous mastitis present with a unilateral mass or area of induration. A few cases of bilateral involvement have been recognized.[13,14] Tenderness and erythema may be present, but are not consistent features. The mass effect varies from 0.5 cm to 8 cm and is frequently moderately large, about 3 to 6 cm in diameter. The location of the mass is not specific and is not consistently subareolar.[11] Skin edema, skin retraction, nipple retraction, and fixation to the chest wall are reported and increase clinical suspicion of breast carcinoma. The xeromammographic appearance of one case of granulomatous mastitis has been published, which resembled changes of inflammatory breast cancer, including a diffuse central mass density and associated nipple re-

Table 14-1 **Differential features of granulomatous breast lesions**

	Caseating granulomas	Microabscesses	Foam cells	Lobular involvement
Duct ectasia/ plasma cell mastitis	0	0	+	0
Tuberculosis	+	0	0	+
Granulomatous mastitis	0	+	0	+
Sarcoidosis	0	0	0	+

traction and skin thickening.[15] One 36-year-old patient had a negative mammogram described with a clinical area of erythema and induration.[15] In over 50% of reported cases, the working diagnosis has been breast cancer.[11,14]

Excision of granulomatous breast lesions has been described for some patients with good results. However, some women develop complications of wound infection, skin ulceration, and draining fistulas.[13,14] These problems suggest an infectious cause by tuberculosis, fungus, aerobic, or anaerobic agents. Appropriate cultures and stains must be performed to exclude an organism requiring specific therapy. Moreover the recent successful use of high-dose steroid therapy for refractory cases mandates exclusion of an infectious etiology.[12,13,15]

Diagnosis of granulomatous mastitis is possible by fine needle aspiration cytology. Culture of aspirated material for *Mycobacterium*, fungi, aerobic, and anaerobic organisms is recommended.[17] It is also appropriate to exclude the diagnosis of sarcoidosis by Kveim test, chest radiographs, and serum levels of both angiotensin-converting enzyme and lysozyme, because granulomatous mastitis is a diagnosis of exclusion.[14]

Traumatic fat necrosis

Traumatic fat necrosis is an isolated and uncommon occurrence in the female breast. The history of trauma is often remote, unknown, or not remembered. In one series a positive history for trauma was elicited in 40% of women.[31] Traumatic fat necrosis is uncommon in males. In females it occurs between ages 20 to 76 years, with most cases occurring during the fifth decade.[37] Most women with the condition are obese and have fatty pendulous breasts.[37] Clinically occult fat necrosis may be identified mammographically years after the traumatic event.

When a trauma history is given, the injury may be one of many mechanisms. Blunt contusion from a fall, abuse, and a motor vehicle accident are common causes. A steering wheel contusion may occur across the upper surface of both breasts. Trauma due to a shoulder restraint injury varies in position depending on the woman's position in the vehicle (e.g., driver or passenger position) and the level at which the shoulder restraint crosses the breast. Unusual patterns of trauma may occur due to horse bite or other injury.

For many women the cause of traumatic fat necrosis is iatrogenic.[32,38,39] Lipid/oil cysts frequently develop in a biopsy, lumpectomy or postirradiation therapy site.[26,28] It is useful to mark the biopsy scar with an external marker prior to mammography to help correlate any mammographic changes with the surgical site. Other infrequent causes of fat necrosis in the breast are spontaneous necrosis secondary to Coumadin therapy[24] and Weber-Christian disease.[27]

Traumatic fat necrosis often has characteristic mammographic features but occasionally mimics cancer clinically or mammographically. Before preoperative mammography was routine, fat necrosis diagnosed by excisional biopsy accounted for only 0.5% of biopsies.[23] Mammographic appearance of traumatic fat necrosis, when classic for a lipid cyst, is pathognomonic and may preclude a diagnostic tissue sampling.

The clinical presentation of fat necrosis may be that of a firm or hard palpable mass, which may be superficial or subcutaneous in location, particularly in a fatty breast. Redness of the skin, ecchymosis, or skin or nipple retraction may occur. Ecchymosis is a particularly helpful clue that suggests traumatic fat necrosis, but it is an inconsistent feature and it may have resolved. Complaints of tenderness are not typical except when mammary duct ectasia is present. Lymph node enlargement may occur.[37]

The gross and microscopic appearance of fat necrosis varies depending on the age of the lesion. Lesions that have been present for some time show a more fibrous response. A typical area of fat necrosis is variegated in appearance and poorly circumscribed. It is firm, often gritty, and yellow-white in color. Areas of hemorrhage, recent or old, and necrosis with softening or liquefaction may be found. The gross appearance is often mistaken for carcinoma.

Histologically, fat necrosis also shows varied characteristics. Typical necrotic adipocytes with granular and eosinophic rather than clear cytoplasm may be present. Mononuclear cells and hemosiderin are frequently seen. Multinucleated giant cells, calcification, and fibrosis are often found and vary in prominence according to the age of the lesion. The diagnosis of fat necrosis may be made with fine needle aspiration.

Extensive hemorrhagic gangrenous necrosis of the breast has been reported after Coumadin therapy. This differs from the classic fat necrosis in a number of ways and is characterized histologically by extensive hemorrhage, venous thrombosis, and acute inflammation of small- and medium-sized arteries.[35] Extensive necrosis has necessitated mastectomy in some cases. Clinically the lesion, although rare, usually is seen in middle-aged to older patients and begins to develop shortly after the onset of Coumadin treatment. The cause may be the induction of a short-lived hypercoaguable state caused by a transient rapid fall in protein C plasma levels before levels of other clotting factors decrease.[29]

The imaging features of traumatic fat necrosis are commonly pathognomonic of the entity. A lipid or oil cyst develops with a low-density fat center surrounded by a thin smooth fibrous wall. Single or multiple lesions may be present. The size of the lesion varies from several millimeters to 5 cm in diameter.[34] Most lipid cysts are between 0.5 and 1.5 cm. Liponecrosis microcytic calcificans describes ring-like calcification of oil cysts up to a few millimeters in size.[40] The contents of the cyst are liquefied fats. An oil cyst produces a classic sonolucent appearance by ultrasound examination.[34] However, because the mammographic appearance of benign lipid cyst is so classic, breast ultrasound examination is not necessary. If the cyst contents are not homogeneous, it is possible to define a fat/fluid level on a horizontal beam radiograph.[30] Rarely the cyst contents may change from lipid to solid or contain a fibrin ball.[30]

Calcifications are known to occur in traumatic fat necrosis. Typically, the calcifications are eggshell or thin circumspherical plaque-like calcifications in the fibrotic wall surrounding the low-density center.[25,26,30,36] This calcification pattern need not be biopsied when both the mammographic appearance and the history are classic for traumatic fat necrosis (Box 14-3). Infrequently the calcification that develops in traumatic fat necrosis consists of thin linear, branching, and bizarre forms. Unusual cases of fat necrosis that mimic the calcification pattern of adenocarcinoma have been reported.[25,27] If there is any doubt concerning the diagnosis, a biopsy is recommended.[28]

Traumatic fat necrosis may also cause a fibrotic response in the breast. This process may manifest as irregular, ill-defined, or spiculated margins to an oval or round mass. This imaging appearance would be impossible to differentiate from cancer unless an unequivocal area of lipid cyst as well as a clearly related trauma history is present. Caution is advised since some cancers may infiltrate, surround, and entrap fat. The difficulty in differential diagnosis may be particularly problematic in women who have been treated by lumpectomy and radiation therapy.[28] Cancer may coexist with fat necrosis. Tissue diagnosis is recommended.

BOX 14-3 CLUES TO DIAGNOSIS OF TRAUMATIC FAT NECROSIS

Ecchymosis
Superficial location in a fatty breast
Location correlating with trauma or surgery
Classic lipid cyst with or without calcifications

In summation, classic lipid cysts are pathognomonic for fat necrosis. However, traumatic fat necrosis may mimic both clinical and mammographic features of invasive breast cancer.[25,33,36] When the lesion is more circumscribed in appearance, the working diagnosis may be papilloma, fibroadenoma, or abscess.[36]

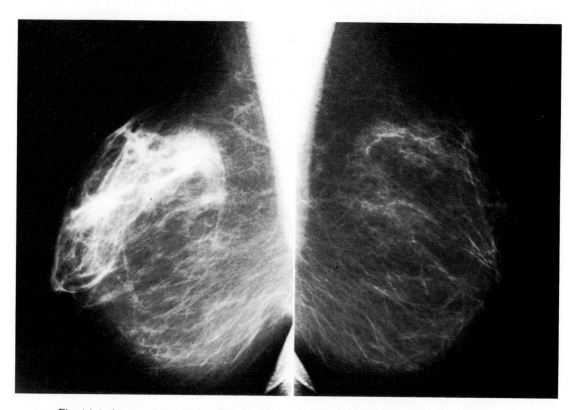

Fig. 14-1 Acute mastitis produced the diffuse asymmetric density in the upper outer quadrant of the right breast. The asymmetry resolved after a course of antistaphylococcal antibiotics.

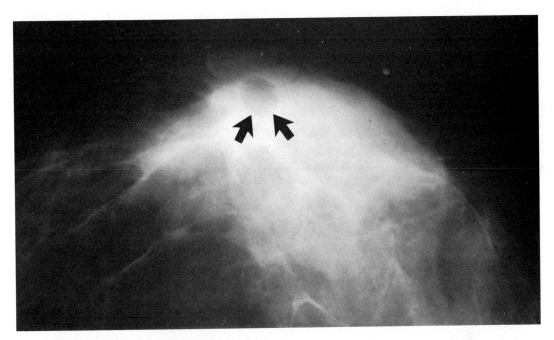

Fig. 14-2 Recurrent abscess despite prior incision. A 1-cm air-containing pocket (*arrows*) noted beneath the areola represents abscess cavity 2 days after spontaneous drainage of pus through perioareolar fistula.

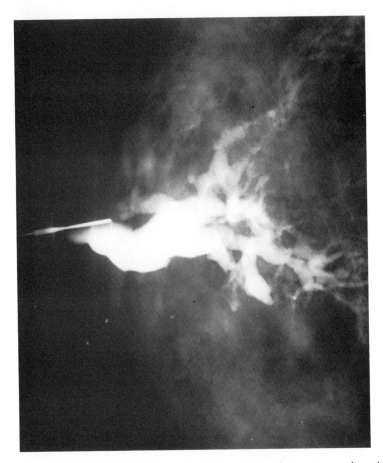

Fig. 14-3 Ectasia of a central duct demonstrated by iodinated contrast on a lateral projection galactogram.

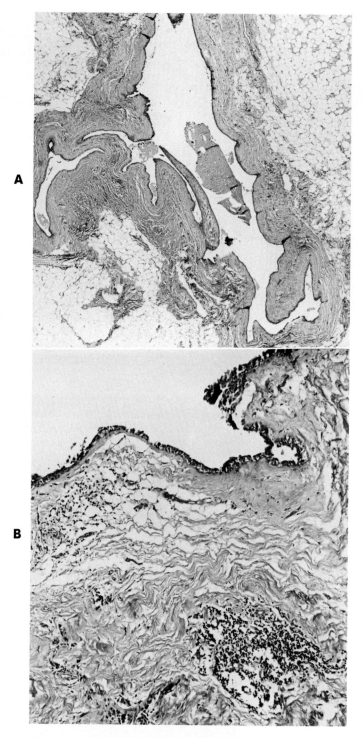

Fig. 14-4 Duct ectasia. Duct ectasia involves larger, more centrally located ducts in the breast. The ducts are dilated, frequently contain amorphous material, and often periductal fibrosis is present **(A)**. At higher magnification the periductal fibrosis and a mononuclear cell infiltrate can be seen. Preserved epithelial duct lining can be seen at the top of the photomicrograph **(B)**.

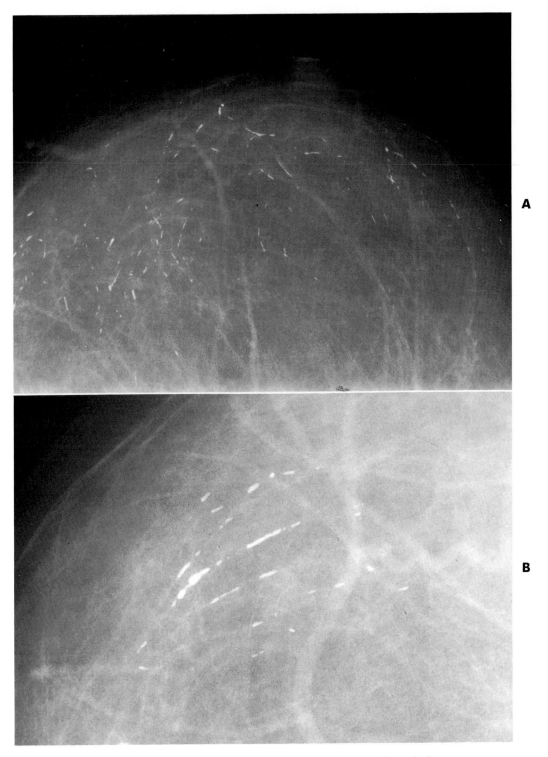

Fig. 14-5 Secretory duct calcifications. **(A)** A typical case of secretory duct calcification causes diffuse coarse linear calcifications oriented towards the nipple. **(B)** The regular size and density of these secretory duct calcifications distinguish them from pleomorphic casting type calcifications.

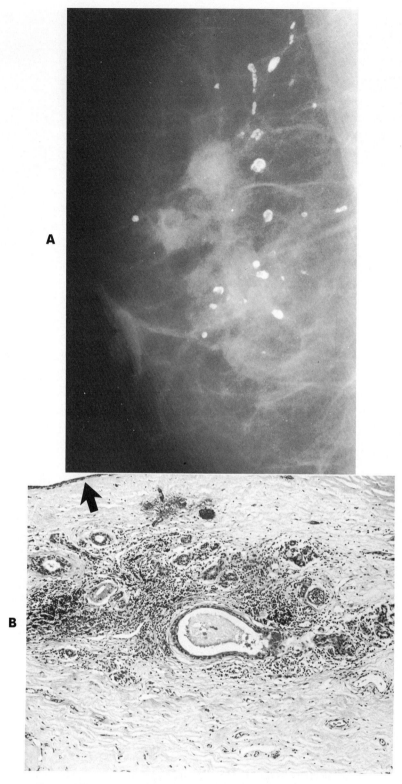

Fig. 14-6 Plasma cell mastitis. **(A)** Plasma cell mastitis produces typical coarse and ring-shaped calcifications associated with ill-defined rounded masses and chronic nipple retraction. **(B)** The mononuclear cell infiltrate seen in plasma cell mastitis usually contains lymphocytes as well as numerous plasma cells. The infiltrate seen here is involving a breast lobule as well as the wall of the adjacent ectatic duct *(arrow)*.

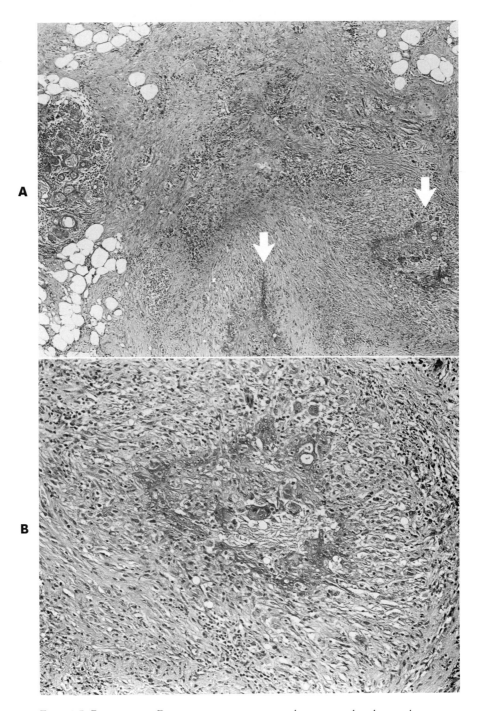

Fig. 14-7 Duct ectasia. Duct ectasia may sometimes be associated with granulomatous inflammation. The characteristic dilated major ducts are present, helping to distinguish the granulomas from those caused by infectious agents or sarcoidosis. The low-magnification photomicrograph **(A)** shows a lobule with chronic inflammation (*far left*) and extensive fibrosis and granulomas (*arrows*). **(B)** At higher magnification a granuloma with numerous giant cells and histocytes is illustrated.

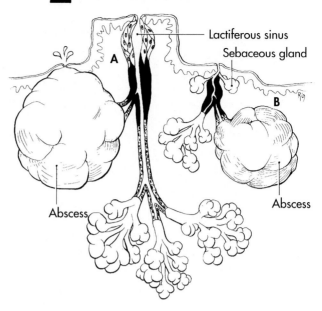

Fig. 14-8 Squamous metaplasia of lactiferous ducts may involve lactiferous ducts of the breast **(A)** or ducts of the glands of Montgomery, **(B)** which empty onto the areola rather than the nipple. In both sites, the duct lumina may become obstructed by keratinaceous debris leading to abscess formation. The abscesses may eventually drain onto the skin of the areola. The process may occur commonly in the glands of Montgomery, where the tortuous nature of the ducts make them more susceptible to obstruction.

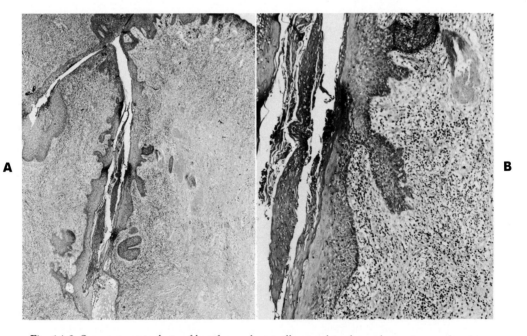

Fig. 14-9 Squamous metaplasia of lactiferous duct is illustrated in these photomicrographs. At low magnification **(A)** the nipple epidermis is at the very top of the photograph. Metaplastic squamous epithelium lines the duct below the level of the lactiferous sinus, where normally one would find a columnar epithelial lining. Keratinaceous debris partially fills the lumen. At higher magnification **(B)** the squamous epithelial lining and intraluminal keratin can be seen better, as well as the inflammatory cell infiltrate that surrounds the duct.

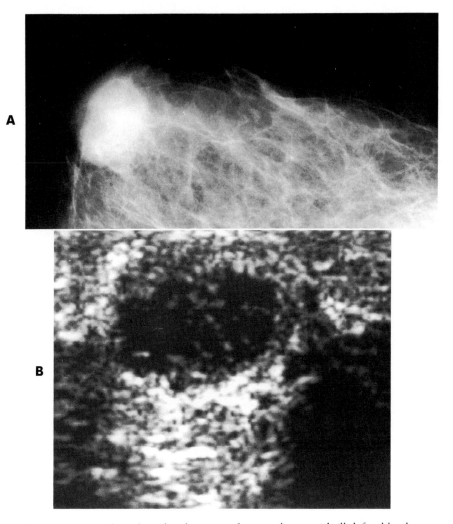

Fig. 14-10 (A) This subareolar abscess is a 3-cm oval mass with ill-defined borders on the MLO projection. (B) Breast ultrasound examination shows a fluid-filled mass containing internal echoes that suggest debris.

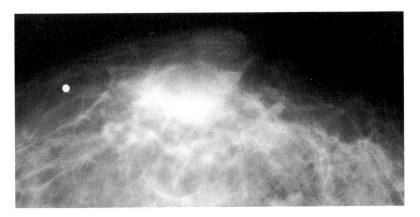

Fig. 14-11 Subareolar abscess is best demonstrated with the nipple in profile as mass with ill-defined margins immediately subareolar. Skin marker indicates that the lesion was palpable.

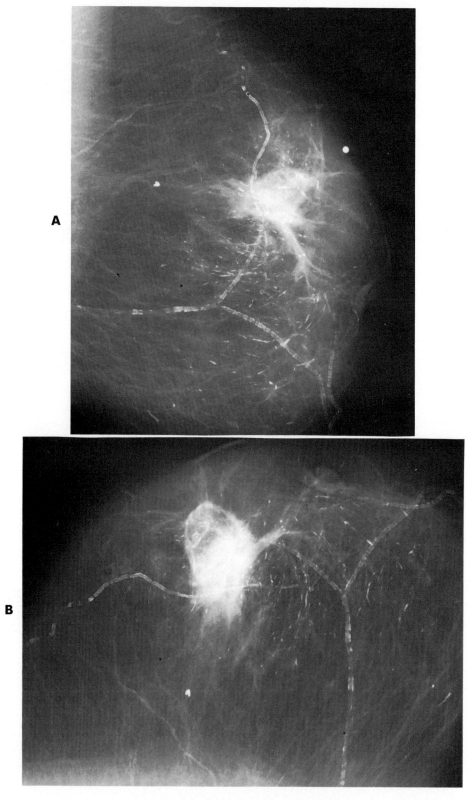

Fig. 14-12 Fat necrosis. **(A)** This oval, ill-defined mass with spiculated margins is relatively superficial in the MLO projection. **(B)** The low-density (fat) center of the mass indicates the diagnosis of fat necrosis and is better visualized in the craniocaudad view.

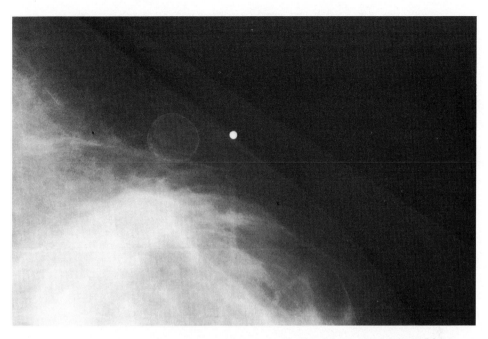

Fig. 14-13 Typical eggshell calcification and low-density mass of fat necrosis is imaged by a tangential view to the bb marking the palpable mass.

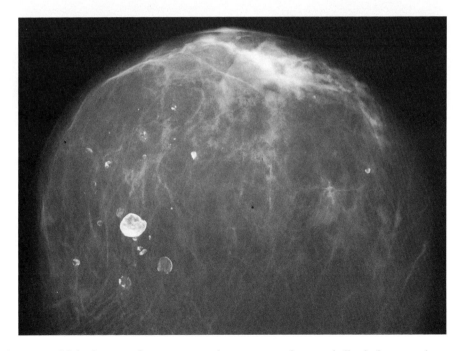

Fig. 14-14 Multiple areas of post-traumatic fat necrosis produce eggshell calcifications of varying size in this woman with a history of bruising due to steering wheel contusion during a motor vehicle accident.

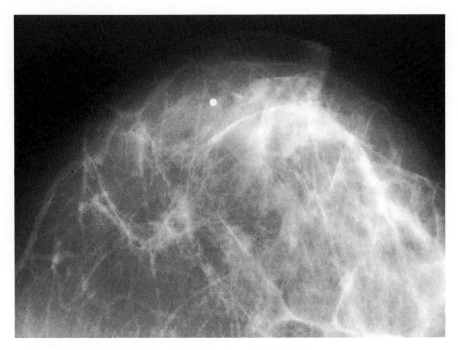

Fig. 14-15 Fat necrosis causes a hypodense round mass with ill-defined margins, secondary to recent biopsy procedure. Skin bbs mark the end of the surgical incision.

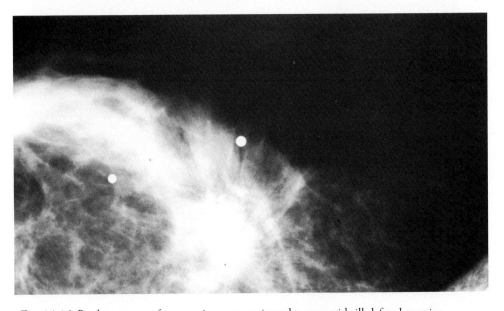

Fig. 14-16 Postlumpectomy fat necrosis causes an irregular mass with ill-defined margins.

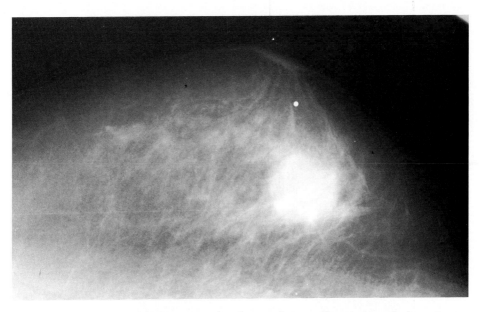

Fig. 14-17 Fat necrosis in this patient produced a round mass with a circumscribed margin anteriorly and an obscured margin posteriorly, mimicking a cyst or fibroadenoma.

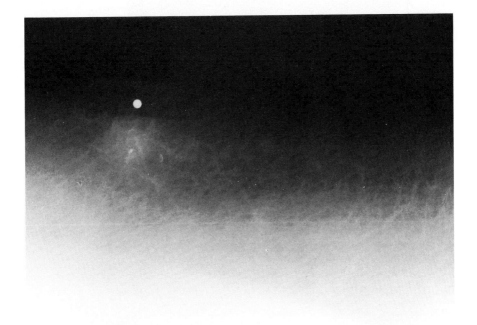

Fig. 14-18 Fat necrosis in this older patient mimicked an invasive breast cancer (an irregular mass with ill-defined margins) in the superficial tissues of the upper outer quadrant, imaged in this MLO projection.

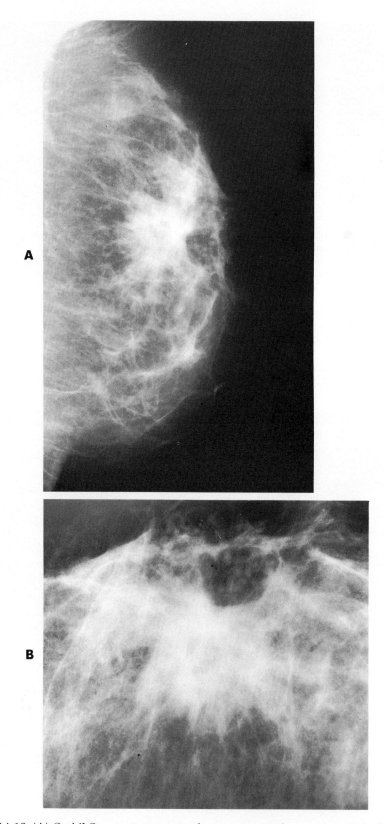

Fig. 14-19 (A) On MLO projection, invasive breast cancer produces an irregularly shaped mass with spiculated margins in the deep tissues of the left breast. Central-entrapped fat, best seen on craniocaudad view **(B),** mimics area of fat necrosis.

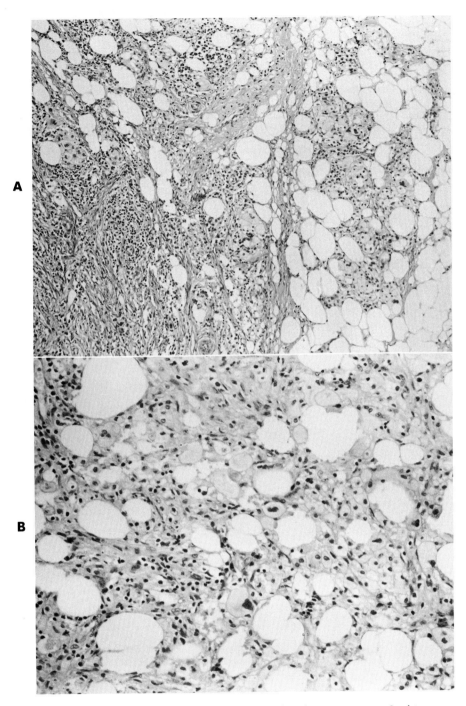

Fig. 14-20 Fat necrosis. Fat necrosis presents a varied histologic appearance. In this photomicrograph **(A)**, viable and necrotic fat cells are interspersed with inflammatory cells, fibroblasts, and giant cells. At higher magnification **(B)**, necrotic fat cells can be recognized by their pale but visible cytoplasm, contrasting with the empty cytoplasm of viable adipocytes.

Fig. 14-21 Fat necrosis. Fat necrosis may be associated with considerable fibrosis as well as inflammation. In this low-magnification photomicrograph **(A)** the fibrosis gives the area of fat necrosis a nodular appearance. At higher magnification **(B),** bands of fibrous tissue are intermixed with fat cells, multinucleated giant cells, and mononuclear inflammatory cells. **(C)** Focally, small lakes of necrotic fat may be seen *(arrow)*. These may lead to the formation of lipid cysts.

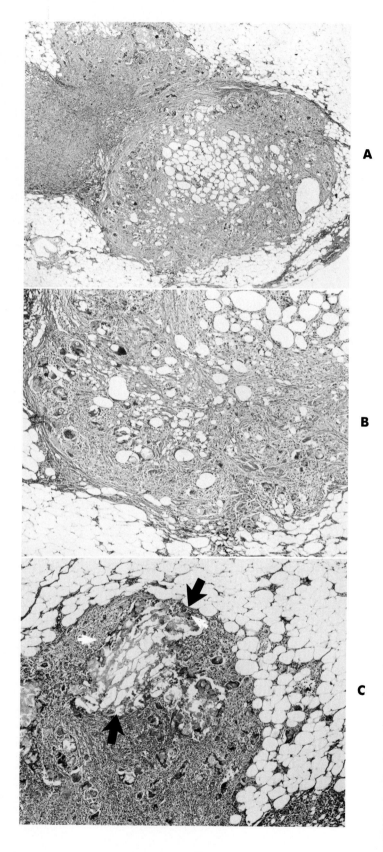

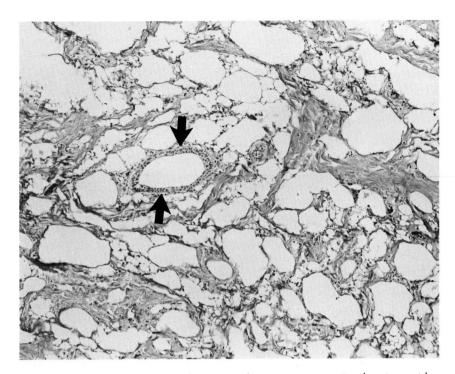

Fig. 14-22 Silicone granulomas. Silicone granulomas, seen in occasional patients with breast implants, may be confused histologically with fat necrosis. The varying-sized vacuoles are not fat cells, however. Giant cells are often present, and fibrosis is sometimes marked. In this photomicrograph a normal mammary duct can be identified (*arrows*).

SYSTEMIC INFLAMMATORY CONDITIONS

Certain diseases may involve the breast as one organ in a more generalized systemic disease process affecting many sites. Some of the infectious diseases previously mentioned fall into this category. Three other conditions, sarcoidosis, Wegener's granulomatosis, and amyloidosis, are discussed in this section.

Sarcoidosis of the breast

Sarcoidosis involving the breast is a very unusual condition even in series of substantial numbers of patients with systemic sarcoidosis. The clinical presentation is varied. The diagnosis may be an incidental finding in tissue biopsied for another reason.[41] In some women, coalescing granulomas form a palpable nodule, which may be 1.0 to 3.5 cm in diameter.[45,47] The diagnosis of sarcoid granulomas of the breast is based on compatible histology and careful exclusion of tuberculosis and fungal disorders. The diagnosis of sarcoidosis of the breast is on firmer ground if it is associated with signs or symptoms of systemic illness, either preceding or following the diagnosis of breast involvement.[44]

The number of accepted reports in the literature of sarcoidosis of the breast varies depending on the criteria used to exclude infectious causes of granulomatous processes. It has been stressed that negative histochemical stains for acid-fast bacilli in histologic sections are not sufficient to exclude a diagnosis of tuberculosis.[47] Similarly, although "hard" histiocytic granulomas with a notable absence of caseation are required for a diagnosis of sarcoidosis, absence of caseation does not exclude a diagnosis of tuberculosis. A negative intermediate-strength purified protein derivative (tuberculin) (PPD) skin test is required by many authors to rule out tuberculosis as a cause of multiple noncaseating epithelioid granulomas.[46,47]

There are other causes of noncaseating granulomas in the breast in addition to sarcoid and tuberculosis[46] (see Table 14-2). Most of these organisms are unusual. An immunosuppressed patient may be more prone to such uncommon infections. Foreign body reaction should also be considered. Use of polarized light to examine the histopathologic section is suggested. As mentioned, late-stage duct ectasia may also cause noncaseating granulomas.[49]

The sarcoid masses may be subcutaneous in location.[45,48] Fixation to the skin has been reported, mimicking breast cancer.[45] Many sarcoid breast lesions are painless; however, occasionally tenderness to palpation is noted.[45] Multiple or bilateral masses are sometimes present simultaneously.[45,47] Coexisting breast carcinoma does occur, even in young women.[46] Therefore even in patients with known systemic sarcoidosis, biopsy is recommended for dominant or suspicious breast masses.

Appropriate testing to support a presumptive diagnosis of sarcoid includes a chest radiograph to assess hilar and paratracheal lymphadenopathy, a Kveim-Stiltzbach test, and serum concentrations of both lysozyme and angiotensin-converting enzyme, which are often elevated in cases of active sarcoidosis. Although fine needle aspiration cytology may suggest a diagnosis of sarcoid of the breast in an appropriate clinical setting as previously emphasized, special stains, cultures, and skin testing are recommended to exclude tuberculosis and fungal and other unusual infections.[42]

The mammographic appearance of sarcoid of the breast mirrors the variable clinical presentation. Few reports describe the x-ray appearance. Skin thickening alone has been described in one patient.[45] In another patient, the xeromammographic appearance of sarcoid was illustrated as an indeterminate nonpalpable oval isodense mass with lobulated and partially obscured margins.[43] Because sarcoid may be an illness of young women, a palpable mass may be appropriately biopsied without mammographic assessment.

Table 14-2 **Some causes of noncaseating granulomas of the breast**

Foreign bodies
  Silicone
  Talc
  Sutures
  Beryllium

Bacteria
  Tuberculosis
  Leprosy
  Brucellosis
  Typhoid

Fungi
  Histoplasmosis
  Blastomycosis
  Cryptococcosis
  Phycomycosis
  Sporotrichosis

Parasites
  Hydatid disease
  Cysticercosis
  Filariasis
  Oxyuria infection

Adapted from Gansler TS and Wheeler JE: Mammary sarcoidosis: two cases and literature review, *Arch Pathol Lab Med* 108:673, 1984.

Wegener's granulomatosis

Wegener's granulomatosis is a systemic disease characterized by necrotizing granulomatous inflammation and vasculitis. The condition involves veins, capillaries, and both small and large arteries. The disease usually affects both the respiratory tract and kidneys, and the classic triad is generalized vasculitis, glomerulonephritis, and necrotizing granulomas of the upper respiratory tract. However, involvement of less common organs, such as the skin, eyes, and breasts, does occur. The first case of Wegener's granulomatosis involving the breast was reported by Elsner and Harper in 1969.[51] Since that time, about 10 cases have been reported.[52] The recognition of Wegener's granulomatosis presenting as a breast mass is important because of the prognostic implications of the diagnosis. That is, the disease may be fatal but can be effectively treated in some patients with corticosteroids and immunosuppressive medications.

Wegener's granulomatosis of the breast has been reported in women age 36 to 59 years of age.[52] The lesion usually causes a unilateral palpable breast mass 2 to 3 cm in diameter. Skin edema (peau d'orange) and skin tethering have been described.[50,53] The mammographic findings are those of a dense round or irregular mass with spiculated or ill-defined margins.[50] Calcifications have not been described. The working diagnosis based on the clinical presentation and mammographic appearance is most often carcinoma of the breast. When bilateral simultaneous masses occur, the working diagnosis has been lymphoma or metasta-

Table 14-3 Vasculitis involving the breast

	Giant cells	Small arteries	Large arteries	Veins and capillaries
Wegener's granulomatosis	+	+	+	+
Giant cell arteritis	+	0	+	0
Polyarteritis nodosa	0	++	0	0

Adapted from Jordan JM, Rowe WT, Allen NB: Wegener's granulomatosis involving the breast: report of three cases and review of the literature, Am J Med 83:159, 1987.

ses.[50,52] Excisional biopsy has been reported as consistent with fat necrosis if the diffuse vasculitic process is not appreciated.[52] Diagnosis of Wegener's granulomatosis is possible by fine needle aspiration cytology.[50] Biopsy of oral, nasal, or orbital tissues may be confirmatory. The clinical recognition of Wegener's granulomatosis of the breast is a challenge. The breast mass may present early in the course of the disease when clinical symptoms of the renal or respiratory tract involvement are minimal or not appreciated.[52,53]

Mild symptoms of coryza, sinusitis, otitis media, malaise, and nonproductive cough (bronchitis) are common complaints but may be the early symptoms of this systemic vasculitis.[50,52] The physician should search for oral mucosal or tongue ulceration and for clinical and laboratory signs of glomerulonephritis. Treatment with corticosteroids and immunosuppressives is effective in causing resolution of breast masses due to Wegener's granulomatosis.[50,52]

Wegener's granulomatosis in the breast may be distinguished histologically from other types of granulomatous inflammation by the vasculitis, the extensive necrosis in the areas of granulomatous inflammation, and the involvement of upper respiratory tract and kidneys. Vasculitis may be marked, and fibrinoid necrosis of vessel walls may be seen. Giant cells are usually not found within affected vessels, although they may be present within granulomas. This finding is helpful in distinguishing Wegener's granulomatosis from the rare cases of giant cell arteritis which have involved the breast.[54] The necrotizing granulomatous inflammation may involve all parts of the breast parenchyma including ducts and lobules (Table 14-3).

Another type of granulomatous inflammation with associated vasculitis that may involve the breast is a recently described lesion termed *granulomatous angiopanniculitis*.[55] This lesion, which begins in subcutaneous adipose tissue but may involve underlying breast tissue, is probably a variant of Weber-Christian disease. The granulomas are nonnecrotizing, and the vasculitis is a lymphocytic angiitis involving small vessels; therefore, confusion with Wegener's granulomatosis should be minimal.

Amyloid

Amyloid deposits in the breast may be associated with a breast cancer[61,62] or may produce a primary localized amyloid tumor. The localized tumoral form is an uncommon cause of a clinical breast mass. Both the clinical and mammographic presentations may simulate breast carcinoma. Amyloid deposits produce amorphous eosinophilic masses with routine hematoxylin and eosin staining. Congo red staining with examination by polarized light gives an apple-green birefringence that is characteristic of amyloid. The elastosis associated with carcinomas and radial scars may be confused with amyloid and also stains with

Congo red. Page and Anderson suggest that this confusion may be eliminated by using the alkaline Congo red staining method.[60]

Primary localized amyloid has a benign course and is differentiated from both secondary amyloidosis and primary systemic amyloidosis. Diffuse secondary amyloidosis is described in association with chronic inflammatory diseases such as rheumatoid arthritis, tuberculosis and osteomyelitis, and certain neoplasms. Primary systemic amyloidosis is not preceded by any disease but in many cases signals a plasma cell neoplasm. Primary localized or tumoral amyloid is more commonly described in the respiratory tract, eyes, or skin than in the breast.[58]

Primary localized amyloid tumor of the breast may present in a postmenopausal woman as a firm painless palpable mass, often 2 to 5 cm in diameter.[56,58,63] The patient's age and the firmness of the lesion make breast carcinoma the primary consideration. Localized amyloid deposits occasionally cause bilateral breast cancer masses.[57]

By mammography the mass or masses may be ill defined or obscured by dense parenchyma.[59,63] Calcifications have been described. Coarse calcifications and more clustered suspicious microcalcifications have both been reported in primary amyloid of the breast.[56,57] Skin changes (retraction and peau d'orange) are reported.[58,59] A preoperative diagnosis of amyloid tumor of the breast may be made by fine needle aspiration and a high index of suspicion.[63] Generally the diagnosis of amyloid breast tumors remains elusive since the clinical and radiographic findings mimic breast cancer, particularly in the elderly woman.[59,63]

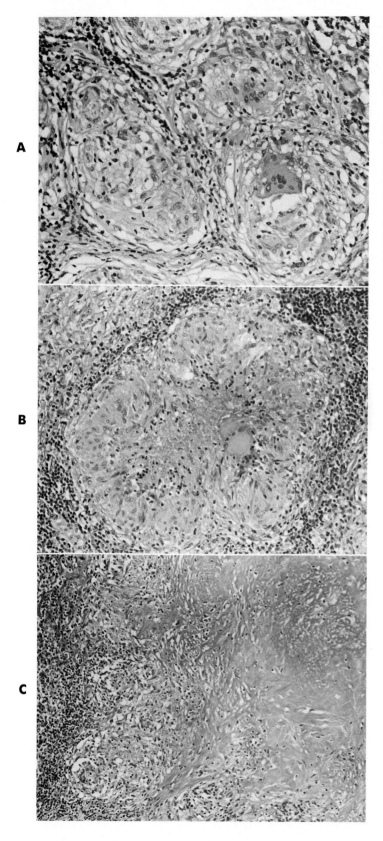

Fig. 14-23 Granulomas in the breast. **(A)** Sarcoidosis. The granulomas of sarcoidosis characteristically are small, composed of multinucleated giant cells and epithelioid cells and are "hard," meaning that they do not exhibit central necrosis. Several granulomas are illustrated in this photomicrograph. **(B)** Tuberculosis. In contrast, the granulomas of tuberculosis typically show central caseation necrosis, as illustrated in this photomicrograph. **(C)** Occasionally the granulomas of tuberculosis are characterized by extensive necrosis, as shown in this photograph. Only a small amount of the granulomatous inflammation is seen at lower left.

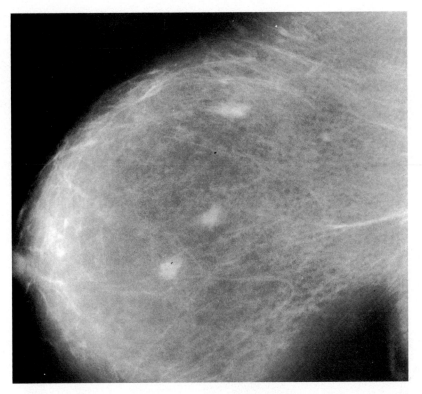

Fig. 14-24 Sarcoidosis of the breast produces multiple clinically occult irregular nodules with ill-defined margins. (Case courtesy of Dr. Susan Williams, Omaha, Nebraska.)

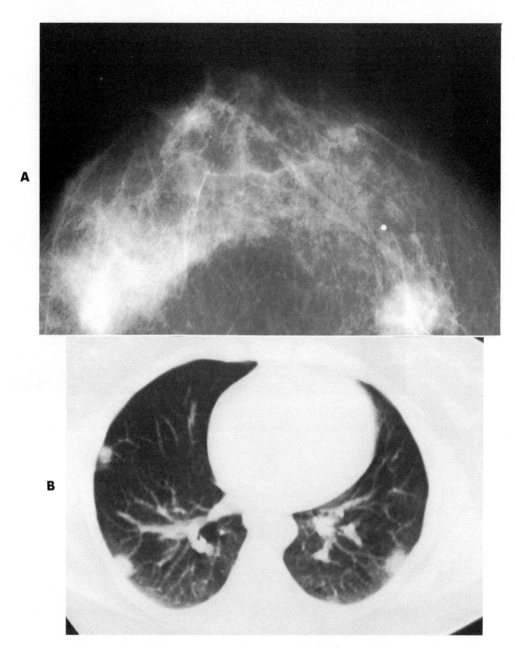

Fig. 14-25 **(A)** Systemic Wegener's granulomatosis produced this round mass of equal density with ill-defined margins in the medial breast on this craniocaudad view. **(B)** The pulmonary lesions are of similar size and shape as demonstrated by CT scan of the chest. (Courtesy of Hugh Hyre, Petersburg, VA).

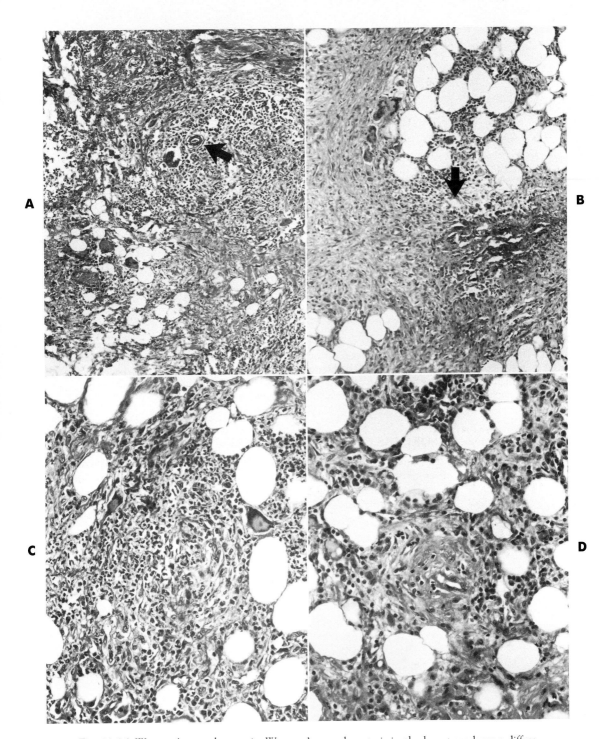

Fig. 14-26 Wegener's granulomatosis. Wegener's granulomatosis in the breast produces a diffuse inflammatory mass with loose granulomas. **(A)** The inflammatory process involves parenchyma and lobules with some preserved small ducts *(arrow)*. **(B)** Wegener's granulomatosis is also characterized by areas of necrosis *(arrow)* that may aid in distinguishing it from other inflammatory processes. **(C)** Wegener's is also associated with vasculitis. **(D)** Walls of affected vessels may exhibit fibrinoid necrosis. (Courtesy of Dr. Manuel Gonzales, Petersburg, Virginia.)

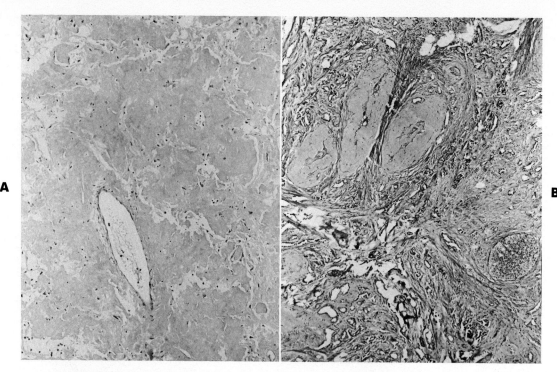

Fig. 14-27 (A) Amyloid can present in the breast as a tumorlike mass of amorphous material that can replace normal mammary parenchyma, as illustrated in this photomicrograph. A normal blood vessel can be identified. **(B)** Elastosis, commonly associated with breast cancer and benign lesions such as radial scars, should not be misdiagnosed as amyloid in the breast. This example of elastosis is associated with a tubular carcinoma.

DISORDERS OF THE MALE BREAST

Pathologic disorders of the male breast include gynecomastia, breast cancer, and other entities, including inflammatory conditions, benign tumors, and metastatic neoplasms. Although some are very rare, any condition reported in the female breast may also occur in the male.[66] The most common clinical disorder in the male breast is gynecomastia.

Gynecomastia

Gynecomastia, a term indicating female type breasts in the male, is often used loosely to describe enlargement of the male breast.[66] In many males breast enlargement is due entirely to fatty tissue deposits and is not considered a disease. Clinical gynecomastia is defined as the presence of a subareolar palpable disk of breast tissue at least 2 cm or greater in diameter in either breast.[76] Differentiation of palpable breast tissue from fat may be difficult, and mammography may be used to confirm the clinical suspicion of gynecomastia (Box 14-4). A technique for measuring the button of subareolar tissue has been reported. The use

---

BOX 14-4 INDICATIONS FOR MALE MAMMOGRAPHY

Breast enlargement, recent or rapid
Breast tenderness, recent onset
Palpable breast mass
Previous mastectomy
Nipple discharge or nipple ulcer-
ation

From Dershaw DD: Male mammography. *AJR Am J Roentgenol* 146:127, 1986.

of the anterior axillary fold, which contains only skin and fat, is recommended as a baseline against which to determine the consistency of the subareolar tissue.[87]

Pseudogynecomastia is breast enlargement from another cause such as lipoma, hemangioma, or neurofibromatosis.[76]

Physiologic versus pathologic gynecomastia. At certain ages (neonatal and pubertal) gynecomastia is considered normal. In the infant male breast, enlargement is a response to placental estrogens and usually regresses within weeks.[66] At puberty 60% to 70% of males develop gynecomastia within 1.2 years of enlargement of the testes (ages 12 to 15 years). Asymmetry is common.[85] Pubertal gynecomastia usually regresses within 2 years after the time of onset.[88]

Prepubertal gynecomastia occurs rarely, is not physiologic, and should raise suspicion of an underlying cause[77] (Box 14-5). *Senescent gynecomastia* is common (30% to 40% prevalence) in aging men.[67] Palpable breast enlargement in the older male correlates with increasing body mass index (BMI) and is usually asymptomatic. Palpable gynecomastia is noted in 80% of men with a BMI of 25 kg/m^2 or greater.[87] Clinical evaluation of senescent gynecomastia is not indicated unless the condition is painful, rapidly enlarging, or associated with an eccentric breast mass or a testicular mass.[87]

Pathophysiologic mechanisms of *pathologic gynecomastia* generally relate to one of four categories: (1) estrogen excess (Table 14-4); (2) androgen deficiency (Box 14-6); (3) drug-induced (Table 14-5); and (4) systemic disorders with idiopathic mechanisms (Box 14-7). In general gynecomastia requires no special therapy except treatment of the underlying etiology, as appropriate. If drug-induced, another drug may be substituted that does not produce gynecomastia. In a minority of men, danazol or surgical excision may be prescribed for exceptional tenderness or for cosmetic concerns.[91]

The typical clinical presentation of gynecomastia is unilateral or bilateral painful or tender breast enlargement. Rarely nipple retraction occurs with gynecomastia.[71] Reports of unilateral nipple discharge in the male usually indicate another process such as carcinoma, papilloma, abscess, or ductal ectasia.[73] Galactography may assist with preoperative planning for excision of the discharging duct. Presence of a palpable mass or asymmetric thickening eccentric to the nipple should raise concern for male breast cancer.

The histologic appearance of gynecomastia is quite characteristic. There is an increase in ductal structures surrounded by a loose edematous cellular stroma, which is reminiscent of a fibroadenoma. Ducts show a variable amount of hyperplasia of the epithelium. This hyperplasia is an expected component of gynecomastia and may be quite florid.[65] Squamous metaplasia may occur within the ducts.[75] Lobules are rarely found in the male breast, even in the setting of gynecomastia.[65]

In the senescent form of gynecomastia, the prominent pattern is stromal fibrosis. Hyperplasia is not usually prominent in this pattern of gynecomastia.

BOX 14-5 CAUSES OF PREPUBERTAL GYNECOMASTIA

Adrenal carcinoma
Testicular tumor
11β-hydroxylase deficiency
Familial gynecomastia
Tuberous sclerosis
Sexual precocity

From Haibach H, Rosenholtz MJ: Prepubertal gynecomastia with lobules and acini: a case report and review of the literature, *Am J Clin Pathol* 80:252, 1983.

Table 14-4 **Gynecomastia: estrogen excess**

A. Gonadal source
1. True hermaphroditism (Van Niekerk, 1976)
2. Gonadal stromal tumors (Hendry et al, 1984)
   a. Leydig cell (Emory et al, 1984; Conway, et al, 1988; Mellor and McCutchan, 1989)
   b. Sertoli cell (Hopkins and Parry, 1969)
   c. Granulosa-theca cell (Laskowski, 1952; Stephanas et al, 1978)
3. Germ cell tumors (Stephanas et al, 1978)
   a. Choriocarcinoma
   b. Seminoma, teratoma
   c. Embryonal carcinoma
B. Nontesticular tumors (Korenman, 1986)
1. Skin: giant pigmented nevus, neurofibromatosis (Leung, 1985)
2. Adrenal cortical neoplasms (Hayles, et al, 1966; Desai and Kapadia, 1988)
3. Lung carcinoma or other malignancy with hCG elevation (Groveman, 1985)
4. Hepatocellular carcinoma
5. Hypernephroma
6. Gastric carcinoma
7. Lymphoma
C. Endocrine disorders
1. Hyperthyroidism (Chopra, 1975)
2. Hypothyroidism (Aranout et al, 1987)
D. Diseases of the liver (Cavanaugh et al, 1990)
1. Alcoholic cirrhosis
2. Nonalcoholic cirrhosis
E. Nutrition alteration states
1. Malnutrition
2. Refeeding (Klatskin, 1947)
3. Paraplegic (Groveman, 1985)
F. Estrogen ingestion
1. Therapeutic
   a. Prostate cancer therapy
   b. Sex change
2. Accidental (Groveman, 1985)
   a. Birth control pills
   b. Estrogen creams
   c. Meat contamination

Adapted from Bland KI, Page DL: In Bland KI, Copeland EM, editors: *The breast: comprehensive management of benign and malignant diseases*, Philadelphia, 1991, WB Saunders.

BOX 14-6 GYNECOMASTIA: ANDROGEN DEFICIENCY

A. Senescent
B. Hypogonadism
  1. Primary testicular failure
    a. Klinefelter's syndrome (XXY) (Cole, 1976)
    b. Reifenstein's syndrome (XY)
    c. Rosewater, Gwinup, Hamwi familial gynecomastia (XY)
    d. Kallmann's syndrome
    e. Kennedy's syndrome with gynecomastia
    f. Congenital anorchia
    g. Hereditary defects of androgen biosynthesis
    h. Adrenocorticotropic hormone deficiency
  2. Secondary testicular failure
    a. Trauma
    b. Orchitis/mumps
    c. Cryptorchidism
    d. Irradiation/chemotherapy
    e. Hydrocele
    f. Varicocele
    g. Spermatocele
    h. Leprosy, granulomatous disease
C. Renal failure

Adapted from Bland KI, Page DL: In Bland KI and Copeland EM, editors: *The breast: comprehensive management of benign and malignant diseases.* Philadelphia, 1991, Saunders.

Table 14-5 Drugs related to gynecomastia

Amiodarone	Isoniazid (another antituberculous drugs)
Amphetamine	Insulin
Anabolic steroids	Ketoconazole
Androgens	Marijuana (cannabis)
Antiandrogens (cyproterone, spironolactone)	Methadone
Bumetanide	Methotrexate
Busulfan	Metronidazole
Chlorambucil	Methyldopa
Cimetidine	Metaclopramide
Corticosteroids	Nifedipine
Cyclophosphamide	Nitrosureas
Cyproterone acetate	Phenothiazine
Diazepam (valium)	Prednisone
Diethylpropion hydrochloride	Procarbazine
Digitalis	Ranitidine
Dilantin	Reserpine
D-Penicillamine	Spironolactone
Domperidone	Sulindac
Estrogen therapy	Theophylline
Ethionamide	Thiacetazone
Flutamide	Thiazide
Furosemide	Tricyclic antidepressants
Griseofulvin	Verapamil
Heroin	Vincristine

BOX 14-7 GYNECOMASTIA: IDIOPATHIC MECHANISMS

A. Nonneoplastic diseases of the lung—cystic fibrosis
B. Trauma (chest-wall)
   1. Blunt trauma
   2. Thoracoplastic surgery
C. CNS-related causes from anxiety and stress
D. AIDS

Adapted from Bland KI, Page DL: In Bland KI, Copeland EM, editors: *The breast: comprehensive management of benign and malignant diseases,* Philadelphia, 1991, Saunders.

Cancer of the male breast

Cancer of the male breast is uncommon, accounting for 1% to 2% of all breast cancers. Because lobular structures are rare in the male breast, most cancers are of ductal origin. Special types of ductal carcinoma may occur as well as sarcomas, lymphomas, leukemia and metastases, which parallel the histopathology seen in females (Table 14-6). Lobular carcinoma in the male breast is distinctly uncommon.[104]

Male breast cancer has been reported in men from ages 5 through 93 years. The average age of diagnosis is 59.6 years.[93] On the average men are 5 to 10 years older than women at the time of diagnosis and risk increases with age.[95] Bilateral breast cancer was diagnosed in only 1.4% of 2217 cases of male breast cancer.[93] An association with Klinefelter's syndrome has been reported and a proposed risk of 3% is estimated.[92,96,98]

The clinical presentation of male breast cancer is most frequently that of mass or palpable thickening in the subareolar area or in the upper outer quadrant[94,95] (Box 14-8). A duration of symptoms of 10 to 18 months is common, caused by patient delay in seeking medical attention.[93] Because the male breast is usually smaller than the female breast, skin ulceration, fixation, or peau d'orange skin changes may be noted at the time of presentation.[82] Clinical presentation with Paget's disease has been reported. Bloody nipple discharge or nipple ulceration or retraction may be the chief complaint. Associated clinical gynecomastia is not a common feature and is described in less than 2% of cases.[101,108]

Over 90% of male breast carcinomas are infiltrating ductal carcinoma. Only 7% are in situ intraductal carcinoma.[107] Lobular carcinoma is uncommon (less than 2% of total cases). A diagnosis of lobular carcinoma suggests a hyperestrogenic state such as Klinefelter's syndrome.[104] In a community hospital study of 45 men with breast cancer, 55% had stage I cancer at the time of presentation. Overall the current thinking is that the prognosis of male breast cancer is *not* less favorable than that of the female patient, stage for stage.[108]

The radiographic appearance of male breast cancer is similar to that of female breast cancer.[115] Mammography helps to differentiate subareolar gynecomastia from an eccentrically placed carcinoma. Many male breast cancers are in the upper outer quadrant. They may be well defined (65% of cases).[103] Microcalcifications have been reported in 13% to 30% of masses.[94,103] Calcifications, when present, may be punctate rather than pleomorphic.[94] Any eccentric mass in a male, no matter how well defined, should be considered suspicious for carcinoma. Carcinoma and radiographic gynecomastia may coexist.[94,102]

Ultrasonography of masses in the male breast may be misleading. The cancer may produce only subtle shadowing, making it difficult to distinguish the lesion from the background echogenicity of fat or gynecomastia.[99]

Table 14-6 **Special types of malignant neoplasm in the male breast**

Tubular carcinoma	(Taxy, 1975)
Inflammatory carcinoma	(Treves, 1953)
Medullary carcinoma	(Crichlow, 1972)
Papillary carcinoma	(Crichlow, 1972)
Leiomyosarcoma	(Hernandez, 1978)

BOX 14-8 CLINICAL FEATURES OF MALE BREAST CANCER (NOT FOUND IN GYNECOMASTIA)

Eccentric mass
Bloody nipple discharge
Fixation on palpation
Skin ulceration or thickening
Axillary adenopathy

Adapted from references 76, 82, 93, 94.

Other male breast disorders

The male breast may develop any of the many benign conditions described in the female breast. In clinical practice the more common conditions other than gynecomastia are abscess, lipoma, and papilloma.

Inflammatory conditions of the male breast. Inflammatory conditions of the male breast are most often acute abscess or mastitis. These clinical presentations and mammographic appearance are similar to the same conditions in the female breast. Breast abscess in the male may cause a nipple discharge and produce an eccentric mass that could be mistaken for breast carcinoma based on imaging studies of mammography or ultrasonography. A history of diabetes should be searched for as a possible underlying cause. Diffuse mastitis and periductal mastitis with ductal ectasia in the male breast have been described but are less common than breast abscess.[119]

Another uncommon inflammatory condition of the male breast is squamous metaplasia of lactiferous ducts (described in detail earlier in this chapter). The clinical presentation is that of recurrent draining fistulas in periareolar tissues. A total ductal excision is curative. It is not associated with an increased risk of malignancy. There are no recognized mammographic findings, other than subareolar ductal shadows. The radiographic finding of a benign epithelial inclusion cyst has also been reported.[114]

Benign breast lesions in the male. Any of the benign conditions that occur in the female may occur in the male. Those associated with lobule formation are distinctly rare unless there is evidence for chronic exposure to estrogen. Most are included in Table 14-7; the most common benign lesions are lipoma and papilloma.

Lipoma is common in the breast or chest wall area. The mass is usually somewhat soft and smooth and corresponds to fatty tissue on mammography. A thin capsule may be imaged radiographically. The ultrasonographic appearance is distinct from gynecomastia and is described as a solid mass with smooth margins and well-defined weakly echogenic areas.[111]

Solitary intraductal papilloma in the male breast may cause unilateral serous or bloody discharge. Galactography may be performed to help localize the ductal

Table 14-7 **Male breast disorders other than gynecomatia and carcinoma**

Hematoma/contusion
Inflammatory conditions
    Abscess/mastitis (Detraux et al, 1985; Greganus et al, 1989)
    Squamous metaplasia of lactiferous ducts (Gottfried, 1986)
    Chronic granulomatous disease (Kapdi and Parekh, 1983)
    Tuberculosis, syphilis (Greganus et al, 1989)
Benign conditions
    Lipoma (Cole-Beuglet et al, 1982)
    Papilloma (Detraux et al, 1985)
    Papillomatosis (Waldo et al, 1975; Bannayan and Hajdu, 1972)
    Fibroadenoma (Anash-Boatneg and Tavassoli, 1989)
    Fibroadenomatoid hyperplasia (Nielsen, 1990)
    Sclerosing adenosis (Biagotti and Kasznica, 1986)
    Apocrine change
    Duct ectasia (Detraux et al, 1985)
    Skin lesions (inclusion cyst) (Kalisher and Peyster, 1975)
Other lesions
    Lymphoma
    Leukemia, chloroma (Anash-Boatneg and Tavassoli, 1992)
    Phyllodes tumor (Reingold and Ascher, 1970)
    Metastases
        Melanoma
        Renal carcinoma
        Lung carcinoma
        Prostate cancer (Salyer and Salyer, 1973)

---

filling defect to guide excisional biopsy.[73] Intraductal carcinoma may produce the same symptom and cannot be differentiated from a solitary papilloma by galactography. Surgical excision is required to establish a pathologic diagnosis.

Other neoplastic conditions are listed in Table 14-7. Of these, lymphoma and metastases to the breast are perhaps the most common. Special histochemical and other studies may be needed to establish a correct diagnosis (see Chapter 13). If the breast is the only site of involvement, electron microscopy may help to confirm a diagnosis of large cell lymphoma.[100] Chloroma may be confirmed by staining for nonspecific esterase. The presence of prostatic specific antigen helps differentiate metastatic prostate adenocarcinoma from a primary breast adenocarcinoma.

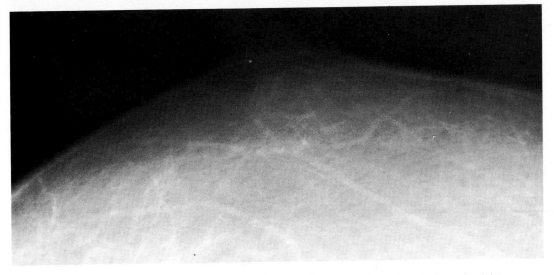

Fig. 14-28 Normal male breast. Craniocaudad views demonstrate fatty tissue and no glandular elements.

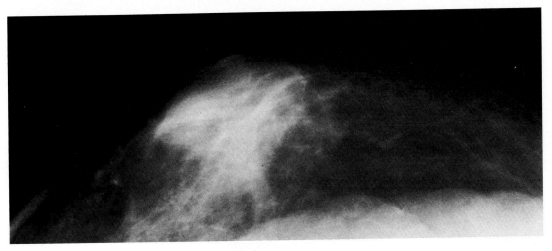

Fig. 14-29 Gynecomastia. Subareolar glandular tissue extends into the central breast area in this male with bilateral gynecomastia. Scalloped border to pectoral muscle is clearly visualized on this craniocaudad projection.

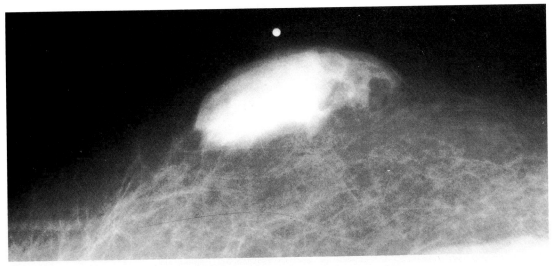

Fig. 14-30 Gynecomastia. Subareolar glandular tissue is quite focal or discoid in this male with drug-induced unilateral gynecomastia.

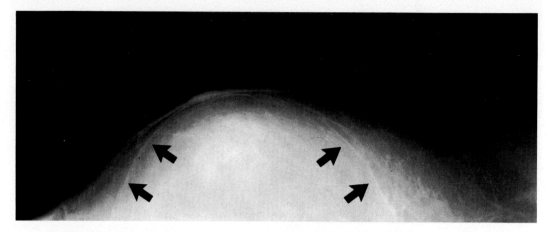

Fig. 14-31 Lipoma. Mammography helps to identify the fatty tumor producing clinical pseudo-gynecomastia in this older man. The capsule is marked by arrows.

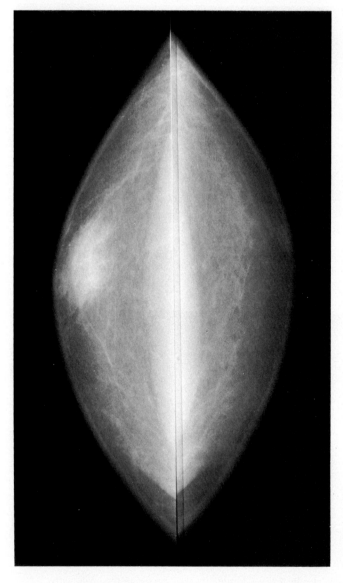

Fig. 14-32 Drug-induced gynecomastia. Bilateral craniocaudad mammograms indicate unilateral gynecomastia, which is most often seen as a side effect from a medication.

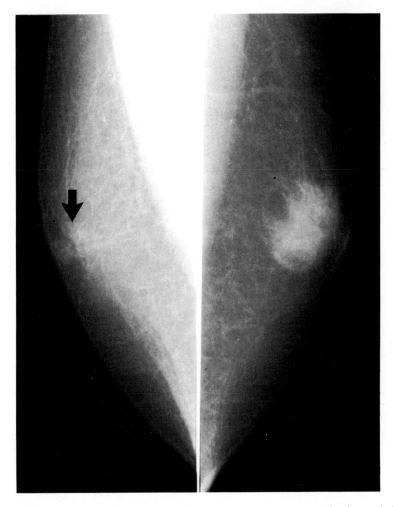

Fig. 14-33 Asymmetric gynecomastia. Asymmetric gynecomastia may be detected if bilateral mammograms are obtained. It is not unusual to identify mild subareolar ductal prominence *(arrow)* in the asymptomatic breast.

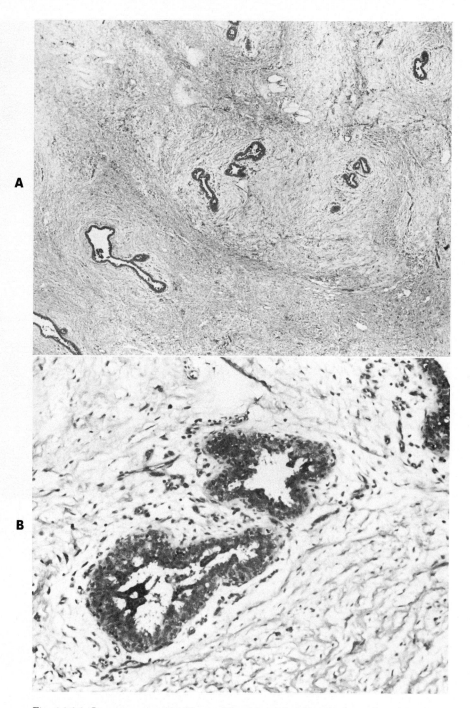

Fig. 14-34 Gynecomastia. **(A)** The proliferation of ductular elements that characterize gynecomastia is often accompanied by an increase in loose periductal connective tissue. **(B)** The ducts themselves frequently exhibit varying degrees of intraductal epithelial hyperplasia.

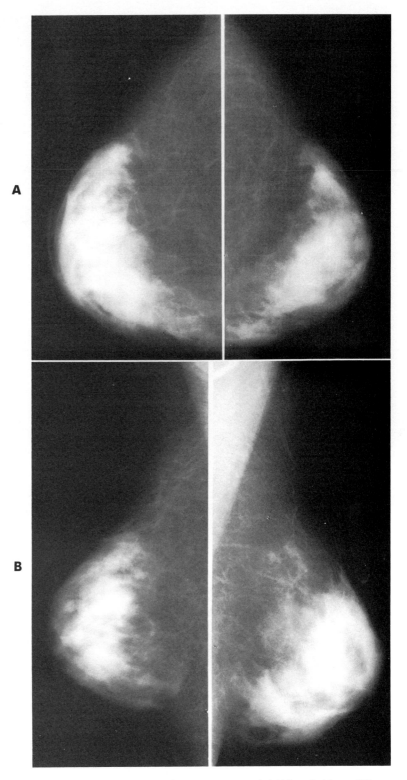

Fig. 14-35 Gynecomastia related to sex change. Craniocaudad **(A)** and oblique **(B)** bilateral mammograms demonstrate marked glandular hypertrophy in this male-to-female sex change patient receiving high-dose exogenous estrogen therapy.

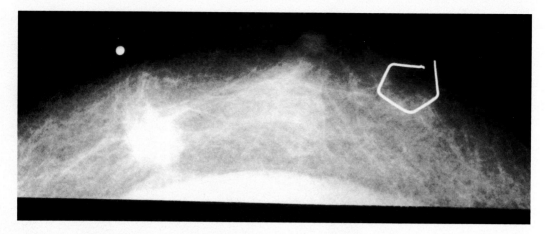

Fig. 14-36 Male breast cancer. A palpable firm mass in the upper outer quadrant of the left breast was proven to be cancer by FNA cytology.

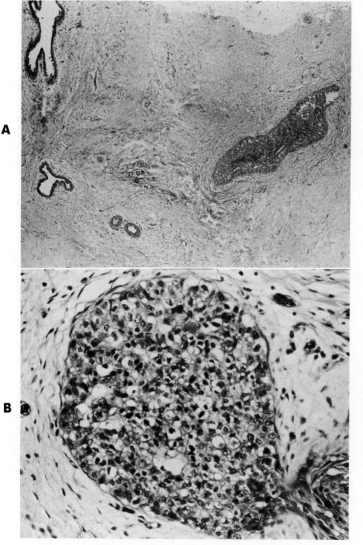

A

B

Fig. 14-37 Ductal carcinoma in situ (DCIS) of the male breast. DCIS can occur in the male breast in the absence of invasive cancer. **(A)** A duct involved by DCIS is seen at right, and the remainder of the biopsy shows gynecomastia. **(B)** This higher magnification photomicrograph of another male patient with DCIS shows the solid proliferation of neoplastic cells filling a duct.

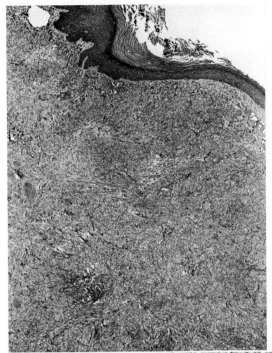

A

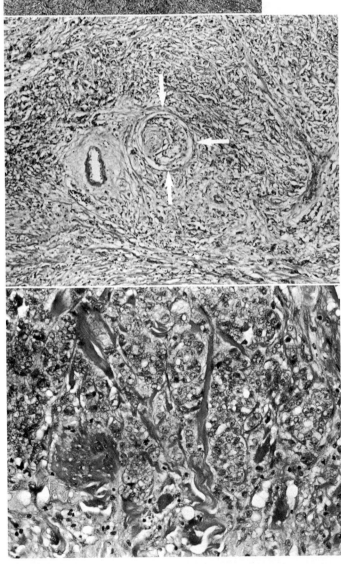

B

C

Fig. 14-38 Invasive carcinoma of the male breast. (A) This poorly differentiated invasive ductal carcinoma extends to the skin in this male patient. The epidermis is seen at the top of the photograph. (B) At higher magnification a preserved duct can be seen. Next to this, a small nerve shows perineural invasion by tumor cells (arrows). (C) At high magnification the anaplastic tumor cells invade in solid sheets between collagen bands.

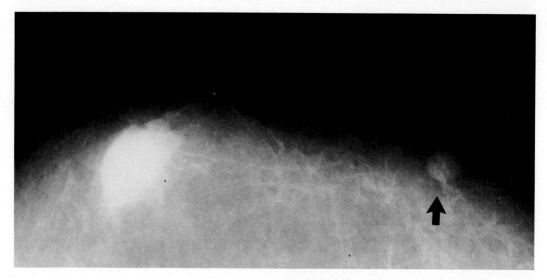

Fig. 14-39 Breast abscess in the male patient. A subareolar mass was associated with pain, redness, and purulent nipple drainage. A reactive lymph node (biopsy proven) is seen more peripherally (*arrow*).

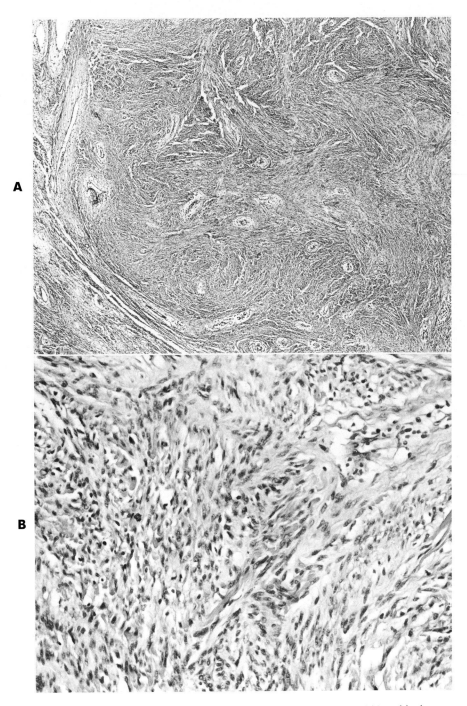

Fig. 14-40 Malignant fibrous histiocytoma in the male breast. Low- **(A)** and high-magnification **(B)** photomicrographs from this malignant fibrous histiocytoma presenting as a breast mass in a 70-year-old man show a spindle cell tumor with a swirled pattern and occasional mitoses. This case illustrates that virtually any lesion found in the female breast may occur in the male. (Case courtesy of Dr. Gary Shapira, Richmond, Indiana.)

REFERENCES
Inflammatory conditions of the breast

Duct ectasia

1. Bundred NJ, Dixon JM, Lumsden AB, et al: Are the lesions of duct ectasia sterile? *Br J Surg* 72:844, 1985.
2. Dixon JM, Anderson TJ, Lumsden AB, et al: Mammary duct ectasia, *Br J Surg* 70:601, 1983.
3. Kopans DB: *Breast imaging.* Philadelphia, 1989, JB Lippincott, p 279.
4. Levitan LH, Witten DM, Harrison EG: Calcification in breast disease: mammographic-pathologic correlation, *AJR Am J Roentgenol* 92:29, 1964.
5. Rees BI, Gravelle IH, Hughes LE: Nipple retraction in duct ectasia, *Br J Surg* 64:577, 1977.
6. Sickles EA: Breast calcifications: mammographic evaluation, *Radiology* 160:289, 1986.

Squamous metaplasia of lactiferous ducts

7. Abboud SL, Powell DE, Sachatello CR: Unpublished observations.
8. Habif DV, Perzin KH, Lipson R, Lattes R: Subareolar abscess associated with squamous metaplasia of lactiferous ducts, *Am J Surg* 119:523, 1970.
9. Powell BC, Maull KL, Sachatello CR: Recurrent subareolar abscess of the breast and squamous metaplasia of lactiferous ducts: a clinical syndrome, *South Med J* 70:935, 1977.

Unusual infections and granulomatous mastitis

10. Campbell FC, Eriksson BL, Angorn IB: Localized granulomatous mastitis: an unusual presentation of typhoid: a case report, *S Afr Med J* 57:793, 1980.
11. Cohen C: Granulomatous mastitis: a review of 5 cases, *S Afr Med J* 52:14, 1977.
12. DeHertogh DA, Rossof AH, Harris AA, Economou SG: Prednisone management of granulomatous mastitis, *N Engl J Med* 303:799, 1980.
13. Fletcher A, Magrath IM, Riddell RH, Talbot IC: Granulomatous mastitis: a report of seven cases, *J Clin Pathol* 35:941, 1982.
14. Going JJ, Anderson TJ, Wilkinson S, Chetty U: Granulomatous lobular mastitis, *J Clin Pathol* 40:535, 1987.
15. Jorgensen MB, Nielsen DM: Diagnosis and treatment of granulomatous mastitis, *Am J Med* 93:97, 1992.
16. Kessler E, Wolloch Y: Granulomatous mastitis: a lesion clinically simulating carcinoma, *Am J Clin Pathol* 58:642, 1972.
17. Macansh S, Greenberg M, Barraclough B, Pacey F: Fine needle aspiration cytology of granulomatous mastitis: report of a case and review of the literature, *Acta Cytol* 34:38, 1990.
18. Mirza NB, Pamba HO, O'Leary P: Hydatid cyst of the breast: case report. *East Afr Med J* 56:235, 1979.
19. Osborne BM: Granulomatous mastitis caused by histoplasma and mimicking inflammatory breast carcinoma, *Human Pathol* 20:47, 1989.
20. Seymour EQ: Blastomycosis of the breast, *AJR Am J Roentgenol* 139:822, 1982.
21. Stelling CB: Dracunculiasis presenting as sterile abscess *Am J Roentgenol* 138:1159, 1982.
22. Tabar L, Kett K, Nemeth A: Tuberculosis of the breast, *Radiology* 118:587, 1976.

Traumatic fat necrosis

23. Adair FE, Munzer JT: Fat necrosis of the female breast, *Am J Surg* 74:117, 1947.
24. Baker KS, Stelling CB: Mammographic appearance of Coumadin-induced fat necrosis, *AJR Am J Roentgenol* 158-689, 1992.
25. Bassett LW, Gold RH, Cove HC: Mammographic spectrum of traumatic fat necrosis: the fallibility of "pathognomonic" signs of carcinoma, *AJR Am J Roentgenol* 130:119, 1978.
26. Bassett LW, Gold RH, Mima JM: Nonneoplastic breast calcifications in lipid cysts: development after excision and primary irradiation, *AJR Am J Roentgenol* 138:335, 1982.
27. Bernstein JR: Nonsuppurative nodular penniculitis (Weber-Christian disease): an unusual cause of mammary calcifications, *JAMA* 238:1942.
28. Clark D, Curtis JL, Martinez A, et al: Fat necrosis of the breast simulating recurrent carcinoma after primary radiotherapy in the management of early stage breast carcinoma, *Cancer* 52:442, 1983.
29. Clouse LH, Comp PC: The regulation of hemostasia: the protein C system, *N Engl J Med* 314:1298, 1986.
30. Evers K, Troupin RH: Lipid cyst: classic and atypical appearances, *AJR Am J Roentgenol* 157:271, 1991.
31. Meyer JE, Silverman P, Gandbhir L: Fat necrosis of the breast, *Arch Surg* 113:801, 1978.
32. Miller CL, Feig SA, Fox JW IV: Mammographic changes after reduction mammoplasty, *AJR Am J Roentgenol* 149:35, 1987.

33. Minagi H, Youker JE: Roentgen appearance of fat necrosis in the breast, *Radiology* 90:62, 1968.
34. Morgan CL, Trought WS, Peete W: Xeromammographic and ultrasonic diagnosis of a traumatic oil cyst, *AJR Am J Roentgenol* 130:1189, 1978.
35. Nudelman HL, Kempson RL: Necrosis of the breast: a rare complication of anticoagulant therapy, *Am J Surg* 111:728, 1966.
36. Orson LW, Cigtay OS: Fat necrosis of the breast: characteristic xeromammographic appearance, *Radiology* 146:35, 1983.
37. Sandison AT, Walker JC: Inflammatory mastitis, mammary duct ectasia, and mammillary fistula, *Br J Surg* 50:57, 1962.
38. Sickles EA, Herzog KA: Mammography of the postsurgical breast. *AJR Am J Roentgenol* 136:585, 1981.
39. Stigers KB, King JG, Davey DD, Stelling CB: Abnormalities of the breast caused by biopsy: spectrum of mammographic findings, *AJR Am J Roentgenol* 156:287, 1991.
40. Tabar L, Dean PB: *Teaching atlas of mammography*, New York, 1985, Thieme-Stratton, p. 172.

Systemic inflammatory conditions

Sarcoidosis of the breast

41. Banik S, Bishop PW, Omerod LB, O'Brien TEB: Sarcoidosis of the breast, *J Clin Pathol* 39:446, 1986.
42. Bodo M, Dobrossy L, Sugar J: Boeck's sarcoidosis of the breast: cytologic findings with aspiration biopsy cytology, *Acta Cytol* 22:1, 1978.
43. D'Orsi CJ: "Zebras" of the breast, *Contemp Diagn Radiol* 10:1, 1987.
44. Fitzgibbons PL, Smiley DF, Kern WH: Sarcoidosis presenting initially as a breast mass: report of two cases, *Hum Pathol* 16:851, 1985.
45. Gallimore AP, George CD, Lampert IA: Subcutaneous sarcoidosis mimicking carcinoma of the breast, *Postgrad Med J* 66:677, 1990.
46. Gansler TS, Wheeler JE: Mammary sarcoidosis: two cases and literature review, *Arch Pathol Lab Med* 108:673, 1984.
47. Ross MJ, Merino MJ: Sarcoidosis of the breast, *Hum Pathol* 16:185, 1985.
48. Shah AK, Solomon L, Gumbs MA: Sarcoidosis of the breast coexisting with mammary carcinoma, *NY State J Med* 90:331, 1990.
49. Tavassoli FA: *Pathology of the breast*, New York, Elsevier, 1992, p. 622.

Wegener's granulomatosis

50. Deininger HK: Wegener's granulomatosis of the breast, *Radiology* 154:59, 1985.
51. Elsner B, Harper FB: Disseminated Wegener's granulomatosis with breast involvement: report of a case, *Arch Pathol* 87:544, 1969.
52. Jordan JM, Rowe WT, Allen NB: Wegener's granulomatosis involving the breast: report of three cases and review of the literature, *Am J Med* 83:159, 1987.
53. Pambakian H, Tighe JR: Breast involvement in Wegener's granulomatosis, *J Clin Pathol* 24:343, 1971.
54. Stephenson TJ, Underwood JCE. Giant cell arteritis: an unusual cause of palpable masses in the breast, *Br J Surg* 73:105, 1986.
55. Wargotz ES, Lefkowitz M: Granulomatous angiopanniculitis of the breast, *Hum Pathol* 20:1084, 1989.

Amyloid

56. Fernandez BB, Hernandez FJ: Amyloid tumor of the breast, *Arch Pathol* 95:102, 1973.
57. Hecht AH, Tan A, Shen JF: Case report: primary systemic amyloidosis presenting as breast masses, mammographically simulating carcinoma, *Clin Radiol* 44:123, 1991.
58. Lew W, Seymour AE: Primary amyloid tumor of the breast: case report and literature review, *Acta Cytol* 29:7, 1985.
59. O'Connor CR, Rubinow A, Cohen AS: Primary (AL) amyloidosis as a cause of breast masses, *Am J Med* 77:981, 1984.
60. Page DL, Anderson TJ: *Diagnostic histopathology of the breast*, Edinburgh, 1987, Churchill Livingstone, pp. 69-70.
61. Patil SD, Joshi BG: Amyloid deposit in carcinoma of the breast, *Indian J Cancer* 7:60, 1970.
62. Santini D, Pasquinelli G, Alberghini M, et al: Invasive breast carcinoma with granulomatous response and deposition of unusual amyloid, *J Clin Pathol* 45:885, 1992.
63. Silverman JF, Dabbs DJ, Norris HT, et al: Localized primary (AL) amyloid tumor of the breast, *Am J Surg Pathol* 10:539, 1986.

Gynecomastia

64. Arnaout MA, et al: Galactorrhea, gynecomastia, and hypothyroidism in a man (letter). *Ann Intern Med* 106:779, 1987.
65. Banayan GA, Hajdu SI: Gynecomastia: clinicopathologic study of 351 cases, *Am J Clin Pathol* 57:431, 1972.
66. Bland KI, Page DL: In Bland KI, Copeland EM, editors: *The breast: comprehensive management of benign and malignant diseases*, Philadelphia, 1991, WB Saunders.

67. Braunstein GD: Gynecomastia, *N Engl J Med* 328:490, 1993.
68. Cavanaugh J, Niewoehner CB, Nuttall FQ: Gynecomastia and cirrhosis of the liver, *Arch Intern Med* 150:563, 1990.
69. Chopra IJ: Gonadal steroids and gonadotropins in hyperthyroidism, *Med Clin North Am* 59:1109, 1975.
70. Conway GS, MacConnell T, Wells G, Slater SD: Importance of scrotal ultrasonography in gynaecomastia, *Br Med J* 297(2):1176-7, 1988.
71. Dershaw DD: Male mammography, *AJR Am J Roentgenol* 146:127, 1986.
72. Desai MB, Kapadia SN: Feminizing adrenocortical tumors in male patients: adenoma versus carcinoma, *J Urol* 139:101, 1988.
73. Detraux P, Benmussa M, Tristant H, Garel L: Breast disease in the male: galactographic evaluation, *Radiology* 154:605, 1985.
74. Emory TH, Charboneau JW, Randall RV, et al: Occult testicular interstitial-cell tumor in a patient with gynecomastia: ultrasonic detection, *Radiology* 151(2):474, 1984.
75. Gottfried MR: Extensive squamous multaplasia in gynecomestia, *Arch Pathol Lab Med* 110:971, 1986.
76. Groveman HD: Gynecomastia. In Taylor RT, editor: *Difficult diagnosis,* Philadelphia, 1985, WB Saunders.
77. Haibach H, Rosenholtz MJ: Prepubertal gynecomastia with lobules and acini: a case report and review of the literature, *Am J Clin Pathol* 80:252, 1983.
78. Hayles AB, Hahn HB, Sprague RC, et al: Hormone-secreting tumors of the adrenal cortex in children, *Pediatrics* 37:19, 1966.
79. Hendry WS, Garview WHH, Ah-See AK, Bayliss AP: Ultrasonic detection of occult testicular neoplasms in patients with gynecomastia, *Br J Radiol* 57:571, 1984.
80. Hopkins GB, Parry HD: Metastasizing Sertoli cell tumor, *Cancer* 23:463, 1969.
81. Klatskin G, Saltin WT, Humm FD: Gynecomastia due to malnutrition. *Am J Med Sci* 213:19, 1947.
82. Korenman SG: The endocrinology of the abnormal male breast, *Ann NY Acad Sci* 464:400, 1986.
83. Laskowski J: Feminizing tumors of the testis: general review with case report of granulosa cell tumor of the testis, *Endokrynol Pol* 3:337, 1952.
84. Leung AKC: Gynecomastia, *Am Fam Physician* 39(4):215, 1989.
85. Mahoney CP: Adolescent gynecomastia differential diagnosis and management, *Pediatr Clin North Am* 37(6):1389, 1990.
86. Mellor SG, McCutchan JDS: Gynaecomastia and occult Leydig cell tumour of the testis, *Br J Urol* 63:420, 1989.
87. Niewoehner CB, Nuttall FQ: Gynecomastia in a hospitalized male population, *Am J Med* 77:633, 1984.
88. Nydick M, et al: Gynecomastia in adolescent boys, *JAMA* 178:449, 1961.
89. Stephanas AV, Samaan NA, Schultz PN, et al: Endocrine studies in testicular tumor patients with and without gynecomastia, *Cancer* 41:369, 1978.
90. Van Niekerk WA: True hermaphroditism: an analytic view with a report of three new cases, *Am J Obstet Gynecol* 126:890, 1976.
91. Webster DJT: Benign disorders of the male breast, *World J Surg* 13:726, 1989.

Disorders of the male breast

Cancer of the male breast

92. Cole EW: Klinefelter syndrome and breast cancer, *Johns Hopkins Med J* 138:102, 1976.
93. Crichlow RW: Carcinoma of the male breast, *Surg Gynecol Obstet* 134:1011, 1972.
94. Dershaw DD, Borgen PI, Deutch BM, Liberman L: Mammographic findings in men with breast cancer, *AJR Am J Roentgenol* 160:267, 1993.
95. Donegan WL: Cancer of the breast in men, *CA* 41:339, 1991.
96. Evans DB, Crichlow RW: Carcinoma of the male breast and Klinefelter's syndrome: is there an association *CA-A Cancer Journal for Clinicians* 37:246, 1987.
97. Hernandez FJ: Leiomyosarcoma of male breast originating in the nipple, *Am J Surg Pathol* 2:299, 1978.
98. Jackson AW, Muldah IS, Ockey CH, O'Connor PJ: Carcinoma of male breast in association with the Klinefelter syndrome, *Br Med J* 1:223, 1965.
99. Jackson VP, Gilmor RL: Male breast carcinoma and gynecomastia: comparison of mammography with sonography, *Radiology* 149:533, 1983.
100. Johnson RL: The male breast and gynecomastia. In Page DL, Anderson TJ, editors: *Diagnostic histopathology of the breast,* Edinburgh, 1987, Churchill Livingstone.
101. Meyskens FL, Tormey DC, Neifeld JP: Male breast cancer: a review, *Cancer Treat Rev* 3:83, 1976.
102. Michels LG, Gold RH, Arndt RD: Radiography of gynecomastia and other disorders of the male breast, *Radiology* 122:117, 1977.
103. Ouimet-Oliva D, Hebert G, Ladouceur J: Radiographic characteristics of male breast cancer, *Radiology* 129:37, 1978.

104. Sanchez AG, Villaneuva AG, Redondo C: Lobular carcinoma of the breast in a patient with Klinefelter's syndrome, *Cancer* 57:1181, 1986.
105. Taxy JB: Tubular carcinoma of the male breast: report of a case, *Cancer* 36:462, 1975.
106. Treves V: Inflammatory carcinoma of the breast in the male patient, *Surgery* 34:810, 1953.
107. Vercoutere AL, O'Connell TX: Carcinoma of the male breast: an update, *Arch Surg* 119:1301, 1984.
108. Yap HY, et al: Male breast cancer: a natural history study, *Cancer* 44:748, 1979.

Other male breast disorders

109. Anash-Boatneg Y, Tavassoli FA: Fibroadenoma and cystosarcoma phyllodes of the male breast, *Mod Pathol* 5:114, 1992.
110. Biagotti G, Kasznica J: Sclerosing adenosis in the breast of a man with pulmonary oat cell carcinoma, *Hum Pathol* 17:861, 1986.
111. Cole-Beuglet C, et al: Ultrasound mammography for male breast enlargement, *J Ultrasound Med* 1:301, 1982.
112. Gottfried MR: Extensive squamous metaplasia in gynecomastia, *Arch Pathol Lab Med* 110:971, 1986.
113. Greganus DE, Parks DS, Farrell EG: Breast disorders in children and adolescents, *Pediatr Clin North Am* 36:601, 1989.
114. Kalisher L, Peyster RG: Xerographic manifestations of male breast disease, *AJR Am J Roentgenol* 125:656, 1975.
115. Kapdi CC, Parekh NJ: The male breast, *Radiol Clin North Am* 21(1):137, 1983.
116. Nielsen BB: Fibroadenomatoid hyperplasia of the male breast, *Am J Surg Pathol* 14:774, 1990.
117. Reingold IM, Ascher GS: Cystosarcoma phyllodes in a man with gynecomastia, *Am J Clin Pathol* 53:852, 1970.
118. Salyer WR, Salyer DC: Metastases of prostatic cancer to the breast, *J Urol* 109:671, 1973.
119. Tedeschi LG, McCarthy PE: Involutional mammary duct ectasia and periductal mastitis in a male, *Hum Pathol* 5:232, 1974.
120. Waldo EO, Sidhu GS, Hu AW: Florid papillomatosis of the male nipple after diethylstilbesterol therapy, *Arch Pathol* 99:364, 1975.

Index